Reoperative Oral and Maxillofacial Surgery

Guest Editors

LUIS G. VEGA, DDS
RUI FERNANDES, DMD, MD

ORAL AND MAXILLOFACIAL SURGERY CLINICS OF NORTH AMERICA

www.oralmaxsurgery.theclinics.com

Consulting Editor
RICHARD H. HAUG, DDS

February 2011 • Volume 23 • Number 1

SAUNDERS an imprint of ELSEVIER, Inc.

W.B. SAUNDERS COMPANY
A Division of Elsevier Inc.

1600 John F. Kennedy Blvd. • Suite 1800 • Philadelphia, PA 19103-2899

www.oralmaxsurgery.theclinics.com

ORAL AND MAXILLOFACIAL SURGERY CLINICS OF NORTH AMERICA Volume 23, Number 1
February 2011 ISSN 1042-3699, ISBN-13: 978-1-4557-0476-7

Editor: John Vassallo; j.vassallo@elsevier.com
Developmental Editor: Jessica Demetriou

Oral and Maxillofacial Surgery Clinics of North America (ISSN 1042-3699) is published quarterly by Elsevier Inc., 360 Park Avenue South, New York, NY 10010-1710. Months of issue are February, May, August, and November. Business and Editorial Offices: 1600 John F. Kennedy Blvd., Suite 1800, Philadelphia, PA 19103-2899. Periodicals postage paid at New York, NY and additional mailing offices. Subscription prices are $329.00 per year for US individuals, $490.00 per year for US institutions, $147.00 per year for US students and residents, $383.00 per year for Canadian individuals, $583.00 per year for Canadian institutions, $441.00 per year for international individuals, $583.00 per year for international institutions and $200.00 per year for Canadian and foreign students/residents. To receive student/resident rate, orders must be accompanied by name or affiliated institution, date of term, and the *signature* of program/residency coordinator on institution letterhead. Orders will be billed at individual rate until proof of status is received. Foreign air speed delivery is included in all *Clinics* subscription prices. All prices are subject to change without notice. **POSTMASTER:** Send address changes to *Oral and Maxillofacial Surgery Clinics of North America,* Elsevier Periodicals Customer Service, 11830 Westline Industrial Drive, St. Louis, MO 63146. Tel: 1-800-654-2452 (U.S. and Canada); 314-447-8871 (outside U.S. and Canada). Fax: 314-447-8029. E-mail: journalscustomerservice-usa@elsevier.com (for print support); journalsonlinesupport-usa@elsevier.com (for online support).

Reprints. For copies of 100 or more, of articles in this publication, please contact the Commercial Reprints Department, Elsevier Inc., 360 Park Avenue South, New York, NY 10010-1710. Tel.: 212-633-3812; Fax: 212-462-1935; Email: reprints@elsevier.com.

Oral and Maxillofacial Surgery Clinics of North America is covered in MEDLINE/PubMed (*Index Medicus*).

Printed and bound by CPI Group (UK) Ltd, Croydon, CR0 4YY

Transferred to Digital Print 2011

Contributors

CONSULTING EDITOR

RICHARD H. HAUG, DDS
Carolinas Center for Oral Health
Charlotte, North Carolina

GUEST EDITORS

LUIS G. VEGA, DDS
Assistant Program Director, Oral and
Maxillofacial Residency Program; Assistant
Professor, Division of Oral and Maxillofacial
Surgery, Department of Surgery, University of
Florida, Health Science Center at Jacksonville,
Jacksonville, Florida

RUI FERNANDES, DMD, MD
Assistant Professor, Division of Oral and
Maxillofacial Surgery, Department of Surgery,
University of Florida, Health Science Center
at Jacksonville, Jacksonville, Florida

AUTHORS

**JULIO ACERO, MD, DMD, PhD,
FDSRCS, FEBOMFS**
Associate Professor of Surgery,
Department of Oral and Maxillofacial
Surgery, Gregorio Marañon Hospital,
Complutense University; Head of the
Department, Quirón University Hospital,
Madrid, Spain

JOHN F. CACCAMESE, DMD, MD, FACS
Associate Professor and Residency
Program Director, Department of Oral
and Maxillofacial Surgery, University of
Maryland Medical System, Baltimore,
Maryland

MATTEO CHIAPASCO, MD
Professor and Head, Unit of Oral Surgery,
Department of Medicine, Surgery and
Dentistry, San Paolo Hospital, University of
Milan, Milan, Italy

NATHAN EBERLE, MD, DMD
Resident, Division of Oral and Maxillofacial
Surgery, Department of Surgery, University
of Florida College of Medicine, Jacksonville,
Florida

TIRBOD FATTAHI, MD, DDS, FACS
Associate Professor of Surgery and Chief,
Division of Oral and Maxillofacial Surgery,
University of Florida, Health Science Center
at Jacksonville, Jacksonville, Florida

RUI FERNANDES, DMD, MD
Assistant Professor, Division of Oral and
Maxillofacial Surgery, Department of Surgery,
University of Florida, Health Science Center
at Jacksonville, Jacksonville, Florida

ELOY GARCÍA, MD, FEBOMFS
Consultant Specialist, Department of Oral
and Maxillofacial Surgery, Clinic i Provincial
and San Juan de Dios Hospitals, Central
University, Barcelona, Spain

RAJESH GUTTA, BDS, MS
Assistant Professor, Division of Oral and
Maxillofacial Surgery, Department of Surgery,
University of Cincinnati, Cincinnati, Ohio

JACOB HAIAVY, MD, DDS, FACS
Director of General Cosmetic Surgery
Fellowship, Inland Cosmetic Surgery, Rancho
Cucamonga; Assistant Clinical Professor of
Oral and Maxillofacial Surgery, Loma Linda,
California

SIMON HOLMES, BDS, MBBS, FDSRCS, FRCS
Consultant Oral and Maxillofacial Surgeon, Barts and the London NHS Trust, The Royal London Hospital, Whitechapel, London, United Kingdom

JUAN CARLOS LÓPEZ-NORIEGA, DDS
Professor, Department of Oral and Maxillofacial Surgery, Faculty of Dentistry, Universidad Nacional Autónoma de México, Ciudad Universitaria, Mexico

PATRICK LOUIS, DDS, MD
Professor, Program Director, Oral and Maxillofacial Residency Program, Department of Oral and Maxillofacial Surgery, School of Dentistry, University of Alabama at Birmingham, Birmingham, Alabama

FARIDEH M. MADANI, DMD
Clinical Professor of Oral Medicine, Department of Oral Medicine, Robert Schattner Center, School of Dental Medicine, University of Pennsylvania, Philadelphia, Pennsylvania

MANSOOR MADANI, DMD, MD
Chairman, Department of Oral and Maxillofacial Surgery, Capital Health Regional Medical Center, Trenton, New Jersey; Associate Professor of Oral and Maxillofacial Surgery, Temple University Hospital, Philadelphia; Director, Center for Corrective Jaw Surgery, Bala Institute of Oral and Facial Surgery, Bala Cynwyd, Pennsylvania

DANIEL PETRISOR, DMD, MD
Fellow, Division of Oral and Maxillofacial Surgery, Department of Surgery, University of Florida, Health Science Center at Jacksonville, Jacksonville, Florida

DMITRY PEYSAKHOV, DMD
Resident of Oral and Maxillofacial Surgery, Temple University Hospital, Philadelphia, Pennsylvania

PHIL PIRGOUSIS, MD, DMD, FRCS, FRACDS(OMS)
Previous Fellow, Division of Oral and Maxillofacial Surgery, Department of Surgery, University of Florida, Health Science Center at Jacksonville, Jacksonville, Florida

JOHAN P. REYNEKE, BChD, MChD, FCMFOS (SA), PhD
Honorary Professor, Department of Maxillofacial and Oral Surgery, University of the Witwatersrand, Johannesburg, South Africa; Clinical Professor, Department of Oral and Maxillofacial Surgery, University of Oklahoma, Oklahoma City, Oklahoma; Clinical Professor, Department of Oral and Maxillofacial Surgery, University of Florida, Gainesville, Florida; Department of Oral and Maxillofacial Surgery, University of Monterrey, Monterrey, Mexico; Private Practice, Sunninghill Hospital, Johannesburg, South Africa

RAFAEL RUIZ-RODRÍGUEZ, DDS
Professor, Department of Oral and Maxillofacial Surgery, Faculty of Dentistry, Universidad Nacional Autónoma de México, Ciudad Universitaria, Mexico

ANDREW R. SALAMA, DDS, MD
Assistant Professor, Department of Oral and Maxillofacial Surgery, Henry Goldman School of Dental Medicine, Boston University, Boston, Massachusetts

LUIS G. VEGA, DDS
Assistant Program Director, Oral and Maxillofacial Residency Program; Assistant Professor, Division of Oral and Maxillofacial Surgery, Department of Surgery, University of Florida, Health Science Center at Jacksonville, Jacksonville, Florida

PETER D. WAITE, MPH, DDS, MD
Professor and Chair, Department of Oral and Maxillofacial Surgery, University of Alabama School of Dentistry, University of Alabama at Birmingham, Birmingham, Alabama

ROBIN S. YANG, DDS
Resident, Department of Oral and Maxillofacial Surgery, University of Maryland Medical System, Baltimore, Maryland

MARCO ZANIBONI, DDS
Assistant, Unit of Oral Surgery, Department of Medicine, Surgery and Dentistry, San Paolo Hospital, University of Milan, Milan, Italy

Contents

> Dental rehabilitation with oral implants has become a routine treatment modality in
> the last decades, with reliable long-term results. However, insufficient bone volume
> or unfavorable intermaxillary relationships may render implant placement impossible
> or incorrect from a functional and esthetic viewpoint. Among the different methods
> for the reconstruction of deficient alveolar ridges, the use of autogenous bone blocks
> represents the most frequently used treatment modality both for limited and
> extended bone defects. Prerequisites for a successful outcome are represented
> by accurate preoperative planning, proper reconstructive procedure, and adequate
> prosthetic rehabilitation. Even if all these principles are followed, complications
> involving the grafts may occur, such as dehiscence, infection, or relevant resorption
> of the graft. The aim of this article is to present an updated overview on the inci-
> dence, prevention and treatment of these complications.

> Enophthalmos is a complex and unpredictable condition to treat secondarily, and
> this is likely to remain a difficult challenge. Modern imaging technology and the
> aggressive stance taken on appropriate primary repair make it likely that surgeons
> will see fewer minor cases and increased numbers of major cases. The choice of re-
> constructive material should be evidence-based rather than based on surgical pref-
> erence. Of crucial importance to the management of all traumas, particularly in
> revisional surgery, is attention to the soft tissue envelope, which adds to the postop-
> erative result, and may camouflage minor degrees of enophthalmos.

> Reoperative midface surgery can be challenging. Although well-established surgical
> principles are still the basis of surgical approaches and techniques, the advent of
> new materials and technologies brings about opportunities to achieve the best pos-
> sible outcomes with bony reconstruction and more precise results. Soft tissue defor-
> mities continue to be some of the most challenging, especially as they relate to the
> orbit, but continually evolving techniques offer improved results for volume correc-
> tions to treat enophthalmos and diplopia. Conventional orthognathic and recon-
> structive rhinoplasty techniques can also be applied to great effect and with
> satisfying results to treat posttraumatic malocclusions and nasal deformities.

> Mandibular fractures are one the most common maxillofacial injuries. Diagnostic
> errors, poor surgical technique, healing disorders, or complications may lead to

the establishment of posttraumatic mandibular deformities. Nonunion, malunion/ malocclusion, or facial asymmetry can be found early during the healing process or as long-term sequelae after the initial mandibular fracture repair. Although occasionally these problems can be solved in a nonsurgical manner, reoperations play an important role in the management of these untoward outcomes. This article discusses the reoperative techniques used for the management of these deformities.

Tirbod Fattahi

Trauma remains the leading cause of death in the first 4 decades of life and is surpassed only by cancer and atherosclerotic disease as the overall leading causes of death in the United States. Many of the injuries involve the facial region, including soft tissue trauma. This article highlights the current available modalities used in the management of unsightly scars or those scars whose location and appearance compromise function.

Johan P. Reyneke

The best time to perform orthognathic surgery for the correction of dentofacial deformities is the first time. However, complications requiring reoperation do occur. A thorough understanding of how to avoid intra- and postoperative complications, and how to manage these problems successfully, is mandatory. This article discusses some of the most common complications, how to avoid these complications, and how to treat complications when they do occur. General surgical complications during and after surgery, such as hemorrhage and infection, are outside the scope of this article.

Peter D. Waite

Reoperation of the nose is challenging and sometimes emotionally difficult for the surgeon and patient. There are multiple pitfalls to be avoided and it is always best to carefully diagnose and establish a surgical treatment plan. Even among the best of plans and surgical techniques, revision may be necessary. The patient and surgeon should understand the limitations of the surgical techniques and the individual anatomy.

Tirbod Fattahi

This article is intended to deal with the difficult subject matter of revision rhinoplasty. Since there is consensus that rhinoplasty is one of the most difficult aesthetic surgery procedures, one would make the inference that a revision rhinoplasty should also be one of the more difficult revision surgeries. The intent of this article is to share with the readers a few pearls and lessons learned dealing with revision rhinoplasty.

Jacob Haiavy

The complexity of the reoperative facelift or neck lift is directly related to the way the primary procedure was performed. Regardless of the primary technique used, the secondary procedure should be directed to the specific problems that the patient exhibits, such as scars, earlobe deformity, hair pattern changes, laxity in the upper face or neck, jowling, or deepening of the nasolabial folds. Contour should be restored within the deep layer support via the elevation of the superficial musculoaponeurotic system and platysma rather than rotating skin flaps in an exaggerated manner in a cephalad direction, producing a tight unnatural look.

TMJ surgeries are not always successful. Many potential pitfalls can occur during any phase of the treatment and can lead to complications, less than desirable results, and short- or long-term failures. Unsatisfactory results can occur for multiple reasons, including misdiagnosis of the original pathologic condition, incorrect selection of surgical technique, technical failures, complications, systemic disease, and unrealistic expectations. This article focuses on the reoperation of the TMJ primarily in cases of internal derangement and discusses TMJ arthrocentesis, arthroscopy, modified condylotomy, and open joint procedures.

Reoperative reconstruction of the midface is a challenging issue because of the complexity of this region and the severity of the aesthetic and functional sequela related to the absence or failure of a primary reconstruction. The different situations that can lead to the indication of a reoperative reconstructive procedure after previous oncologic ablative procedures in the midface are reviewed. Surgical techniques, anatomic problems, and limitations affecting the reoperative reconstruction in this region of the head and neck are discussed.

Ideal reconstruction of the mandible is important for a multitude of reasons and has been and continues to be among the most common surgical challenges for reconstructive surgeons of the head and neck. Historically, pedicle flaps, such as the pectoralis major and deltopectoral myocutaneous flaps, were workhorse flaps for lower facial third head and neck reconstruction. This article outlines the relevant anatomy of the perimandibular region, reconstructive options including second free flaps, relevant workup, and complications pertaining to reoperative mandibular surgery.

Approximately 36,000 people in the United States will be diagnosed with oral or oropharyngeal cancer in 2010. In more than 90% of the cases of oral cavity and oropharyngeal cancers, histopathologic examination reveals squamous cell carcinoma (SCCA). Despite appropriate initial treatment, oral SCCA recurs in 25% to 48% of cases. Several studies have shown that most cancers recur within about 2 years after the initial treatment. Hence, close follow-up of patients is important for the timely detection of recurrences. This article discusses the types of recurrence and the surveillance and treatment of recurrent oral SCCA.

Oral and Maxillofacial Surgery Clinics of North America

THE CLINICS ARE NOW AVAILABLE ONLINE!
Access your subscription at:
www.theclinics.com

Preface
Reoperative Oral and Maxillofacial Surgery

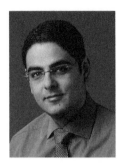 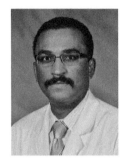

Luis G. Vega, DDS   Rui Fernandes, DMD, MD
Guest Editors

Surgery is not about what you do now but about what you do next...
—*Robert Ord, DMD, MD*

We are very pleased to be guest editors for this *Oral and Maxillofacial Surgery Clinics* dedicated to "Reoperative Oral and Maxillofacial Surgery."

Whether we are seasoned surgeons or recent graduates, we are all faced with patients needing reoperative interventions. The term "reoperative surgery" is often perceived negatively due to its connotation of complication and blame. As a result, surgeons are often reluctant to discuss their experiences, forgoing opportunities for shared learning.

Reoperative surgery has different meanings for different surgeons. It may encompass touchup procedures for cleft lip and palate patients, redoing a facelift due to continued aging and its sequelae, multistage maxillofacial reconstructive procedures, correction of an unsatisfactory orthognathic result, complications from bone grafts for dental implants, or a reoperation due to a positive margin or recurrence of initial disease. Reoperative maxillofacial surgery is often more difficult than the initial surgery due to the inherent scarring and altered anatomy. Equally, the surgeon must dedicate significant time to planning to minimize the need for yet another intervention in the future.

We have sought to recruit leaders in our specialty to contribute their collective experiences in dealing with these difficult processes. We hope that within this text the reader will find pearls of wisdom shared by our contributors that will better their clinical practices and minimize the need for reoperative procedures.

To our contributors, we offer our sincere thanks for your time and effort. We recognize that you have busy professional and personal lives and we are deeply grateful for your commitment to this project. We would like to extend our thanks to the editor, Mr John Vassallo, for his patience and commitment throughout this project. Last, we would like to thank our families: Marina and Eva Vega, and Candace, Gabriela, and Alessandro Fernandes, for their continued support and love, without which we could not do what we love.

Luis G. Vega, DDS
Rui Fernandes, DMD, MD

Division of Oral and Maxillofacial Surgery
Department of Surgery
University of Florida
Health Science Center at Jacksonville
653-1 West 8th Street
Jacksonville, FL 32209, USA

E-mail addresses:
luis.vega@jax.ufl.edu (L.G. Vega)
rui.fernandes@jax.ufl.edu (R. Fernandes)

Oral Maxillofacial Surg Clin N Am 23 (2011) xi
doi:10.1016/j.coms.2010.12.004
1042-3699/11/$ – see front matter © 2011 Elsevier Inc. All rights reserved.

Failures in Jaw Reconstructive Surgery with Autogenous Onlay Bone Grafts for Pre-implant Purposes: Incidence, Prevention and Management of Complications

Matteo Chiapasco, MD*, Marco Zaniboni, DDS

KEYWORDS

- Alveolar ridge augmentation • Oral implant
- Autogenous bone • Preprosthetic surgery
- Bone transplantation • Revascularized free flap
- Failure • Complication

Dental rehabilitation of partially or totally edentulous patients with oral implants has become a routine treatment modality in the last decades, with reliable long-term results.[1–12] However, unfavorable local conditions of the alveolar ridge, due to atrophy, periodontal disease, trauma, and tumor resection sequelae, may provide insufficient bone volume or unfavorable vertical, horizontal, and sagittal intermaxillary relationships, which may render implant placement impossible or incorrect from a functional and esthetic viewpoint.

Among the different methods for the reconstruction of deficient alveolar ridges, which include osteoinduction with growth factors such as bone morphogenetic proteins (BMPs),[13,14] guided bone regeneration,[15–18] distraction osteogenesis,[19–22] reconstruction with allografts,[23,24] reconstruction with autogenous bone grafts,[12,25–49] and reconstruction with revascularized free flaps, the use of autogenous bone blocks represents the most frequently used treatment modality for both limited and extended bone defects.[12,25–49]

A recent literature review by Chiapasco and colleagues[50] in 2009, including articles related to autogenous bone grafts taken from intraoral or extraoral sites, with samples of a minimum of 10 patients followed at least for 1 year after the start of prosthetic loading of implants placed in the reconstructed areas, provided 26 articles fulfilling the aforementioned criteria.[12,25–49] Overall, 893 patients presenting with alveolar defects of the jaws were treated by means of autogenous bone grafts followed by placement of 4390 implants; the prosthetic rehabilitation was started on average 4 to 6 months after implant installation. Uneventful healing/consolidation of both intraoral and extraoral grafts occurred in the majority of patients. The survival rate of implants placed in reconstructed maxillae and mandibles ranged from 60% to 100%, with a median value of

The authors have nothing to disclose.

Unit of Oral Surgery, Department of Medicine, Surgery and Dentistry, San Paolo Hospital, University of Milan, Via Beldiletto 1/3, 20142 Milan, Milan, Italy

* Corresponding author.

E-mail address: matteo.chiapasco@unimi.it

Oral Maxillofacial Surg Clin N Am 23 (2011) 1–15

doi:10.1016/j.coms.2010.10.009

91.5%. These data appear to demonstrate that high percentages of success of the reconstructive procedure and high survival rates of the implants placed in the reconstructed areas can be expected. Prerequisites for a successful outcome of reconstructions using autogenous bone grafts are represented by accurate preoperative planning, proper reconstructive procedure, and adequate prosthetic rehabilitation.

Accurate preoperative planning includes: (a) clinical and radiographic evaluation of the area to be rehabilitated, including standard radiographs such as panoramic radiograph, lateral cephalometric radiograph, intraoral radiographs, and computed tomography; (b) evaluation of systemic diseases or habits that may contraindicate reconstructive procedures and implant-supported restorations, such as immune system disorders, severe renal or liver diseases, heavy smoking or alcohol abuse, or no compliance by patients; (c) evaluation of local factors that may contraindicate reconstructive procedures and related implant-supported rehabilitation, such as periodontal disease to residual dentition, poor oral hygiene, hypovascularized or scarry intraoral tissues as a consequence of previous and failed attempts of implant therapy (in particular subperiosteal implants), or irradiation in the head and neck area (in particular when doses exceed 48 Gy).

A good vascular condition of the recipient bed is an important prerequisite for success. In fact, the revascularization and integration process of a bone graft is highly dependent on a good blood supply of the recipient bed, including the residual bone and the surrounding soft tissues. Bone grafts, in fact, behave as a dead scaffold, which must be substituted by new bone formation. Therefore, scarry and hypovascularized soft tissues in the area to be reconstructed, irrespective of the extension of the defect, may preclude adequate revascularization and consequent integration of the graft.[50,51]

A proper reconstructive procedure includes: (a) surgery under sterile conditions; (b) antibiotic coverage; (c) correct choice of bone donor site; (d) adequate modeling and fixation of the grafts to the recipient sites; (e) a tension-free, watertight suture of the flaps covering the grafts; (f) no load of the reconstructed areas in the postoperative period; (g) timing of implant placement and loading with prosthetic superstructures.

The first 2 aspects are obvious and do not deserve particular comments. It is worth noting only that although implants placed in native bone might not need antibiotic coverage, in the vast majority of the available publications antibiotic prophylaxis is suggested, in order to prevent infection following bacterial contamination of the graft.[50,51]

As far as the donor site is concerned, it must be underlined that, as a general principle, intraoral sites are used for the reconstruction of defects of limited size (partial edentulism involving 1 to 3–4 teeth gaps), whereas extraoral grafts are generally used for the reconstruction of extended defects (both partial and total edentulism involving one or both jaws). Intraoral donor sites are mainly represented by the mandibular symphysis and the mandibular ramus. These sites offer good bone with a dense, cortical layer that is generally less exposed to bone resorption over time as compared with cancellous bone.

Extraoral sites are mainly represented by the iliac crest and the calvarium, and to a lesser extent, the tibia. The iliac crest offers relevant quantities of bone but, due to its relevant cancellous component, is exposed to a higher risk of resorption over time. The calvarium, on the contrary, offers relevant quantities of highly corticalized bone, which has been demonstrated to be less prone to resorption. The only limit is generally represented by a more difficult acceptance by patients, although morbidity is much lower than that related to iliac crest.[50,51]

Adequate modeling and fixation of the grafts to the recipient sites is also a fundamental step to obtain a successful integration. Imprecise adaptation to the recipient site and absence of stability may lead to connective tissue growth between the graft and the recipient site, thus leading to partial or nonintegration of the graft and eventually to its loss. As a perfect adaptation of a bone block to the often irregular shape of the recipient site may be difficult, any "void" between the bone graft and the recipient site should be filled with autogenous bone chips.

A tension-free, watertight suture of the flaps covering the grafts is one of the most important phases of the reconstructive procedure. Periosteal releasing incisions are therefore fundamental in preventing early dehiscence of the surgical wound, which exposes to the risk of graft failure.

To prevent wound dehiscence, it is highly recommended to avoid any loading on the operated area with removable prostheses for at least 8 weeks after surgery. After that period, if necessary, removable prostheses relined with soft materials may be allowed. The best solution for partially edentulous patients is represented by provisional fixed prostheses supported by neighboring teeth, but with no contact with the reconstructed area.[50,51]

The timing of implant placement in reconstructed areas is still under debate: both implant placement in conjunction with bone grafting and implant placement after consolidation of bone grafts have been proposed. Those who advocate simultaneous implant placement[12,26,29,30,33,34,37,39,46] do so based on the fact that resorption of an onlay graft over time is not a linear process but is most pronounced soon after its transplantation.[34] Simultaneous implant placement shortens the waiting time before rehabilitation, thus potentially reducing the risk of bone resorption.

Those who advocate delayed placement[31,35,38,40,41,43,44,45,49] think that simultaneous placement of implants may expose the patient to some risks, which can be summarized as follows: (1) in the case of wound dehiscence, exposure and infection/necrosis of the bone graft may occur and lead to partial or total loss of the graft; (2) immediate implants are placed into avascular bone, which increases the risk of nonintegration.

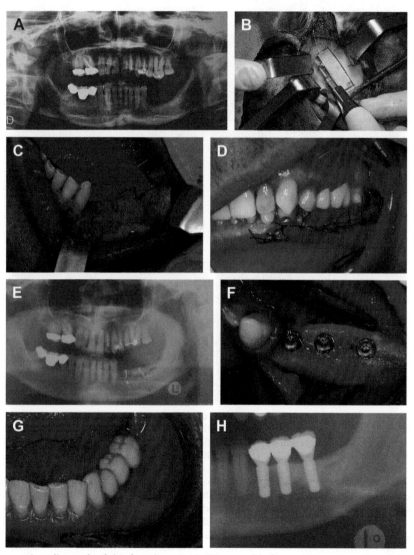

Fig. 1. (*A*) Panoramic radiograph of this female patient, 55 years old, shows relevant atrophy of the posterior left mandible with no more than 4 mm between the alveolar crest and the alveolar nerve: there is a clear indication for correcting the deficient ridge in order to place implants of adequate dimensions. (*B*) Bone harvesting from the calvarium (parietal bone) by means of piezosurgery. (*C*) Reconstruction of the mandible with calvarial bone blocks in both the horizontal and vertical dimensions. (*D*) A hermetic suture is fundamental to prevent exposure of the graft and potential infection. (*E*) Postoperative control demonstrating the correction obtained. (*F*) Six months later, after an uneventful healing, the grafted bone appears well integrated in the recipient site and 3 implants are installed in the reconstructed area. (*G, H*) Final result showing excellent integration of both bone graft and implants in the reconstructed area.

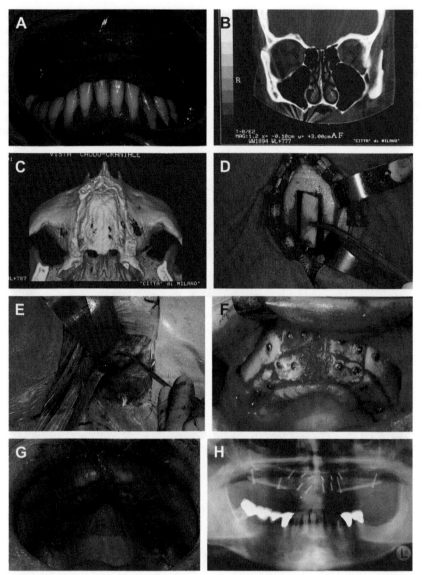

Fig. 2. (*A–C*) Initial clinical and radiographic situation of this 35-year-old female patient shows an edentulous maxilla affected by severe tridimensional resorption of the alveolar ridge with expanded maxillary: this situation renders implant placement in the residual bone impossible. (*D, E*) Bone harvesting is performed from both the calvarium (parietal bone) and anterior iliac crest. (*F*) The severely atrophic maxilla is reconstructed with onlay grafts stabilized with titanium microscrews to correct the vertical, horizontal, and anterior-posterior deficit. (*G*) A hermetic suture is obtained after adequate releasing incisions of the periosteum, despite the relevant increase of bone volume. (*H*) Postoperative radiographic control demonstrates the correction obtained. (*I, J*) Five months later, after an uneventful healing, the grafted bone appears well integrated in the recipient site and 8 implants are installed in the reconstructed maxilla. (*K, L*) Final result showing excellent integration of both bone graft and implants in the reconstructed area.

Conversely, when a delayed protocol is performed it is possible to place implants (albeit partly) in a revascularized graft. Because the regenerative capacity of bone is determined by the presence of vessels, bone marrow, and vital bone surfaces, a delayed approach permits better integration of implants (higher values of bone-implant contact) and better stability of implants, as compared with immediate implant placement.

Despite these considerations, however, much controversy still exists as far as timing of implant placement in grafted areas is concerned, and no conclusions can be drawn.

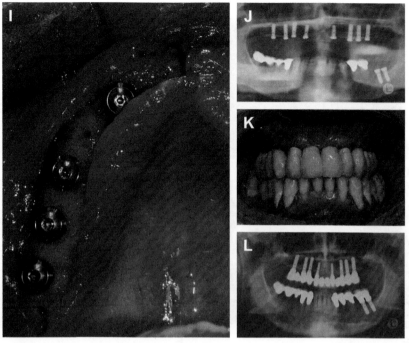

Fig. 2. (*continued*)

Finally, loading times of implants placed in grafted areas is also still controversial: although no conclusive recommendations can be made, due to the wide range of waiting times proposed and to the different characteristics of macro-, micro-, and nanogeometry of different implant systems (which may influence osseointegration times), most investigators suggest waiting times similar to those proposed for implants placed in nonreconstructed bone (3–6 months), with no detrimental effects on osseointegration.[50,51] However, it is worth noting that, although limited, there is also evidence that early or immediate loading of implants placed in reconstructed areas may lead to successful integration.[43,52]

Some clinical cases with successful outcome are presented in **Figs. 1** and **2**.

COMPLICATIONS RELATED TO BONE GRAFTING AND MANAGEMENT

Even if all these principles, including surgery under sterile conditions, antibiotic coverage, adequate modeling and fixation of the grafts to the recipient sites, a watertight suture of the flaps covering the grafts, and finally no load of the reconstructed areas in the postoperative period, are followed, complications involving the grafts may occur.

The systematic review by Chiapasco and colleagues[49] in 2009 reported partial loss of the graft caused by wound dehiscence/infection in 3.3% of the cases while total loss of the graft

occurred in 1.4% of the cases, the majority being related to extensive reconstructions of atrophic maxilla with iliac grafts.

In more detail, the following represents the main complications, which may involve a reconstruction with autogenous bone grafts:

1. Dehiscence with exposure of the bone graft but without clinical evidence of infection
2. Infection of the graft with or without dehiscence of the flap
3. Relevant resorption of the graft.

It is worth noting that the treatment modalities presented in this article are derived from clinical experience of the authors and not by standardized protocols, because to the authors' knowledge no standardized treatment modalities have ever been published in the literature.

Dehiscence with Exposure of the Bone Graft but Without Clinical Evidence of Infection

Even if a hermetic and tension-free suture of the flap overlying the graft has been performed at the end of the reconstruction, dehiscence of the suture may occur at any time after surgery (days, weeks, or even months afterwards). Dehiscence can be very limited (just a few millimeters) or extended. The management of a dehiscence and its evolution is mainly related to the development or nondevelopment of infection.

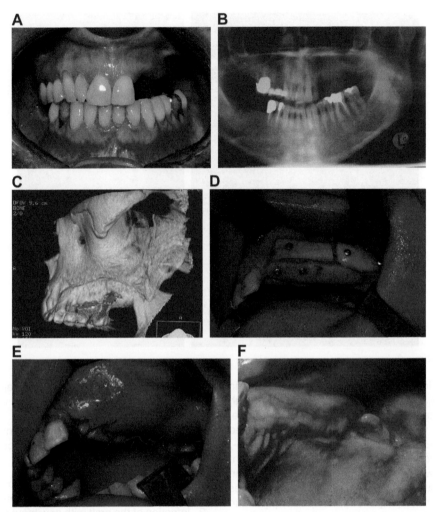

Fig. 3. (A–C) Initial clinical and radiographic situation of this 40-year-old female patient shows an edentulous left maxilla with insufficient alveolar bone to host implants caused by horizontal and vertical bone resorption in association with maxillary sinus expansion. (D, E) Reconstruction of the edentulous area with calvarial bone blocks in both the horizontal and vertical dimensions, in association with sinus floor elevation and grafting. (F) Despite a hermetic suture 3 weeks after the reconstruction, a small dehiscence appeared in the posterior part of the reconstructed area. (G) After 4 weeks of weekly controls and infection control with chlorhexidine mouth rinses, a spontaneous closure of the dehiscence occurred, with no signs of infection; postoperative control demonstrating the correction obtained. (H) Five months later, no bone loss was detected and 4 implants were inserted in the reconstructed area. (I, J) Final result showing excellent integration of both bone graft and implants in the reconstructed area.

If a dehiscence occurs within a few days after surgery (1–3 days), an attempt to resuture the flap can be performed, but it must be remembered that contamination by oral bacteria has already occurred and the risk of promoting growth of bacteria and consequent infection in a secluded and noncontrollable site is high. The authors think that it is safer to leave the wound open and to proceed as follows.

In the case of absence of clinically detectable infection (no presence of purulent secretions, no pain or local swelling, no relevant inflammation of

soft tissues covering the graft), the first treatment modality includes antibiotic coverage and chlorhexidine mouth rinses or gel applications over the exposed area. This basic treatment can be associated to a "wait and see" strategy (in particular for limited graft exposures [few millimeters] or to the creation of multiple perforations of the exposed bone graft) with a small round burr assembled on a low-speed handpiece with constant irrigation with cold sterile saline, until bleeding from the recipient blood is obtained. In such a way, granulation tissue may develop

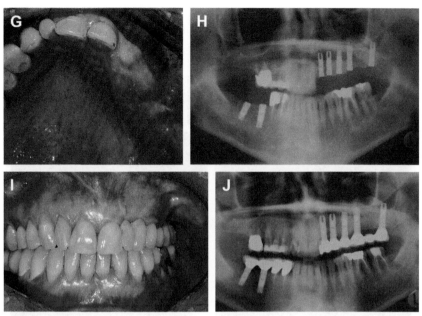

Fig. 3. (*continued*)

through the perforations starting from the recipient bed and secondary healing leading to spontaneous coverage of the exposed graft may occur, eventually rescuing the graft. This procedure can be repeated some days or weeks afterwards if the coverage of the graft is incomplete. Two clinical examples are reported in **Figs. 3** and **4**.

If this treatment modality appears to be ineffective, a second chance can be represented by surgical curettage of both the exposed bone and the margins of surrounding soft tissues, to remove the superficial part of the contaminated bone in association with or without further perforations. This approach leads to a reduction of the initial volume of the graft, but may facilitate a secondary healing.

If the exposure persists but without signs of infection, the patient can be followed with periodic controls until the time of implant placement, when bone integration of the graft has occurred (3–4 months for intraoral grafts, 3 months on average for iliac grafts, and 5–6 months when calvarium is used). At that time, whichever treatment has been adopted, the following scenarios can be found:

> Preservation of the majority of the original graft bone volume
> Partial loss of the graft
> Total loss of the graft.

In the first event, the patient is treated with a standard protocol, including raising a flap, removal of the screws/plates used to stabilize the graft, and implant placement according to the original prosthetically driven plan, with the aid of surgical templates.

In the second situation, if the loss of part of the graft is limited, the original planning of implant placement can be modified and the surgeon may try to place implants in the well-consolidated parts of the graft, ignoring the compromised parts. Of course, this type of approach can be performed in cases of limited bone losses in extended reconstructions. In the case of partial loss of the graft in a single tooth gap, this strategy cannot be applied.

Finally, despite absence of clinical evidence of infection, the exposed graft may appear nonintegrated at the time of implant placement. In such a situation the only possibility is to remove the graft. Reintervention with a new graft may be proposed to the patient, but it is strongly recommended to wait a reasonable period of time until healing of the area has occurred through spontaneous closure of the surgical wound. A clinical example is reported in **Fig. 5**.

Infection of the Graft With or Without Dehiscence of the Flap

If a clinically detectable infection of the graft occurs, with or without dehiscence of the flap (pain, swelling, purulent secretion, fever, and so forth), despite antibiotic treatment the chances of rescuing the graft are low, and in the majority of cases part of the graft or the complete graft must be removed so as to avoid diffusion of the infection

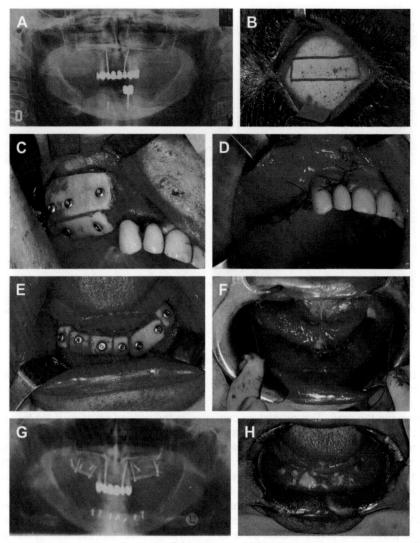

Fig. 4. (*A*) Preoperative panoramic radiograph of this 55-year-old female patient shows sequelae of malpractice, with some very narrow implants still in function and some fractured. Another 10 implants (4 in the mandible and 6 in the maxilla) had been removed by her dentist before this consultation. The maxilla shows both right and left edentulous ridges with relevant alveolar bone resorption and sinus expansion, which render implant installation difficult or impossible. (*B–D*) The maxilla has been reconstructed by means of calvarial blocks in association with sinus grafting, with particulated bone taken from the calvarium: great attention was dedicated toward obtaining a tension-free hermetic closure of the flaps. (*E, F*) During the same surgical session, the failing implants placed in the mandible were removed and the heavily resorbed anterior mandible was reconstructed with calvarial bone blocks as well: again, great care was dedicated toward obtaining a watertight closure. (*G*) Postoperative radiographic control shows the correction of the maxillomandibular deficits. (*H, I*) Although the healing process of the mandibular reconstruction was uneventful, 8 weeks after the reconstruction a small dehiscence occurred in the right maxilla, with no detectable signs of infection. (*J*) The exposed bone was perforated with a burr to promote the formation of granulation tissue and to favor secondary healing. (*K*) Four weeks later, a complete closure of the dehiscence was obtained. (*L*) After another 3 months, it was possible to insert implants in the reconstructed areas.

and eventually major complications, such as osteomyelitis to the native bone. In such a situation, the sooner the treatment is done the fewer are the problems encountered, and a rapid regression of signs and symptoms of infection will generally occur.

If only part of the graft is removed, there is still a possibility to place implants in the residual "healthy" part of the graft (if enough bone is present) without any regrafting procedure (**Fig. 6**). If the bone loss is more extended or it includes the whole graft, regrafting can be proposed to the

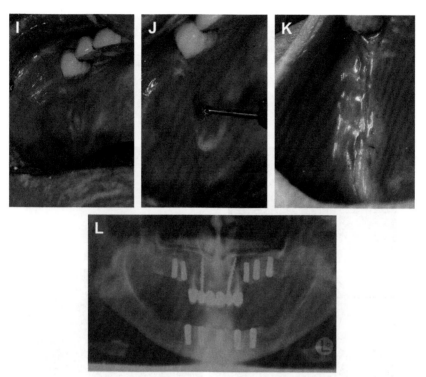

Fig. 4. (*continued*)

patient, but it is highly suggested not to perform it immediately: there is a high probability of residual infection in the recipient site, which may lead to a quick failure of the regrafting procedure.

In the case of total failure of reconstructions of extremely atrophic jaws, with or without the presence of scarry and/or hypovascularized tissues, the risk of another failure of a new graft is possible. In such cases, the use of free vascularized flaps can be adopted instead of a graft. The rationale of this type of transplant is that the bone can immediately survive thanks to its vascular pedicle, and it does not need revascularization and substitution as occurs with bone grafts. Therefore, vascularized bone transplants may survive also in recipient beds presenting with poor local conditions, such as hypovascularized, scarry tissues. Among the different flaps, the fibula free flap is considered the most suitable for the reconstruction of extremely atrophic jaws and for implant-supported prosthetic rehabilitation, thanks to its reliability and adaptability, the length of the vascular pedicle, the large amount of bone tissue provided, and the diameter and good quality of its cortical component.[53–56]

Relevant Resorption of the Graft

Even if no dehiscence/infection of the graft occurs, the bone graft may undergo dimensional contraction, with relevant and often unpredictable variations among patients, as demonstrated by several publications.[12,27,32,33,35,38,39,42,44,46]

Results reported in the literature, however, are contradictory, due to relevant differences in observation periods, type and site of reconstruction, timing of implant loading, use or nonuse of provisional dentures on reconstructed sites, and last but not least, the site of bone harvesting.[50,51]

With regard to bone resorption of onlay grafts the following conclusions can be drawn, despite the limits caused by the paucity of available data[50,51]:

1. Bone resorption is greater in the first year after the reconstruction and in the first year after loading of implants, with a significant reduction in the following years.
2. Relevant differences in bone resorption were found according to donor sites. In the case of iliac grafts, resorption rates of the initial graft height 1 to 5 years after loading of implants ranged from 12% to 60%. In the case of intraoral grafts, there are insufficient data to draw any meaningful conclusion. The best results were found for vertical reconstruction with calvarial grafts, where resorption rates ranged from 0% to 15% of the initial graft height. This finding seems to indicate that cortical thickness and density of donor bone are factors that might influence the resorption pattern.

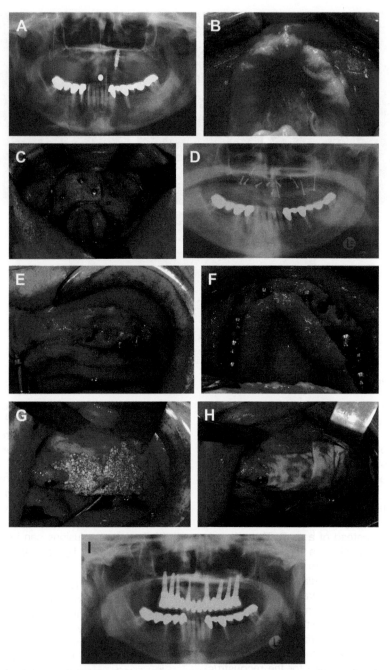

Fig. 5. (*A*) Preoperative panoramic radiograph of this 40-year-old female patient shows sequelae of malpractice, with only 1 implant (out of 8 originally placed) still in place but with loss of osseointegration and chronic infection. A severe bone loss of the alveolar ridge involves all of the maxilla. (*B*) After removal of the residual implant, a very compromised alveolar ridge was present, with impossibility of placing implants of adequate dimensions. (*C, D*) A tridimensional reconstruction of the maxilla including bilateral sinus grafting and iliac onlay grafts. (*E*) Despite an apparently uneventful healing, at the time of implant placement an area of relevant bone resorption was found in the left maxilla. (*F–H*) Eight implants were inserted in the areas not affected by resorption, while the area affected by graft loss was filled with bovine bone mineral and covered with collagen membranes. (*I*) Radiographic control 1 year after the completion of prosthetic rehabilitation shows good integration of the implants in the reconstructed areas (some bone resorption has nevertheless developed around some implants).

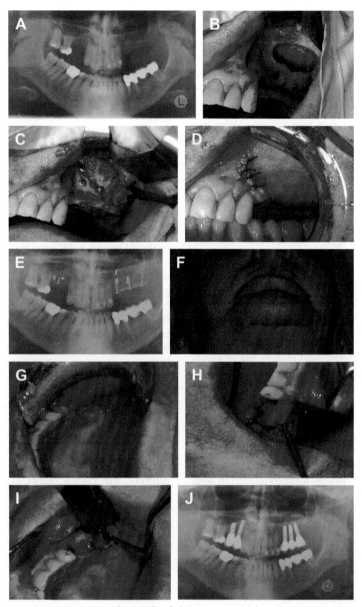

Fig. 6. (*A*) The preoperative panoramic radiograph of this 60-year-old female patient shows a partially edentulous maxilla with insufficient bone volume on the left maxilla to host implants of adequate dimensions, due to horizontal and vertical resorption of the alveolar ridge in association with maxillary sinus expansion. (*B, C*) The reconstructive procedure consisted of sinus grafting in association with vertical and horizontal bone grafts taken from the anterior iliac crest. (*D*) Great care was dedicated toward obtaining a watertight closure. (*E*) The postoperative radiographic control shows the bone augmentation obtained. (*F, G*) Twelve weeks after surgery the patient showed facial swelling and intraoral suppuration, despite an absence of clinically detectable dehiscence. (*H, I*) The patient was immediately treated by removal of the distal part of the graft, which appeared nonvital and nonintegrated, while the rest of the graft was left in situ after a careful surgical curettage. (*J*) Two months later it was possible to complete the treatment with installation of implants in the residual and well-integrated graft followed by final prosthetic rehabilitation.

3. Oversized grafts should be harvested to maintain enough graft volume after the initial resorption phase.
4. If autogenous bone grafts are used, it is highly recommended to use corticocancellous bone blocks. Cancellous bone alone and particulated bone, if not associated with membranes of titanium meshes, do not provide sufficient rigidity to withstand tension from the overlying soft tissues or from the compression by provisional

removable dentures, and may undergo almost complete resorption.

5. There is some evidence that the coverage of autogenous bone grafts with low-resorption rate bone substitutes and resorbable membranes may reduce the risk of bone resorption.[57–59]

It is worth noting that these conclusions are mainly related to onlay grafts used for vertical augmentation, whereby measurements of vertical modifications of the initial bone volume are easily performed on panoramic radiographs or intraoral radiographs, both before and after implant placement. On the contrary, modifications of horizontal augmentations are more difficult to measure, as computed tomography scans are needed, concomitant with increased economic and biologic costs.

Recent publications have also advocated the use of autogenous pericranium, harvested alone or in association with calvarial grafts, to be placed over the grafts at the end of the reconstructive procedure. This approach seems to reduce the exposure of bone grafts (and related risk of infection) also in the case of wound dehiscence.[60–62]

DISCUSSION

Data from the literature appear to demonstrate that the use of autogenous bone grafts to allow implant installation in deficient alveolar ridges is a predictable and reliable technique.[50,51] In less than 5% of the cases, however, exposure/infection of the grafts, which may eventually lead to bone graft loss, may occur. Yet it has been demonstrated also that in cases where these complications occur, in the majority of the cases it is still possible to install implants (besides cases of total loss or single tooth gaps). In case of relevant loss, regrafting followed by delayed implant placement or implant placement in association with guided bone regeneration procedures is a common method to solve these problems.

However, the pros and cons of bone transplantation must be carefully weighed, as far as economic and biologic costs (morbidity) are concerned. In particular, the size and the site (maxilla or mandible) of the defect must be carefully evaluated.

In the case of moderate to severe atrophy in partially edentulous patients, other surgical options, such as distraction osteogenesis, guided bone regeneration, and sagittal osteotomies, which may present less morbidity, should be taken into consideration. Moreover, it is necessary to consider the area where atrophy has occurred. In

recent years, an increasing number of articles related to the use of short implants with apparently acceptable survival rates after the start of prosthetic loading have been published.[63–70] In particular, the atrophic posterior areas, for which esthetic problems are frequently not as relevant (with the exception of patients with gummy smile), may be treated with short implants without any previous reconstruction, albeit taking into account that longer superstructures may represent a prosthetic and functional compromise. By contrast, the atrophic maxilla does not appear to be "the right candidate" for the use of short implants, as long teeth may represent an unacceptable solution for the majority of patients. Therefore, patients' expectations should be carefully evaluated preoperatively before a decision is made.

In the case of severely atrophied edentulous maxillae, relevant resorption of the alveolar process and the presence of nasal and paranasal cavities (maxillary sinuses) lead to a clinical situation that is not compatible with implant placement, because of insufficient quantity and low quality of the residual bone. In these cases, onlay grafts (with or without associated sinus grafts) are one of the few options that permit the recreation of a more favorable environment for implant placement. Conversely, the edentulous mandible, although severely atrophied, may present local conditions that are also compatible with safe implant placement without reconstruction. It has also been demonstrated that in the case of severe atrophy, the dense highly corticalized bone of the mandibular symphysis is able to support the functional demands of removable or fixed implant–supported prostheses, also when short implants (less than 8 mm) are used, with high survival rates of implants (>90% after observation periods of at least 5 years).[71,72] Therefore, reconstruction of the atrophic edentulous mandible should be limited to cases presenting with extreme atrophy, when the residual available bone is insufficient for harboring even implants of reduced dimensions.

REFERENCES

1. Albrektsson T, Zarb G, Worthington P, et al. The long term efficacy of currently used dental implants: a review and proposed criteria of success. Int J Oral Maxillofac Implants 1986;1(1):11–25.
2. van Steenberghe D. A retrospective multicenter evaluation of the survival rate of osseointegrated fixtures supporting fixed partial prostheses in the treatment of partial edentulism. J Prosthet Dent 1989;6(2):217–23.

3. van Steenberghe D, Lekholm U, Bolender C, et al. The applicability of osseointegrated oral implants in the rehabilitation of partial edentulism: a prospective multicenter study of 558 fixtures. Int J Oral Maxillofac Implants 1990;5(3):272–81.

4. Lekholm U, Gunne J, Henry P, et al. Survival of the Brånemark implant in partially edentulous jaws: a 10-year prospective multicenter study. Int J Oral Maxillofac Implants 1999;14(5):639–45.

5. Lindquist LW, Carlsson GE, Jemt T. A prospective 15-year follow-up study of mandibular fixed prostheses supported by osseointegrated implants. Clinical results and marginal bone loss. Clin Oral Implants Res 1996;7(4):329–36.

6. Buser D, Mericske-Stern R, Beranrd JP, et al. Long-term evaluation of non-submerged ITI implants. Part I: 8-year life table analysis of a prospective multicenter study with 2359 implants. Clin Oral Implants Res 1997;8(3):161–72.

7. Arvidson K, Bystedt H, Frykholm A, et al. Five-year prospective follow-up report of Astra Tech Implant System in the treatment of edentulous mandibles. Clin Oral Implants Res 1998;9(4):225–34.

8. Weber HP, Crohin CC, Fiorellini JP. A 5-year prospective clinical and radiographic study of non-submerged dental implants. Clin Oral Implants Res 2000;11(2):144–53.

9. Brocard D, Barthet P, Baysse E, et al. A multicenter report on 1,022 consecutively placed ITI implants: a 7-year longitudinal study. Int J Oral Maxillofac Implants 2000;15(5):691–700.

10. Leonhardt A, Grondahl K, Bergstrom C, et al. Long-term follow-up of osseointegrated titanium implants using clinical, radiographic and microbiological parameters. Clin Oral Implants Res 2002;13(2):127–32.

11. Esposito M, Worthington HV, Thomsen P, et al. Interventions for replacing missing teeth: different times for loading dental implants. Cochrane Database Syst Rev 2004;3:CD003878.

12. Becktor J, Isaksson S, Sennerby L. Survival analysis of endosseous implants in grafted and nongrafted edentulous maxillae. Int J Oral Maxillofac Implants 2004;19(1):107–15.

13. Urist MR. Bone: formation by autoinduction. Science 1965;150:893–9.

14. Reddi AH, Weintroub S, Muthukumaram N. Biologic principles of bone induction. Orthop Clin North Am 1987;18(2):207–12.

15. Dahlin C, Linde A, Gottlow J, et al. Healing of bone defects by guided tissue regeneration. Plast Reconstr Surg 1988;81(5):672–6.

16. Dahlin C, Andersson L, Linde A. Bone augmentation at fenestrated implants by an osteopromotive membrane technique. A controlled clinical study. Clin Oral Implants Res 1991;2(4):159–65.

17. Hämmerle CH, Jung RE, Feloutzis A. A systematic review of the survival of implants in bone sites augmented with barrier membranes (guided bone regeneration) in partially edentulous patients. J Clin Periodontol 2002;29(Suppl 3):226–31.

18. Burchardt H. The biology of bone graft repair. Clin Orthop Relat Res 1983;174:28–42.

19. Ilizarov GA. The tension-stress effect on the genesis and growth of tissues: Part I. The influence of stability of fixation and soft tissue preservation. Clin Orthop Relat Res 1989;238:249–81.

20. Iizarov GA. The tension-stress effect on the genesis and growth of tissues: Part II. The influence of the rate and frequency of distraction. Clin Orthop Relat Res 1989;239:263–85.

21. Jensen OT, Cockrell R, Kuhlke L, et al. Anterior maxillary alveolar distraction osteogenesis: a prospective 5-year clinical study. Int J Oral Maxillofac Implants 2002;17(1):52–68.

22. Chiapasco M, Consolo U, Bianchi A, et al. Alveolar distraction osteogenesis for the correction of vertically deficient edentulous ridges: a multicenter prospective study on humans. Int J Oral Maxillofac Implants 2004;19(3):399–407.

23. Barone A, Varanini P, Orlando B, et al. Deep-frozen allogeneic onlay bone grafts for reconstruction of atrophic maxillary alveolar ridges: a preliminary study. J Oral Maxillofac Surg 2009;67(6):1300–6.

24. Contar CM, Sarot JR, Bordini J, et al. Maxillary ridge augmentation with fresh-frozen bone allografts. J Oral Maxillofac Surg 2009;67(6):1280–5.

25. Adell R, Lekholm U, Gröndahl K, et al. Reconstruction of severely resorbed edentulous maxillae using osseointegrated fixtures in immediate autogenous bone grafts. Int J Oral Maxillofac Implants 1990;5(3):233–46.

26. Jensen J, Sindet-Pedersen S. Autogenous mandibular bone grafts and osseointegrated implants for reconstruction of the severely atrophied maxilla: a preliminary report. J Oral Maxillofac Surg 1991;49(12):1277–87.

27. Donovan MG, Dickerson NC, Hanson LJ, et al. Maxillary and mandibular reconstruction using calvarial bone grafts and Brånemark implants: a preliminary report. J Oral Maxillofac Surg 1994;52(6):588–94.

28. Mc Grath CJ, Schepers SH, Blijdorp PA, et al. Simultaneous placement of endosteal implants and mandibular onlay grafting for treatment of the atrophic mandible. A preliminary report. Int J Oral Maxillofac Surg 1996;25(3):184–8.

29. Åstrand P, Nord PG, Brånemark PI. Titanium implants and onlay bone graft to the atrophic edentulous maxilla. Int J Oral Maxillofac Surg 1996;25(1):25–9.

30. Vermeeren JI, Wismeijer D, van Waas MA. One-step reconstruction of the severely resorbed mandible with onlay bone grafts and endosteal implants.

A 5-year follow-up. Int J Oral Maxillofac Surg 1996; 25(2):112–5.

31. Triplett RG, Schow SR. Autologous bone grafts and endosseous implants: complementary techniques. Int J Oral Maxillofac Surg 1996;54(4):486–94.

32. Schliephake H, Neukam FW, Wichmann M. Survival analysis of endosseous implants in bone grafts used for the treatment of severe alveolar ridge atrophy. J Oral Maxillofac Surg 1997;55(11): 1227–33.

33. van Steenberghe D, Naert I, Bossuyt M, et al. The rehabilitation of the severely resorbed maxilla by simultaneous placement of autogenous bone grafts and implants: a 10-year evaluation. Clin Oral Investig 1997;1(3):102–8.

34. Verhoeven JW, Cune MS, Terlou M, et al. The combined use of endosteal implants and iliac crest onlay grafts in the severely atrophic mandible: a longitudinal study. Int J Oral Maxillofac Surg 1997;26(5):351–7.

35. Lundgren S, Nyström E, Nilson H, et al. Bone grafting to the maxillary sinuses, nasal floor and anterior maxilla in the atrophic edentulous maxilla. Int J Oral Maxillofac Surg 1997;26(6):428–34.

36. Widmark G, Andersson B, Andrup B, et al. Rehabilitation of patients with severely resorbed maxillae by means of implants with or without bone grafts. A 1-year follow-up study. Int J Oral Maxillofac Implants 1998;13(4):474–82.

37. Keller EE, Tolman DE, Eckert S. Surgical-prosthodontic reconstruction of advanced maxillary bone compromise with autogenous onlay block bone grafts and osseointegrated endosseous implants: a 12-year study of 32 consecutive patients. Int J Oral Maxillofac Implants 1999;14(2):197–209.

38. Chiapasco M, Abati S, Romeo E, et al. Clinical outcome of autogenous bone blocks or guided bone regeneration with e-PTFE membranes for the reconstruction of narrow edentulous ridges. Clin Oral Implants Res 1999;10(4):278–88.

39. Lekholm U, Wannfors K, Isaksson S, et al. Oral implants in combination with bone grafts. A 3-year retrospective multicenter study using the Brånemark implant system. Int J Oral Maxillofac Surg 1999; 28(3):181–7.

40. Bahat O, Fontanessi RV. Efficacy of implant placement after bone grafting for three-dimensional reconstruction of the posterior jaw. Int J Periodontics Restorative Dent 2001;21(3):221–31.

41. Bell RB, Blakey GH, White RP, et al. Staged reconstruction of the severely atrophic mandible with autogenous bone graft and endosteal implants. J Oral Maxillofac Surg 2002;60(10):1135–41.

42. Becktor JP, Eckert SE, Isaksson S, et al. The influence of mandibular dentition on implant failures in bone-grafted edentulous maxillae. Int J Oral Maxillofac Implants 2002;17(1):69–77.

43. Raghoebar GM, Schoen P, Meijer HJ, et al. Early loading of endosseous implants in the augmented maxilla: a 1-year prospective study. Clin Oral Implants Res 2003;14(6):697–702.

44. Jemt T, Lekholm U. Measurements of buccal tissue volumes at single-implant restorations after local bone grafting in maxillas: a 3-year clinical prospective study case series. Clin Implant Dent Relat Res 2003;5(2):63–70.

45. Iizuka T, Smolka W, Hallermann W, et al. Extensive augmentation of the alveolar ridge using autogenous calvarial split bone grafts for dental rehabilitation. Clin Oral Implants Res 2004;15(5):607–15.

46. Nyström E, Ahlqvist J, Gunne J, et al. 10-year follow-up of onlay bone grafts and implants in severely resorbed maxillae. Int J Oral Maxillofac Surg 2004; 33(3):258–62.

47. van der Meij EH, Blankestijn J, Berns RM, et al. The combined use of two endosteal implants and iliac crest onlay grafts in the severely atrophic mandible by a modified surgical approach. Int J Oral Maxillofac Surg 2005;34(2):152–7.

48. Molly L, Quirynen M, Michiels K, et al. Comparison between jaw bone augmentation by means of a stiff occlusive titanium membrane or an autologous hip graft: a retrospective clinical assessment. Clin Oral Implants Res 2006;17(5):481–7.

49. Levin L, Nitzan D, Schwartz-Arad D. Success of dental implants placed in intraoral block bone grafts. J Periodontol 2007;78(1):18–21.

50. Chiapasco M, Casentini P, Zaniboni M. Bone augmentation procedures in implant dentistry. Int J Oral Maxillofac Implants 2009;24(Suppl):237–59.

51. Chiapasco M, Zaniboni M, Boisco M. Augmentation procedures for the rehabilitation of deficient edentulous ridges with oral implants. Clin Oral Implants Res 2006;17(Suppl 2):136–59.

52. Chiapasco M, Gatti C, Gatti F. Immediate loading of dental implants placed in severely resorbed edentulous mandibles reconstructed with autogenous calvarial grafts. Clin Oral Implants Res 2007;18(1): 13–20.

53. Bähr W, Stoll P, Wächter R. Use of the "double barrel" free vascularized fibula in mandibular reconstruction. J Oral Maxillofac Surg 1998;56(1):38–44.

54. Chiapasco M, Gatti C. Immediate loading of dental implants placed in revascularized fibula free flaps: a clinical report on 2 consecutive patients. Int J Oral Maxillofac Implants 2004;19(6):906–12.

55. De Santis G, Nocini PF, Chiarini L, et al. Functional rehabilitation of the atrophic mandible and maxilla with fibula flaps and implant-supported prosthesis. Plast Reconstr Surg 2004;113(1):88–98.

56. Chiapasco M, Romeo E, Coggiola A, et al. Long-term outcome of dental implants placed in revascularized fibula free flaps used for the reconstruction of maxillo-mandibular defects due to extreme atrophy.

Clin Oral Implants Res 2010. DOI:10.1111/
j.1600–0501.2010.01999.x. [Epub ahead of print].

57. Maiorana C, Beretta M, Salina S, et al. Reduction of autogenous bone graft resorption by means of bio-oss coverage: a prospective study. Int J Periodontics Restorative Dent 2005;25(1):19–25.

58. von Arx T, Buser D. Horizontal ridge augmentation using autogenous block grafts and the guided bone regeneration technique with collagen membranes: a clinical study with 42 patients. Clin Oral Implants Res 2006;17(4):359–66.

59. Gielkens PF, Bos RR, Raghoebar GM, et al. Is there evidence that barrier membranes prevent bone resorption in autologous bone grafts during the healing period? A systematic review. Int J Oral Maxillofac Implants 2007;22(3):390–8.

60. Autelitano L, Rabbiosi D, Poggio A, et al. Pericranium graft in reconstructive surgery of atrophied maxillary bones. Minerva Stomatol 2008;57(5):265–74.

61. Gatti F, Chiapasco M, Gatti C. Innesti ossei autologhi di apposizione a scopo implantare. Dentista Moderno 2009;12:32–48.

62. Heberer S, Rühe B, Krekeler L, et al. A prospective randomized split-mouth study comparing iliac onlay grafts in atrophied edentulous patients: covered with periosteum or a bioresorbable membrane. Clin Oral Implants Res 2009;20(3):319–26.

63. ten Bruggenkate CM, van den Bergh JP. Maxillary sinus floor elevation: a valuable pre-prosthetic procedure. Periodontol 2000;1998(17):176–82.

64. Goené R, Bianchesi C, Hüerzeler M, et al. Performance of short implants in partial restorations: 3-year follow-up of osseotite implants. Implant Dent 2005;14(3):274–80.

65. Misch CE, Steignga J, Barboza E, et al. Short dental implants in posterior partial edentulism: a multicenter retrospective 6-year case series study. J Periodontol 2006;77(8):1340–7.

66. Arlin ML. Short dental implants as a treatment option: results from an observational study in a single private practice. Int J Oral Maxillofac Implants 2006;21(5):769–76.

67. Romeo E, Ghisolfi M, Rozza R, et al. Short (8-mm) dental implants in the rehabilitation of partial and complete edentulism: a 3- to 14-year longitudinal study. Int J Prosthodont 2006;19(6):586–92.

68. Renouard F, Nisand D. Impact of implant length and diameter on survival rates. Clin Oral Implants Res 2006;17(Suppl 2):35–51.

69. Maló P, de Araújo Nobre M, Rangert B. Short implants placed one-stage in maxillae and mandibles: a retrospective clinical study with 1 to 9 years of follow-up. Clin Implant Dent Relat Res 2007;9(1):15–21.

70. Anitua E, Orive G, Aguirre JJ, et al. Five-year clinical evaluation of short dental implants placed in posterior areas: a retrospective study. J Periodontol 2008;79(1):42–8.

71. Keller EE. Reconstruction of the severely atrophic edentulous mandible with endosseous implants: a 10-year longitudinal study. J Oral Maxillofac Surg 1995;53(3):305–20.

72. Stellingsma K, Raghoebar GM, Meijer HJ, et al. The extremely resorbed mandible: a comparative prospective study of 2-year results with 3 treatment strategies. Int J Oral Maxillofac Implants 2004;19(4):563–77.

Reoperative Orbital Trauma: Management of Posttraumatic Enophthalmos and Aberrant Eye Position

Simon Holmes, BDS, MBBS, FDSRCS, FRCS

KEYWORDS
- Enophthalmos • Posttraumatic orbital deformities
- Reoperative orbital trauma • Aberrant eye position

The posttraumatic position of the globe within the orbit is a prima facie indicator of severity of facial injury and of the success of surgical reduction. The aesthetic effect of this condition is immense, and patients complain about the shape of the upper eyelid and the reduced degree of eye opening, often referring to their shrunken eye. There are several causes and subtypes of abnormal eye position, and each requires a problem-focused approach to obtain the best clinical result. Causes of late presentation relate either to failure of the patient to access appropriate medical care, or to failure to diagnose in the acute setting. Advances in modern anesthesiology and resuscitation techniques have resulted in a cohort of severely injured patients presenting for primary and secondary craniofacial reconstruction. In these instances, enophthalmos may not be treatable in the primary setting because of massive soft tissue injury, direct globe injury, or inability of the patient to undergo extensive primary surgery (**Fig. 1**).[1]

DEFINITION AND PATHOGENESIS

Enophthalmos can be defined as a posterior position of one eye relative to the other. When a vertical discrepancy between the 2 globes is present, it is described as hypoglobus.

Assessment of enophthalmos in milder cases is difficult, and minor degrees are not obvious to the observer, either to the surgeon or the untrained observer. There is a physiologic variance between normal individuals, and this may be as much as 2 mm. Koo and colleagues[2] showed that observers do not notice changes in eye position of less than 2 mm; 97% of observers will spot enophthalmos when the discrepancy is between 5 and 8 mm. They studied the point at which most observers notice this deformity, which was shown to be between 3 and 4 mm.

The disturbance in the integrity of the orbital floor leading to posttraumatic enophthalmos was recognized toward the end of the nineteenth century. The link between size of the orbital cavity and volume of its contents as a putative mechanism has endured. Modifications and secondary factors have been described, including the Lockwood ligament forming a supportive sling, and herniation of intraconal orbital fat.[3]

The relationship between orbital volume and enophthalmos has led surgeons to postulate that orbital volume may be measured, and that discrepancies between the 2 orbits could be related with the degree of enophthalmos. Although this may seem logical, there is no universal agreement between volume of increase and degree of enophthalmos. Furthermore, the appropriate time span between time of injury and presentation of the deformity is unclear.[4–8]

The bony orbit is often described as a pyramidal structure, and each of the walls has a complex

Barts and the London NHS Trust, The Royal London Hospital, 1st Floor John Harrison House, Whitechapel, London E1 1BB, UK
E-mail address: simon.holmes@bartsandthelondon.nhs.uk

Oral Maxillofacial Surg Clin N Am 23 (2011) 17–29
doi:10.1016/j.coms.2010.10.010

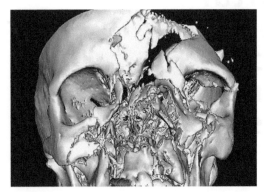

Fig. 1. Gross craniofacial fracture with left orbital disruption and total destruction of all 4 orbital walls. Secondary management of enophthalmos is inevitable.

shape and a direct contribution to the position of the globe. It is expected that new defects, or malunions of these individual walls, could potentially change the position of the globe, which explains why incorrectly reduced zygomatic fractures that may not disturb the orbital floor may contribute to aberrant globe position.

There are 2 key areas within the orbit that have been identified as prime determinants of eye position. The first is the junctional portion between the medial wall and the orbital floor in the posterior third of the orbit, known as Hammer's key area.[9] The second is the S-shaped curvature of the posterior third of the orbital floor, behind the

coronal equator of the globe. The reconstruction of this floor curvature is mimicked by custom-made implants.[10,11]

Consequently, it has been postulated that disturbances in the shape of the key areas, together with the size of the defects, should predispose to enophthalmos. Lee and colleagues[12] studied the relationship between small medial orbital wall fractures and enophthalmos. The study indicated that, even with fractures as small as 0.55 cm, enophthalmos may be observed. The size of the bony defect may not be the only determinant of enophthalmos. Kim and colleagues[13] showed that the height/width ratios of the medial rectus muscle measured in a coronal computed tomography (CT) scan may be a useful parameter to predict enophthalmos in medial orbital wall fractures; furthermore, they suggested that when the ratio was more than 0.7, surgical correction was indicated. Ahn and colleagues[8] showed a positive correlation between late enophthalmos and an increased orbital fracture volume. In addition, they were able to establish a mathematical formula using linear regression to predict that enophthalmos = 0.84 V+0.07 where V is fracture site volume. For every 1.0-mL increase in volume, the amount of enophthalmos was estimated to be 0.84 mm. Enophthalmos of 2 mm or more was predicted with an orbital fracture volume of 2.30 mL.

Enophthalmos caused by soft tissue contraction in the form of fat atrophy is seen in acquired medical conditions, and may be seen particularly

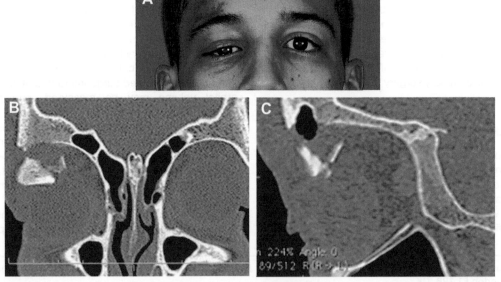

Fig. 2. (*A*) Frontal view of a patient with late-presentation right orbital roof fracture. (*B*) Coronal and (*C*) sagittal CT scan views showing impingement of the bone fragments on the globe itself, causing ophthalmoplegia. This deformity cannot be corrected by manipulation below the globe.

in severe trauma.[14,15] However, this is often disputed.[16,17]

Although less common, enophthalmos/orbital dystopia may also be a function of orbital roof/supraorbital rim disruption (**Fig. 2**).

SURGICAL ANATOMY: BONE

The position of the eye is a function of the anatomy of the hard and soft tissues of the supporting structures. The bone provides a safe and stable platform and protects the eye and adnexal structures. The dimensions of the bony orbit are 50 mm deep by 35 mm wide and 40 mm high, giving a volume of 30 mL. The bony orbit is made up of 7 bones (**Fig. 3**). Within this osteology there are unique properties that dictate the fracture configuration following energy transfer.

Of particular surgical significance is the horizontal process of the palatine bone, which often provides a ledge delineating the posterior margin of the fracture, and is a convenient landmark with which to site the posterior margin of the reconstruction. The junction between the sphenoid and zygomatic bones is an important surgical landmark. The thick nature of the constituent bones is usually maintained, which enables visualization of surgical reduction. This visualization is particularly relevant during revisional surgery in which malunited bone has undergone significant remodeling, thus obscuring the correct anatomic position (**Fig. 4**).

DIAGNOSIS OF ENOPHTHALMOS
History

The cause of orbital floor/wall fractures is usually blunt trauma. Although all mechanisms of trauma

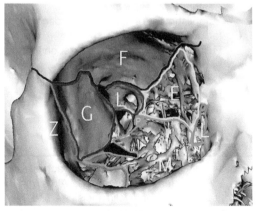

Fig. 3. Osteology of the right orbit, consisting of 7 bones. Note the robust roof and lateral walls. Frontal (F), ethmoid (E), palatine (P), zygomatic (Z), lacrimal (L), maxillary (M), and sphenoid greater (G) and lesser (L) wings.

may cause these injuries, the force is usually applied either to the globe directly, or to the orbital margins.

Enophthalmos presenting at the time of primary injury is unusual, because orbital adnexal swelling and hematoma usually mask the physical signs. If enophthalmos presents early, it usually implies an extremely large orbital fracture.

Patients presenting with disorders of eye position can normally remember a facial injury some months or years previously. The full magnitude of the injury is often underplayed at the time of the primary injury. Prognostic factors for the development of enophthalmos are shown in **Box 1**.

Examination

The diagnosis of established enophthalmos with significant relative differences in anterior globe projection is usually straightforward. The patient notices a shrunken smaller eye compared with the normal side and an increased, or thicker, upper eyelid. The appearance of the upper eyelid with supratarsal hollowing is a typical deformity and is a direct manifestation of the retroposition of the globe within the orbit (**Fig. 5A**). The full extent of the retroposition of the globe is often most evident when the patient is viewed from below, in worm's eye view (see **Fig. 5B**). It is also important to record any impression of inferior positioning of the globe.

Full examination of the position of the orbital margins, zygomatic bone, nasoethmoid, frontal bones, and maxilla must include extraorbital extension of any fracture pattern. It is important to examine and record the level of sensation, particularly of the infraorbital and zygomaticofacial nerves.

Further diagnostic studies complement the clinical examination; an orthoptic and ophthalmologic examination will exclude damage to the globe and interference with conjugate gaze as well as differentiation between mechanical, neurologic, and muscular causes of diplopia (**Table 1**).

Hertel Assessment

Use of the Hertel exophthalmometer provides a noninvasive mechanism of recording globe position with accuracy and objectivity. It also may be used to judge the outcomes of the surgical therapy. Although the use of this instrument has recently attracted criticism, both in terms of reliability compared with other techniques and inter- and intraoperative variability, it remains a valid tool and more objective than simply eyeballing the patient.[18,19]

The observer sits in front of the patient and seats the footplates of the meter on the lateral orbital

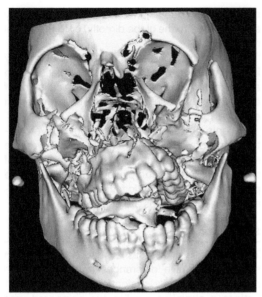

Fig. 4. CT scan three-dimensional reconstruction of a patient with panfacial fractures that allows appreciation of interrelationship of middle third fractures with the orbital margins and thus likely contribution to the pathogenesis of enophthalmos. Lateralization of the bone between the frontozygomatic suture and the floor must be addressed in addition to the internal orbit otherwise aesthetic correction will never be achieved.

margin, which is then measured and recorded to allow reproducibility in the future (**Fig. 6**A). To record the degree of enophthalmos, the blue cone on the meter is then lined up with the longest line on the mirror. The anterior surface of the cornea is measured using the scale on the mirror and the number is recorded and compared with the contralateral eye (see **Fig. 6**B). Although this instrument allows a degree of objectivity, its readings should be interpreted cautiously. It is not usually possible to assess acute injuries in this manner because the swelling precludes seating

---

Box 1
Prognostic factors for development of enophthalmos

- Large floor defect
- Medial wall defect
- Posterior fractures
- Loss of palatine bone shelf
- Orbital roof involvement
- Associated zygomatic fracture
- Damage to ocular muscles
- Damage to lacrimal apparatus
- Damage to globe

---

the footplates. In addition, if there is a contour deficit of the lateral orbital margin, the footplates will not sit in the correct position. These potential problems must be allowed for in the diagnosis and in subsequent treatment planning.

Imaging

Modern CT scanning techniques have revolutionized the diagnosis of facial injuries. Helical CT data acquisition is rapid, and facial scans can be obtained as part of the initial trauma series in the emergency room. Liaison with the radiologist is essential to ensure that the correct data are obtained, particularly to include all parts of the face that are likely to be included in the fracture pattern. This liaison ensures minimal radiation exposure for greatest diagnostic yield. There is increasing evidence for the use of cone beam CT in the diagnosis of orbital wall injuries, allowing for reduced radiation dose.[20] It is essential that the CT scan has adequate resolution in the form of slice thickness. Ideally, the slice thickness should be no greater than 1 mm, particularly if models or navigation techniques are to be used. Coronal, axial, and sagittal views are used for the measurement of the size of the defect. They also help in the establishment of the most important determinant of surgical difficulty: the position of the defect (**Fig. 7**). The position of the globe itself can be seen in a conventional CT scan. The degree of enophthalmos and the volume of the internal orbit can be measured, and this is often cited in the scientific literature to relate and quantify degree of enophthalmos.[6]

PRINCIPLES OF MANAGEMENT

The management of posttraumatic enophthalmos and aberrant eye position is based on:

- Aesthetic access incisions
- Establishment of correct three-dimensional facial skeleton
- Full exploration of orbit and reconstruction of orbital floor and walls
- Correction of the orbital soft tissue deficit
- Reconstruction of supporting facial soft tissues.

Aesthetic Access Incisions

Access to the internal orbit may be achieved by a variety of different approaches. Although the transcutaneous lower eyelid incisions find favor with many, access may be limited particularly to the medial wall. Postsurgical scarring is normally minimal, but may be noticeable in some patients. Visible scars may be seen in more than 40% of

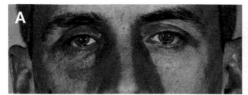
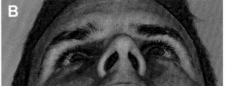

Fig. 5. (*A*) Anterior view of a patient with right enophthalmos secondary to extensive medial and orbital floor fractures. Note the supratarsal hollowing. (*B*) Worm's eye view that shows the full extent of the deformity.

transcutaneous incisions. Most patients with facial trauma are of an age at which lower eyelid skin creases may not be present, and even a well-healed scar may induce asymmetry.

McCord and Moses[21] described exposure of the inferior orbit with a fornix incision and lateral canthotomy in 1979. The obvious proximity of the conjunctiva to the orbital contents, and the excellent aesthetic results achieved, have revolutionized the approach to the complex orbit. Retrospective studies have shown positive outcome of the transconjunctival approach compared with that of the subciliary.[22] Although canthal reconstruction may lead to lid malposition, this is both technique sensitive and largely avoidable with increasing experience. The versatility of the transconjunctival approach has been greatly improved by the addition of the transcaruncular extension, which represents a short additional mucosal incision, but enables the surgeon to expose the medial wall to the orbital apex without interfering with the medial canthal tendon or lacrimal apparatus.[23–26] The author considers that the

McCord lid swing coupled with transcaruncular extension leads to rapid and superb surgical access to all aspects of the orbit subject to pure and impure fractures (**Figs. 8** and **9**).

Advances in endoscope technology, and increased understanding of functional endoscopic sinus surgery techniques, have led to interest in orbital traumatology. Endoscopic visualization of the orbit and fracture elements has been used both diagnostically and therapeutically via both transantral and endonasal approaches.[27,28] Proponents of this approach highlight the stealthy nature of surgical access, the lack of postoperative eyelid complications, and the increased likelihood of anatomic repair.[29,30] However, most fractures may be appropriately accessed and reconstructed with a predictable aesthetic outcome using the approach described earlier. In the author's practice, endoscopic assistance is used rarely, and is particularly reserved for extensive medial wall injuries with proximity to the orbital apex, and fixation of the orbital soft tissues to the nasal septum or the remnant medial wall.

Establishment of Correct Three-dimensional Skeletal Form

The precise surgical approach used depends on the condition of the bony elements, and treatment algorithms are largely either osteotomies or computer-aided design and computer-aided manufacturing replacement using synthetic material.

When enough bone remains from the original injury, reposition using osteotomies and rigid fixation is indicated (**Fig. 10**). Continuity defects of the infraorbital rim can be addressed using alloplastic implants such as Medpore to achieve a smooth margin. The infraorbital rim is a problem area and, unless reconstructed, the final aesthetic appearance of the lower eyelid will be impaired.

On occasion, particularly in cranio-orbital fractures, the remaining cranial or orbital bones are lost or not amenable to segment and move. In those cases, the use of a custom-made implant, such as a polyether ether ketone (PEEK) implant may salvage an otherwise untreatable condition.

Table 1 Enophthalmos diagnostic studies	
Modality	**Diagnostic Yield**
Radiology	Quantification of size of defect
	Position of defect
	Extent of craniofacial extension
	Quantification of eye position
	Presence of foreign bodies within the orbit
Hertel	Position of globe
Ultrasound	Ocular integrity
	Intraocular foreign body
Orthoptist	Assessment of conjugate gaze
	Differentiation between mechanical, neurologic, and muscular causes of diplopia
	Assessment of functional deficit

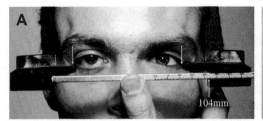
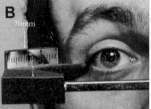

Fig. 6. (A) Hertel exophthalmometer in place (B). Close-up view of the right eye. Note the blue cone lined up with the longest line.

The advantage of PEEK implants is that the material itself may be screwed into, which facilitates fixation to the skull and reattachment of the surrounding muscles (**Fig. 11**).

Full Exploration of Orbit and Reconstruction of Orbital Floor and Walls

Throughout the history of orbital floor fracture management, there has been no universal agreement as to the best material for reconstruction. All materials have significant advantages and significant disadvantages. Materials used can be classified in terms of origin (eg, autogenous or alloplastic). Alloplastic materials can be classified according to structure, biodegradability, manufacture, or even physical form.

In secondary reconstruction, some materials are especially popular. Autogenous bone is often referred to as the gold standard because of its potential for revascularization and its capacity for osteoconduction and osteoinduction. Bone has been used for many years, and different donor sites are said to yield different patterns of resorption.[31] It has been said that cranial bone is the most stable and least likely to resorb, and the most favorable to handle operatively.[32,33] This opinion has being challenged with a direct comparison between cranial and iliac crest bone graft in late enophthalmos management.[34]

Most defects, particularly those treated in the acute phase, may be reconstructed with a wide variety of materials. For established and complex defects, special consideration needs to be given to the use of titanium mesh. Ellis and Tan[35] highlighted the increased accuracy of fit when using titanium compared with cranial bone. Although this improvement relates to the ease of manipulation of the material, they also established that both materials could be successfully used.[35]

Replication of the precise anatomic contours is central to good outcome, but this is extremely

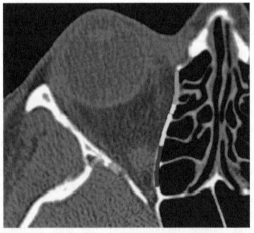

Fig. 7. Surgical access and risk of damage to the optic nerve increase as the fracture approaches the posterior orbit. Axial CT scan view depicting access areas and level of difficulty: green, safe and easy access; yellow, moderate difficulty that requires good surgical exposure; red, difficult access that requires extensive orbital exposure, so consider using custom-made implants or navigation technology.

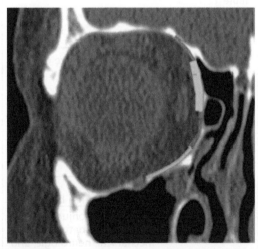

Fig. 8. Coronal CT scan view depicting the required surgical access to the medial orbital wall based on defect location: blue, transconjunctival; red, swinging lid; green, transcaruncular; purple, craniofacial access.

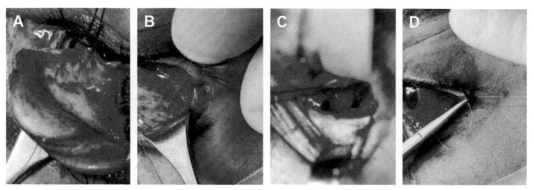

Fig. 9. Surgical approach. (*A*) Traction sutures may be applied to the conjunctiva to enable it to act as a physiologic eye shield. (*B*) To achieve maximum exposure, it is essential to ensure full division of the lower limb of the lateral canthus, shown here intact. (*C*) The use of the transconjunctival incision accompanied with a McCord lateral cantholysis and transcaruncular extension allows visualization of the entire orbit from the frontozygomatic suture to the junction between the anterior skull base and medial orbital wall. (*D*) It is important to maintain the upper limb of the canthus because it greatly simplifies closure at the end of the operation. Two sutures are placed, the first to reconstruct the tendon, the second to close a gray line.

technique sensitive and surgically difficult. The use of stereolithographic models with custom-made titanium constructs leads to an accurate prosthesis and has yielded excellent results.[10] However, this technique is expensive and time consuming, and not suitable for impure orbital injuries. It could be argued that the cost benefits in reduced operating time, reduced manipulating of the orbital tissues, and quality of the results provide an overall cost benefit.

Recent advances in understanding of the commonality of orbital shape across all populations have resulted in the development of preformed anatomic titanium mesh implants for true-to-original reconstruction.[36,37] This mesh enables rapid reconstruction of medial and large orbital floor fractures with almost custom-made accuracy. The S-shaped curvature of the floor is reconstructed reliably and the posterior portion of the implant may sit on the palatine bone, but,

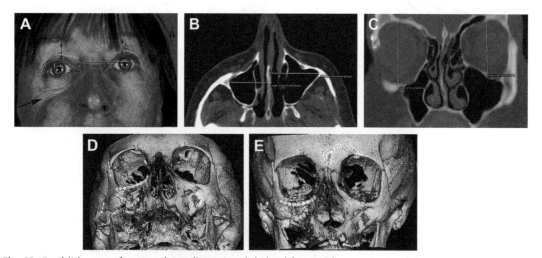

Fig. 10. Establishment of correct three-dimensional skeletal form with osteotomies. (*A*) Frontal view of a patient suffering from right enophthalmos, hypoglobus, upper eyelid supratarsal hollowing, and zygomatic hard and soft tissue depression. (*B, C*) Preoperative axial and coronal CT scan views showing the extent of the deformity. Measurement between fixed points allows precise operative planning of the three-dimensional movements required to achieve symmetry. (*D, E*) Postoperative three-dimensional CT scan reconstruction after osteotomies and orbital reconstruction.

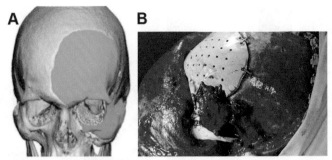

Fig. 11. Establishment of correct three-dimensional skeletal form with custom-made implants. (*A*) Zygomatic and frontal PEEK implants. (*B*) Implant in place; note the reattachment of the temporalis muscle.

in extensive posterior defects, a predictable result can be achieved by cantilevering back (**Fig. 12**). In addition to being strong, they also allow ease of placement and can be used following open reduction or zygomatic osteotomy.

Strategies for Extensive Posterior Defects

These defects are regarded as a high risk with respect to damage to the structures at the orbital apex, and because of potentially poor outcomes because of failure of reconstruction of the

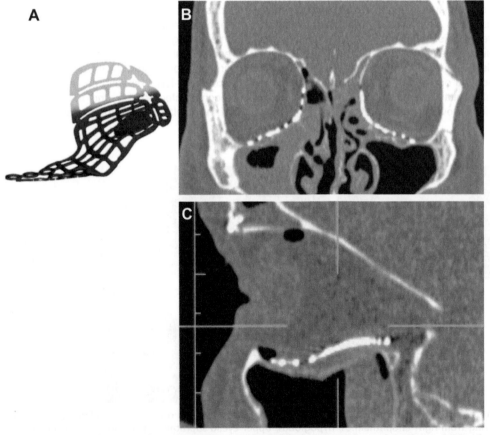

Fig. 12. Establishment of correct three-dimensional skeletal form with preformed implants. (*A*) Preformed anatomic titanium mesh that mimics the fit of custom-made plates. (*B*) Postoperative coronal CT scan view showing the excellent anatomic fit of the mesh. (*C*) Postoperative sagittal view showing the reconstruction of S-shaped curvature of the floor.

posteromedial bulge. Revision orbital injuries are particular difficult because of the additional scarring, making dissection hazardous. In these circumstances, although the extended approach described earlier is useful, adjunctive endoscopic support, either via a transnasal, transantral, or transorbital approach, can aid dissection and check the fit of the implant.[38,39]

Occasionally, intraoperative navigation may be beneficial and it is particularly useful if plain titanium mesh is used.[40] Preformed anatomic titanium mesh implants are also extremely useful; they have the advantage that the position of the plate with respect to the orbital apex is already known, avoiding repeat manipulation of the orbital contents and repeated insertions (**Fig. 13**).

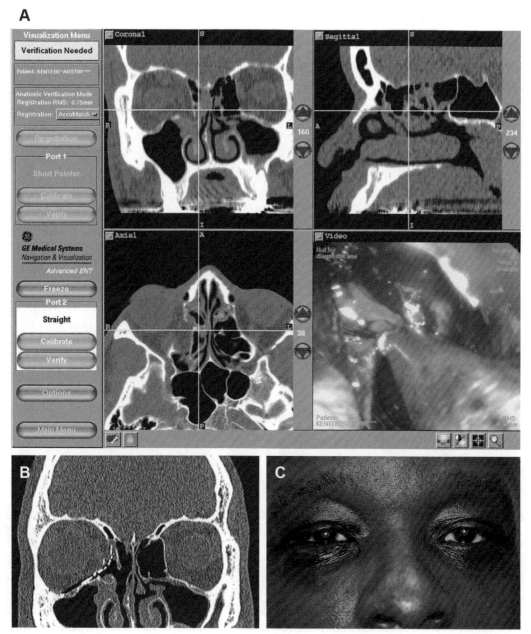

Fig. 13. Extensive posterior defects. (*A*) Navigation-assisted repair of extensive medial wall defect. (*B*) Postoperative CT scan showing the excellent anatomic fit of the implant. (*C*) Postoperative view of the patient 10 days after surgery.

Correction of the Orbital Soft Tissue Deficit

Extensive trauma to the orbit results in damage not only to hard tissues but also to the soft tissues. The interrelationship between orbital trauma and the orbital contents has been well described in the literature.[41] Increased orbital volume, either as a manifestation of imperfect reconstruction or soft tissue loss, may be addressed by alloplastic replacement. In cases of high-energy trauma or penetrating injuries, visual function may be impaired and, aesthetically, the grossly damaged eye represents a considerable challenge. If possible, it is best to retain the globe remnant with or without an ocular prosthesis. If the globe remnant has 15 degrees of movement, the prosthesis and the contact lens will move (**Fig. 14**).

Reconstruction of Supporting Facial Soft Tissues

Even after optimal bone reconstruction, the soft tissue results, and hence the facial appearance, may prove to be disappointing. The cheek fat pad becomes atrophied or depressed and the area might require additional treatment with

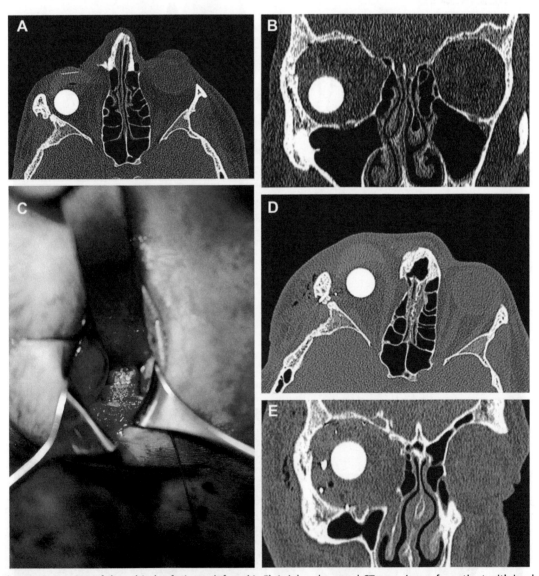

Fig. 14. Correction of the orbital soft tissue defect. (*A, B*) Axial and coronal CT scan views of a patient with inadequate orbital soft tissue augmentation. (*C*) The defect was address using an enophthalmos Medpore wedge and a 6-mm block of Medpore on the lateral orbital wall. (*D, E*) Postoperative axial and coronal CT scan views showing a favorable position of the implant and reduced enophthalmos.

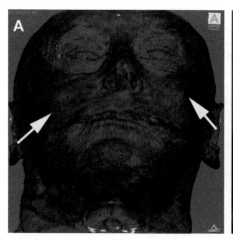
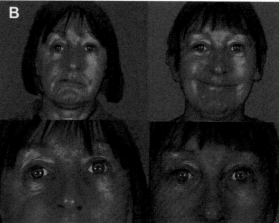

Fig. 15. Reconstruction of supporting facial soft tissues. (*A*) Three-dimensional CT reconstruction of the patient in **Fig. 10** before reoperation. Note the right cheek fat pad depression (*white arrows*). (*B*) Before and after pictures of the same patient after osteotomies, reconstruction of the orbit, and resuspension of the surrounding soft tissues.

placement of facial implants or fat grafting. In addition, it is important to remember that redraping of the facial soft tissues is required and can be achieved via the orbital or coronal approaches with long sutures, fascial slings, or the endotines implants (**Fig. 15**).

SUMMARY

Although the management of enophthalmos is subject to considerable surgeon variance between assessment, access, and materials used, there is universal agreement in the literature that it remains a complex and unpredictable condition to treat secondarily. As expectations increase, and patients survive more significant mechanisms of injury, it is likely that the challenge will remain difficult to meet.

With the imaging technology available today, and the more aggressive stance taken toward appropriate primary repair, it is likely that surgeons will simply see fewer minor cases and increased numbers of the bad ones.

The correct three-dimensional position of the facial skeleton is of paramount importance; without it, any orbital reconstruction is likely to fail.

The choice of reconstructive material should be evidence based rather than based simply on surgical preference, although good surgeons will get good results regardless of what materials are available. Titanium has many advantages compared with bone, and concerns about infection and rejection, and incarceration of soft tissues, do not occur with any convincing frequency in the literature. Cranial bone remains a viable alternative in postinfective cases,

particularly if the graft were taken as part of a coronal access procedure.

Of crucial importance to the management of all traumas, particularly in revisional surgery, is attention to the soft tissue envelope, which adds to the postoperative result, and may camouflage minor degrees of enophthalmos.

REFERENCES

1. Seider N, Gilboa M, Miller B, et al. Orbital fractures complicated by late enophthalmos: higher prevalence in patients with multiple trauma. Ophthal Plast Reconstr Surg 2007;23(2):115–8.
2. Koo L, Hatton M, Rubin P. When is enophthalmos "significant"? Ophthal Plast Reconstr Surg 2006; 22(4):274–7.
3. Clauser L, Galie M, Pagliaro F, et al. Posttraumatic enophthalmos: etiology, principles of reconstruction, and correction. J Craniofac Surg 2008;19(2):351–9.
4. Whitehouse R, Batterbury M, Jackson A, et al. Prediction of enophthalmos by computed tomography after 'blow out' orbital fracture. Br J Ophthalmol 1994;78(8):618–20.
5. Raskin EM, Millman AL, Lubkin V, et al. Prediction of late enophthalmos by volumetric analysis of orbital fractures. Ophthal Plast Reconstr Surg 1998;14(1):19–26.
6. Fan X, Li J, Zhu J, et al. Computer-assisted orbital volume measurement in the surgical correction of late enophthalmos caused by blowout fractures. Ophthal Plast Reconstr Surg 2003;19(3):207–11.
7. Kolk A, Pautke C, Schott V, et al. Secondary posttraumatic enophthalmos: high-resolution magnetic resonance imaging compared with multislice computed tomography in postoperative orbital

volume measurement. J Oral Maxillofac Surg 2007; 65(10):1926–34.

8. Ahn HB, Ryu WY, Yoo KW, et al. Prediction of enophthalmos by computer-based volume measurement of orbital fractures in a Korean population. Ophthal Plast Reconstr Surg 2008;24(1):36–9.

9. Hammer B, Prein J. Correction of post-traumatic orbital deformities: operative techniques and review of 26 patients. J Craniomaxillofac Surg 1995;23(2):81–90.

10. Lieger O, Richards R, Liu M, et al. Computer-aided design and manufacture of implants in the late reconstruction of extensive orbital fractures. Arch Facial Plast Surg 2010;12(3):186–91.

11. Zhang Y, He Y, Zhang ZY, et al. Evaluation of the application of computer-aided shape-adapted fabricated titanium mesh for mirroring-reconstructing orbital walls in cases of late post-traumatic enophthalmos. J Oral Maxillofac Surg 2010;68(9):2070–5.

12. Lee WT, Kim HK, Chung SM. Relationship between small-size medial orbital wall fracture and late enophthalmos. J Craniofac Surg 2009;20(1):75–80.

13. Kim YK, Park CS, Kim HK, et al. Correlation between changes of medial rectus muscle section and enophthalmos in patients with medial orbital wall fracture. J Plast Reconstr Aesthet Surg 2009; 62(11):1379–83.

14. Nasr AM, Ayyash I, Karcioglu ZA. Unilateral enophthalmos secondary to acquired hemilipodystrophy. Am J Ophthalmol 1997;124(4):572–5.

15. Chang BY, Cunniffe G, Hutchinson C. Enophthalmos associated with primary breast carcinoma. Orbit 2002;21(4):307–10.

16. Bite U, Jackson IT, Forbes GS, et al. Orbital volume measurements in enophthalmos using three-dimensional CT imaging. Plast Reconstr Surg 1985;75(4):502–8.

17. Schuknecht B, Carls F, Valavanis A, et al. CT assessment of orbital volume in late post-traumatic enophthalmos. Neuroradiology 1996;38(5):470–5.

18. Nkenke E, Benz M, Maier T, et al. Relative en- and exophthalmometry in zygomatic fractures comparing optical non-contact, non-ionizing 3D imaging to the Hertel instrument and computed tomography. J Craniomaxillofac Surg 2003;31(6):362–8.

19. Nkenke E, Maier T, Benz M, et al. Hertel exophthalmometry versus computed tomography and optical 3D imaging for the determination of the globe position in zygomatic fractures. Int J Oral Maxillofac Surg 2004;33(2):125–33.

20. Zizelmann C, Gellrich NC, Metzger MC, et al. Computer-assisted reconstruction of orbital floor based on cone beam tomography. Br J Oral Maxillofac Surg 2007;45(1):79–80.

21. McCord CD, Moses JL. Exposure of the inferior orbit with fornix incision and lateral canthotomy. Ophthalmic Surg 1979;10(6):53–63.

22. De Riu G, Meloni SM, Gobbi R, et al. Subciliary versus swinging eyelid approach to the orbital floor. J Craniomaxillofac Surg 2008;36(8):439–42.

23. Garcia GH, Goldberg RA, Shorr N. The transcaruncular approach in repair of orbital fractures: a retrospective study. J Craniomaxillofac Trauma 1998; 4(1):7–12.

24. Shorr N, Baylis HI, Goldberg RA, et al. Transcaruncular approach to the medial orbit and orbital apex. Ophthalmology 2000;107(8):1459–63.

25. Goldberg RA, Mancini R, Demer JL. The transcaruncular approach: surgical anatomy and technique. Arch Facial Plast Surg 2007;9(6):443–7.

26. Lee CS, Yoon JS, Lee SY. Combined transconjunctival and transcaruncular approach for repair of large medial orbital wall fractures. Arch Ophthalmol 2009; 127(3):291–6.

27. Lee MJ, Kang YS, Yang JY, et al. Endoscopic transnasal approach for the treatment of medial orbital blow-out fracture: a technique for controlling the fractured wall with a balloon catheter and Merocel. Plast Reconstr Surg 2002;110(2):417–26.

28. Otori N, Haruna S, Moriyama H. Endoscopic endonasal or transmaxillary repair of orbital floor fracture: a study of 88 patients treated in our department. Acta Otolaryngol 2003;123(6):718–23.

29. Strong EB, Kim KK, Diaz RC. Endoscopic approach to orbital blowout fracture repair. Otolaryngol Head Neck Surg 2004;131(5):683–95.

30. Farwell DG, Strong EB. Endoscopic repair of orbital floor fractures. Otolaryngol Clin North Am 2007; 40(2):319–28.

31. Smith JD, Abramson M. Membranous vs endochondrial bone autografts. Arch Otolaryngol 1974;99(3): 203–5.

32. Zins JE, Whitaker LA. Membranous versus endochondral bone: implications for craniofacial reconstruction. Plast Reconstr Surg 1983;72(6): 778–85.

33. Kelly CP, Cohen AJ, Yavuzer R, et al. Cranial bone grafting for orbital reconstruction: is it still the best? J Craniofac Surg 2005;16(1):181–5.

34. Siddique SA, Mathog RH. A comparison of parietal and iliac crest bone grafts for orbital reconstruction. J Oral Maxillofac Surg 2002;60(1):44–50.

35. Ellis E, Tan Y. Assessment of internal orbital reconstructions for pure blowout fractures: cranial bone grafts versus titanium mesh. J Oral Maxillofac Surg 2003;61:442–53.

36. Metzger MC, Schön R, Tetzlaf R, et al. Topographical CT-data analysis of the human orbital floor. Int J Oral Maxillofac Surg 2007;36(1):45–53.

37. Schön R, Metzger MC, Zizelmann C, et al. Individually preformed titanium mesh implants for a true-to-original repair of orbital fractures. Int J Oral Maxillofac Surg 2006;35(11):990–5.

38. Jin HR, Yeon JY, Shin SO, et al. Endoscopic versus external repair of orbital blowout fractures. Otolaryngol Head Neck Surg 2007;136(1):38–44.

39. Ballin CR, Sava LC, Maeda CA, et al. Endoscopic transnasal approach for treatment of the medial orbital blowout fracture using nasal septum graft. Facial Plast Surg 2009;25(1):3–7.

40. Schmelzeisen R, Gellrich NC, Schoen R, et al. Navigation-aided reconstruction of medial orbital wall and floor contour in cranio-maxillofacial reconstruction. Injury 2004;35(10):955–62.

41. al-Qurainy IA, Stassen LF, Dutton GN, et al. The characteristics of midfacial fractures and the association with ocular injury: a prospective study. Br J Oral Maxillofac Surg 1991;29(5):291–301.

Reoperative Midface Trauma

Robin S. Yang, DDS[a], Andrew R. Salama, DDS, MD[b],
John F. Caccamese, DMD, MD[a],*

KEYWORDS

- Reoperation • Complications • Zygoma fractures
- Naso-orbital-ethmoidal fractures • Nasal fractures

Residual facial disharmony caused by traumatic craniomaxillofacial injury can have a profound effect on a patient's quality of life. The consequences might be primarily functional or aesthetic, but both can be debilitating. Whether it is a change in vision, the ability to communicate, masticate, or how one is perceived in society, the cost of facial trauma can far exceed the initial hospitalization and injury.

Maxillofacial trauma is predominantly seen in the younger population (ages 20–40 years), with a male gender predilection; road traffic accidents are the most common cause of injury.[1] Within the realm of facial trauma, the midface, because of its location and projection within the facial sphere, is highly susceptible to injury.

Trauma to the craniomaxillofacial complex requires precise and meticulous surgical intervention. The clinician must have a knowledge of anatomic structures, an understanding of function, as well as an awareness of the normal three-dimensional spatial positioning of the facial bones. Revision surgery is common, because there are frequent factors that limit the ideal management in the acute setting. The primary goal of any reconstructive surgery requires that clinicians recreate, to the best of their abilities, normal and functional physical appearance. The goals of primary traumatic reconstruction of the face include restoration of masticatory, ocular, olfactory, respiratory, sinus, and sensory function, as well as maintaining the most aesthetic physical appearance possible. Adherence to the central tenants of initial fracture management will hopefully limit secondary facial deformity requiring revision surgery.

ANATOMY OF THE MIDFACE REGION

The midfacial portion of the facial skeleton is an integral component of the face, bridging the neurocranium above, with the mandible below, forming a highly specialized and functional central unit. The midface and the neurocranium house the globes, whereas, in combination with the mandible, the midface helps to form the upper aerodigestive complex. The midfacial skeleton and overlying soft tissue is largely responsible for an individual's unique appearance and individual facial fingerprint. The main skeletal components that comprise the midface include the maxilla, zygoma, lateral and medial orbital walls, orbital floor, nasal bones, and the naso-orbital-ethmoid complex. The constructs of the facial skeleton have been described as a series of horizontal and vertical and horizontal buttresses.[2] These areas of primary stability within the facial skeleton help in the accurate reduction of bony fractures and serve as primary areas for the placement of rigid fixation. Specific anatomic points are discussed later. However, it must be emphasized that alterations in the position of any of these basic facial structures will cause downstream distortions or misalignment of other portions of the facial skeleton and potential alterations in function.

[a] Department of Oral and Maxillofacial Surgery, University of Maryland Medical System, 650 West Baltimore Street, Room 1217, Baltimore, MD 21201, USA
[b] Department of Oral and Maxillofacial Surgery, Henry Goldman School of Dental Medicine, Boston University, Boston, MA, USA
* Corresponding author.
E-mail address: jcaccamese@umaryland.edu

Oral Maxillofacial Surg Clin N Am 23 (2011) 31–45
doi:10.1016/j.coms.2010.10.005
1042-3699/11/$ — see front matter © 2011 Elsevier Inc. All rights reserved.

MAXILLARY FRACTURES

Maxillary trauma has been reported to be associated with 14% to 17% of facial injuries.[3] Frequently, the maxilla is fractured in the setting of other facial fractures, most notably the nasal bones and the orbitozygomatic complex. In addition, fractures of the maxilla are associated with a high incidence of concomitant neurologic injury.

The maxilla is the central bony unit of the face and shares skeletal articulations with many of the bones in the craniofacial skeleton. In contrast with the mandible, the maxilla is less dense and houses the paranasal sinuses. It has been suggested that such a design offers an evolutionary advantage in which crumple zones potentially absorb the energy of blunt trauma, preventing direct transmission of forces to the neurocranium. Rene Le Fort[4] in his classification of midface fractures noted specific areas of weakness in the facial skeleton. The articulations of the maxilla with the zygoma and the frontal bones have been proven to be areas of stability and reproducibility. Stabilization of the frontomaxillary and zygomaticomaxillary buttresses (**Fig. 1**) with internal fixation devices can sufficiently restore the projection in the middle third of the face, and, in combination with maxillomandibular fixation of an intact stable mandible, it can also restore the posterior height of the facial skeleton.[5] These anatomic principles are also true for secondary/reoperative maxillary trauma.

Secondary deformities following Le Fort fractures were seen in nearly two-thirds of patients before the introduction of rigid internal fixation, typified by the posterior-superior displacement of the maxilla.[6] Major complications associated with improperly reduced or inadequately fixated maxillary Le Fort fractures include malocclusion with facial asymmetry and poor aesthetics (**Fig. 2**). Nonunion of the maxilla can also occur, but is rare. The porous nature of the maxillary bone and ample blood supply lends itself to quicker healing and decreased rates of infections. Micromovement of the maxilla in patients who prematurely return to full masticatory function can lead to bony nonunion. In addition, Steidler and colleagues[7] reported chronic postoperative sinusitis in 1.7% of patients with midface trauma in their series. Traumatic septal injury and overimpaction of the maxilla can result in deformities of the nasal septum. Morgan and colleagues[8] reported that up to 20% of patients with midface fractures suffered from postoperative septal deviations. Soft tissue complications, including facial fat atrophy, nerve damage, shortening of the upper lip length, and a widened alar base, can be anticipated as postoperative soft tissue complications.

Work-up

Postoperative follow-up of patients with facial trauma should include thorough head and neck examinations and periodic imaging and photographs as circumstances dictate. Careful attention must be paid to the function of the upper aerodigestive system, including occlusion/mastication, airflow, and sinus disorders. Residual tissue edema can mask bony asymmetry, which can be difficult to fully evaluate until the soft tissue redrapes and swelling resolves.

The imaging modalities of choice to evaluate the primary reconstruction of the maxilla are computed tomography (CT) scans in the axial, coronal, and sagittal planes. Three-dimensional CT reconstructions of the standard two-dimensional views may provide a better-generalized overview of improper

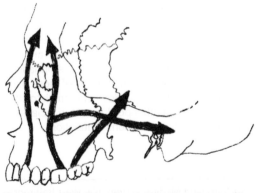

Fig. 1. The vertical maxillary buttresses: nasomaxillary, zygomaticomaxillary, and pterygomaxillary areas of stability. (*From* Betts N, Scully J. Transverse maxillary distraction osteogenesis. In: Fonseca RJ, Marciani R, Turvey T, editors. Oral and maxillofacial surgery. 2nd edition. St Louis (MO): Saunders Elsevier; 2009. p. 227 (v3); with permission.)

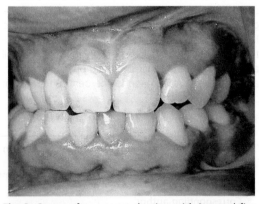

Fig. 2. Status after open reduction with internal fixation of comminuted Le Fort III fractures with postoperative malocclusion.

bony alignment highlighting gross distortions in form and symmetry. Plain films including orthopantomograms (OPG) as well as lateral and anterior-posterior cephalometrics will often provide sufficient information with less detail. Information obtained from these radiographs can be used to plan presurgical movements of the maxilla.

Dental models should be obtained to evaluate the occlusal relationship of the maxilla and mandible when an abnormal maxillomandibular relationship is recognized, especially in the setting of a multipiece maxillary fracture. These models can then be used to fabricate occlusal splints for intraoperative positioning of the jaws. More recently, CT scans combined with laser-scanned dental models have allowed surgical splints to be fabricated with computer-aided design (CAD) and computer-aided manufacturing (CAM) technology, based on virtual planning parameters, performed solely from three-dimensional images. The goals of secondary maxillary reconstruction may not include the reestablishment of the premorbid occlusion, but rather a more ideal/functional relationship of the maxillomandibular complex. Preoperative consultation with an orthodontist might yield the best overall results because, unlike patients having traditional orthognathic surgery, posttraumatic patients may not have had ideally decompensated occlusions premorbidly. Previous dental records and photographs may help with the secondary surgical planning. Any discrepancies should be identified and correlated with the global treatment plan. Neurosensory and motor deficits should also be documented before revision surgery.

Surgical Treatment

Access can be achieved via vestibular incision with or without an anterior maxillary degloving approach, which affords far more generous access to the external nasal framework and zygoma.[9] Scarring from the initial access and repair can distort traditional landmarks, in particular the intranasal soft tissue landmarks required for the midface degloving approach. All previous fracture sites and areas of fixation should be exposed before performing any osteotomies. Hardware that is either mobile or could potentially interfere with osteotomies should be removed. In a series of 266 patients, 33% of patients required maxillary plate removal, predominantly for infections or patient discomfort, whereas 30% were removed for secondary reconstruction/revision surgery.[9] The maxilla should be fully mobilized once planned osteotomies are complete. Mobilization of the osteotomized maxilla can be challenging secondary to fibrosis and scarring and

may require significant but judicious manipulation with Rowe forceps and Tesseir mobilizers. Once the maxilla has been adequately mobilized and passively repositioned, maxillomandibular fixation (MMF) should be applied, with an emphasis on condylar positioning to limit postoperative open bite (**Fig. 3**). The application of rigid fixation may be difficult owing to the presence of traumatic bone voids and screw holes from previously placed rigid internal fixation (**Fig. 4**). Postoperative MMF should be adjunctively used for stability when the fixation is questionable for immediate function. Supplementary bone grafting has been advocated to achieve clinical bony union of the maxilla. It has been suggested that any maxillary bony defects greater than 5 mm should be considered for grafting (see **Fig. 4**).[10]

Fracture patterns involving both the mandible and maxilla require special attention, because the transverse dimension of the maxilla can be directly influenced by the nonanatomic reduction of a concomitant mandible fracture at the time of the initial surgery. An improperly reduced mandible can then directly affect the planned width of the maxilla at the time of revision. The mandible will then necessitate its own reosteotomy and repositioning during the revision procedure to attain the goals set forth for the maxilla and midface. Proper attention should be paid to the anterior nasal spine and the seating of the nasal septum to prevent septal buckling. If indicated, a septoplasty can be performed. Tissue resuspension can be incorporated to prevent soft tissue drooping, especially in the alar base and malar areas.

ZYGOMA FRACTURES

Trauma to the midface often involves fractures of the zygoma and its articulations. A retrospective study of zygoma fractures, extending for a 10-year period,

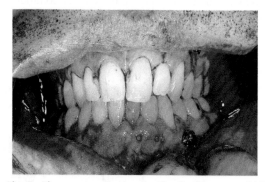

Fig. 3. The same patient as in **Fig. 2** with premorbid occlusion reestablished. The midlines are coincident with normal intercuspation. Maxillomandibular fixation was established with intermaxillary fixation screws.

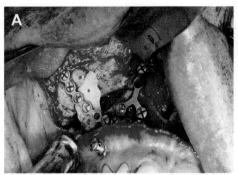
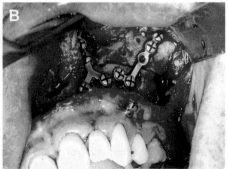

Fig. 4. Intraoperative picture of same patient as in **Fig. 2** at the time of revision Le Fort osteotomy. (*A*) Note the anterior maxillary defects, the need for grafting on the right maxilla. (*B*) The multiple holes in the anterior maxilla from previous fixation.

found that 80% of the injuries were caused by road traffic accidents, and 40% of zygoma injuries were associated with other facial fractures, 30% of which involved the orbital contents. In the same study, 40% of zygoma fractures were treated by an open approach.[11] Ellis and colleagues[12] reported that 43% of all patients with facial trauma suffered orbito-zygomatic fractures. The anatomic complexity of the zygoma and its three-dimensional positioning make reconstruction a challenge. Souyris and colleagues[13] evaluated complications after primary orbitozygomatic repair in a retrospective study involving 1393 patients; 7% had some degree of infraorbital nerve dysfunction, and 12% had malposition of their zygomas resulting in diplopia, enophthalmos, or dystopia. In a more recent study in 2005, Kelley and colleagues[14] showed that only 2% of their postsurgical zygoma complications resulted in late enophthalmos that required intervention with reosteotomies. Kurita and colleagues[15] analyzed satisfaction in 95 patients treated for zygoma fractures with open reduction and rigid internal fixation; complete satisfaction was reported in only 72% of the patients. Pain, parasthesias, deformities, and trismus were the most commonly cited complaints.

Relevant Anatomy

Displaced fractures of the zygoma can cause functional and cosmetic deformities. The position of the zygoma in the midface contributes to the anterior-posterior and transverse projection of the facial skeleton. The zygoma is classically described as a quadrilateral bone that articulates with the temporal, sphenoidal, frontal, and maxillary bones, thus creating 4 different sutures (**Fig. 5**).

These articulations form much of the orbital framework, and thus fractures lend themselves to disruptions of the orbital rim, floor, and lateral walls. The zygoma serves as an anatomic insertion point for several of the muscles of mastication, including the temporalis and masseter muscles, as well as several of the muscles of facial expression. The Whitnall's tubercle lies just medial to the lateral orbital margin, below the frontozygomatic suture. It serves as the attachment of the lateral canthal tendon and Lockwood's suspensory ligament. Properly repositioning this structure is critical for the reestablishment of orbital aesthetics and proper lid position (**Fig. 6**).

Several classification systems for zygomatic fractures have been developed.[16] The authors have

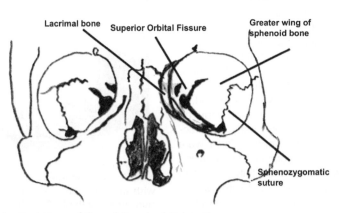

Fig. 5. The bones and articulations of the orbit and orbital cavity.

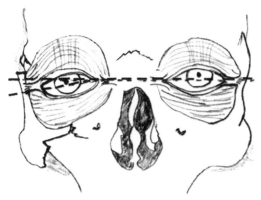

Fig. 6. Orbital dystopia related to zygoma malposition. (*From* D'Addario M, Cunningham L. Management of zygomatic fractures. In: Fonseca RJ, Marciani R, Turvey T, editors. Oral and maxillofacial surgery. 2nd edition. St Louis (MO): Saunders Elsevier; 2009. p. 197 (v2); with permission.)

found classifications to be of limited value in the decision-making process or treatment. Treatment is based on the degree of functional impairment and cosmetic defect. Although traditionally some investigators have advocated closed approaches, the authors collectively use open approaches to maximize anatomic reduction and to optimize strategic placement of rigid internal fixation. Selected isolated zygomatic arch fractures can be treated with closed reduction. Complications and sequelae associated with zygomatic fractures and their repair that are amendable to reoperation can be seen in **Box 1**. This article discusses surgical options for skeletal complications after primary repair.

Enophthalmos can be defined as recession of the globe within the orbit in an anterior-posterior dimension. Clinically, this manifests as a retrograde displacement of the globe that can also be

Box 1
Complications and sequelae associated with zygomatic fractures and their repair

- Soft tissue complications

  Fat atrophy

  Lid retraction

  Ectropion
- Ocular disturbances

  Diplopia
- Enophthalmos
- Malposition of the zygoma

  Orbital dystopia

  Facial asymmetry

  Facial widening

associated with downward displacement (hypoglobus) (**Fig. 7**). Patients are able to perceive differences in globe position and a difference of as little as 3 mm has been associated with patient dissatisfaction.[17] Physical findings associated with enophthalmos include a deep upper eyelid profile or hollowing, poor lid contact with the globe, eyelid asymmetry, as well as possible functional problems such as diplopia, tear pooling or epiphora, or diminished visual fields. There have been many postulates as to what leads to traumatic enophthalmos. Manson and colleagues[18,19] discussed the role of intraconal orbital fat displacement from the muscle cone, whereas others have suggested fat atrophy or scarring as a major causative factor. Even the lack of proper reconstruction of the supporting ligamentous structures of the orbit has been discussed as a possible cause of posttraumatic enophthalmos.[20]

Enophthalmos is commonly caused by gross malpositioning of the zygoma or an orbital wall/floor fracture. Irrespective of mechanism, the increase in orbital volume from fractures of any of the 4 walls is believed to account for the poor support of the globe. Proper treatment involves reestablishment of the orbital volume.

Work-up

The initial work-up of a posttraumatic patient having orbital reconstruction should always include a detailed ophthalmologic evaluation. Posttraumatic visual problems must be delineated and quantified clearly, especially diplopia and visual field defects. It is also helpful to have an accurate assessment of visual acuity, especially if there was a change from baseline after the initial injury. Differences in globe position must be established objectively to allow for the most accurate correction. Swelling and postoperative edema may complicate the postoperative results of an initial surgical procedure and confound the soft tissue analysis as well as the ophthalmologic examination. In this case, it is helpful to obtain postoperative imaging to aid in the evaluation because it may take up to 6 months for full resolution of soft tissue swelling. If gross enophthalmos is evident after the resolution of soft tissue swelling, a CT scan with axial, coronal, sagittal cuts, as well as three-dimensional reformatted reconstructions, can be helpful to evaluate for significant bony displacement. One-millimeter cuts will provide greater detail and can be used for virtual planning and image-guided reconstructions if necessary.

During the last decade, advances in technology have begun to aid the surgeon in treatment planning as well as trouble-shooting intraoperatively when treating complicated midface deformities. Numerous

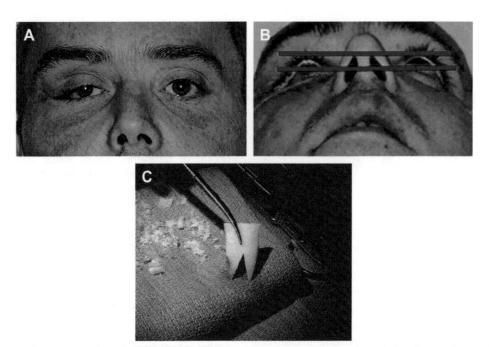

Fig. 7. (*A, B*) Patient with enophthalmos status after comminuted Le Fort III with medial wall as well as roof and floor fractures. (*C*) Porous polyethylene wedge carved and placed into the lateral orbit for enophthalmos correction. The floor was left alone to avoid disturbing the vertical position of the globe.

studies have detailed the use of CT-assisted preoperative planning and intraoperative navagation.[21–25] In the maxillofacial region, this technology has allowed clinicians to transfer two-dimensional data into an accurate three-dimensional stereolithographic model.[22] The model can be used to perform preoperative surgical plate adaptation as well as planning osteotomies and designing guides before going to the operating room. More recently, image guidance has allowed surgeons to intraoperatively navigate and gauge implant placement in real time in addition to guiding the proper realignment of bony anatomy. Gellrich and colleagues[23] incorporated the use of preoperative models as well as intraoperative navigation to accurately restore orbital volume. The main limitation of this technology, which also limits the results of any secondary bony reconstruction, seems to be the in the correction of the soft tissue deformities associated with traumatic/iatrogenic insults.[21]

Surgery

Typically, the surgical approach uses existing scars to prevent additional soft tissue injury or facial scarring. This approach also allows scar revision when necessary. Occasionally, an additional access is required and the most aesthetic route that allows appropriate access should be chosen. Forcing a more aesthetic approach or struggling with

limited access can leave a less complete correction of the deformity or greater soft tissue damage because of excessive retraction.

Vertical dystopia can be corrected with reexploration of the orbital floor and reconstitution of orbital floor height with a reconstruction material of the surgeon's choice (autogonous bone, alloplastic implant, etc). Both bone and alloplastic materials can be incrementally stacked to achieve appropriate vertical position of the globe, and slight clinical overcorrection is often recommended to account for intraoperative edema, although navigation-assisted surgery allows more precise positioning of the implant. The surgeon must always consider the resorption profile of autogenous implants, because this affects long-term outcomes. In cases in which there was inaccuracy or difficulty in finding the posterior ledge of the fracture during primary repair, an endoscopic transantral approach may be helpful in proper positioning of the implant. Prebent orbital plates may obviate the need to locate a posterior ledge, because the plates are rigid enough to be used in a cantilevered configuration and are contoured for appropriate globe support (**Fig. 8**).

Surgical correction of an underprojected zygoma can be achieved by reosteotomizing the zygomatic articulations and repositioning the entire bone (**Fig. 9**). This approach can be met with difficulty because positioning the segment is

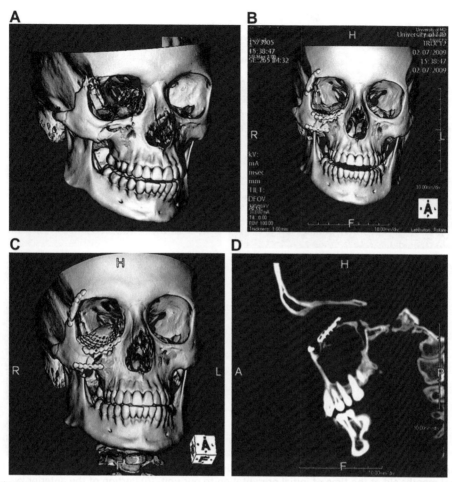

Fig. 8. (*A*) Initial CT scan three-dimensional reconstruction showing the initial zygomatic injury. (*B*) Immediate postoperative CT scan illustrating placement of orbital reconstruction mesh into maxillary sinus. (*C, D*) Postoperative CT scan of the secondary reconstruction using prebend orbital floor mesh with capture of the posterior ledge.

complicated by the absence of reliable bony landmarks. Once again, navigation can be extremely helpful in planning and accurately the repositioning the zygoma. Alternatively, custom-made and stock alloplastic implants (eg, polyetheretherketone [PEEK] and Medpor) can be use to augment projection, volume, or contour, and are preferred by some because of their nonresorbing properties. Both PEEK and Medpor can be customized to patient-specific defects, whereas Medpor has several stock options that can be carved and contoured intraoperatively. Still others have used contoured cranial bone because it is autogenous and the long-term prospect of infection is low. It also has a favorable resorption profile.

Enophthalmos correction can be extremely challenging, primarily because of the difficulty in estimating the soft tissue contribution to the problem once skeletal anatomy has been corrected. Classically, Tessier and colleagues[26]

noted 3 tenets of late treatment of enophthalmos: (1) a complete subperiosteal dissection of the orbit up to 1 cm from the apex to free the periorbita from displaced orbital wall fragments, (2) repositioning of the orbital framework with osteotomies, and (3) reconstruction of the walls and framework by bone grafts. These principles have so far held true, with the exception of the introduction of synthetic implants. One limiting factor is the proper identification of the affected anatomic structures within the orbit, which may prove difficult because of scarring, contractures, and malpositioned grafting materials. Implant placement and volume correction can affect the vertical position of the globe in addition to its anteroposterior position. The challenge is to move the globe forward without introducing vertical dystopia. Implants are generally placed along the floor, behind the equator of the globe, and along the lateral wall of the orbit (see **Fig. 7**C). Careful attention must

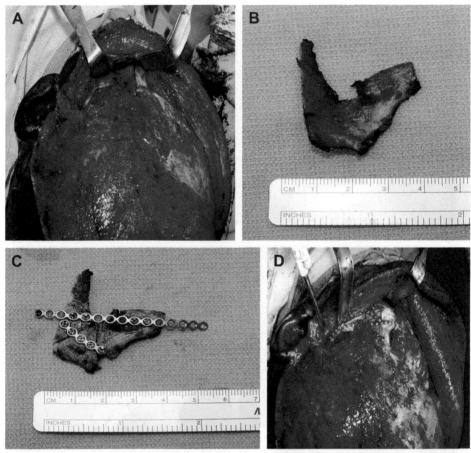

Fig. 9. (*A*) Patient with untreated zygomatic arch fracture with facial deformity and limited opening. The injury was several months old at the time of initial presentation to our unit. (*B*) Portion of the anterior zygoma/zygomatic arch after osteotomy and explantation. (*C, D*) Zygoma after further osteotomy and reshaping on the table and replantation.

then be given to reestablishing canthal position after all of the orbital soft tissue attachments have been liberated. Key areas of symmetry to be evaluated after enophthalmos correction include globe position, canthal position, palpeberal fissure length and shape, as well as upper lid crease fullness. From a functional standpoint, one hopes to have a resolution of diplopia, if present, and possibly an improvement in visual fields.

NASAL BONE FRACTURES

The central location of the nose and its prominence on the facial skeleton make nasal bone fractures the most common facial fracture. They have been estimated to occur in approximately 39% of patients with facial fractures.[26] In view of the reported incidence, it is also considered that nasal fractures are largely underrepresented, because many factures are treated in an office setting, rather at than the trauma center where much of the data is gathered.

Posttraumatic nasal deformity represents one of the primary reasons patients seek septorhinoplasty. The incidence of posttraumatic nasal deformities requiring some form of revision procedure ranges from 14% to 50%.[27,28] Although nasal bone fractures are considered to be a common occurrence, many of the primary treatment modalities remain controversial. The high reoperative rate of nasal fractures can be attributed to the lack of optimal initial reduction or stabilization, instability of the bony and cartilaginous segments caused by the fracture pattern, or delayed presentation for primary treatment.

Correction of a posttraumatic nose involves more than straightening the nose, and requires the surgeon to understand the relevant anatomy as well as current rhinoplasty techniques. First and foremost, the correct diagnosis must be made and an accurate surgical problem list created. Careful anatomic inspection is required to correlate nasal deformity with specific anatomic injuries and functional deficits. Next, standard rhinoplasty techniques are used to address each issue and reconstruct the traumatized nose, restoring not only aesthetics but also an intact nasal airway.

Relevant Anatomy

Proper anatomic knowledge of the complex nasal apparatus is necessary for proper treatment of primary and secondary nasal reconstruction. The nose is a composite osseocartilagenous structure with mucocutaneous coverage and lining. The paired nasal bones articulate with the frontal bone and the maxilla. The bony portion of the nasal septum consists of the perpendicular plate of the ethmoid bone posterosuperiorly and the vomer posteroinferiorly. The nasal septum forms the midline support structure of the nose. The posterior cartilage portion articulates with the ethmoid and the vomer. The more anterior quadrangular cartilaginous portion articulates with the maxilla below and allows for the flexibility of the nasal septum, but is a common location for dislocation after trauma. The septal area can be a key zone for proper anatomic reconstruction.[29] The maxilla and the palatine bones form the bony floor of the nasal cavity.

There are paired upper and lower lateral nasal cartilages that form the internal anatomy of the nose. The upper lateral cartilages are triangular and form attachments with the nasal bones superiorly and with the maxilla laterally. The lower lateral cartilages form medial attachments with the nasal septum and are divided into medial crura, lateral crura, and the domes. Superiorly, they articulate with the upper lateral cartilages via the scroll. The medial crura and the septum participate in formation of the columella. The lateral crura gives support to the alar area, and adjacent to the lateral crus are the sesamoid cartilages embedded within the fibroareolar connective tissue.

Work-up

A proper history of the patient's previous nasal trauma and previous surgeries will give the clinician a better idea about the treatment plan. It is important to discuss pretrauma conditions such as nasal obstruction or septal deviations. A good patient history will also help define the goals of operative treatment. Certain patients may be fixated on impaired nasal breathing, whereas others may be concerned with more cosmetic issues, although it is best to address all relevant complaints and defects at the time of revision, if possible. The physical examination of the patient with a nasal deformity caused by trauma is key

to the establishment of an objective problem list. All relevant angles should be evaluated, such as the nasofrontal ($\sim$135°) and nasolabial angles (90–108°). The brow-nasal tip aesthetic lines should be symmetric, gentle curves with the greatest width at the nasal bony vault and at the tip. Intercanthal distance should be 32 to 34 mm in a white adult. The alar width should correspond with lines dropped from the inner canthus and should be symmetric. Nasal tip elevation and deviation should also be noted. An internal examination should be performed with a headlight and nasal speculum to document synechiae, nasal valve problems, septal deviation, and turbinate issues. The use of topical decongestants can assist in the examination.

Preoperative imaging can be of value in assessing posttraumatic nasal deformity, especially if there are questions following the internal examination. Plain films are of limited value, but CT scans provide a complete view of the relevant nasal anatomy as well as other relevant facial injuries and residual deformity that can contribute to a patient's physical appearance.

A premorbid photograph can help establish a proper template, although patients might not want to be restored to their exact preoperative appearance, and this should be elucidated in the interview.

RESIDUAL NASAL DEFORMITY

Even if the primary nasal repair was suboptimal, sufficient time must be allowed for healing of the initial injury before revision is undertaken. Resolution of inflammation and edema will allow the surgeon a better appreciation of all relevant cosmetic and functional issues to be dealt with at the time of revision. Although potentially distressing to the patient, this will provide a better starting point for the reconstructive surgeon and a more accurate postoperative result.

The role of true closed reduction is not likely an option in secondary revision rhinoplasty. This procedure can occasionally be used in a late presenting nasal bone fracture or in the early postoperative period if residual gross deformity is observed when sufficient edema has resolved. Otherwise, either an endonasal or transcolumellar open approach is more appropriate. Although some believe that endonasal approaches are most suitable for limited problems, experienced rhinoplastic surgeons can achieve excellent results with this method. For many surgeons, the transcolumellar approach is preferred in that it provides direct visualization of all osseocartilagenous anatomy and allows ease of graft placement into all locations of the nose. This approach is particularly useful when simultaneously addressing the reconstruction of the nasal septum, tip, and vaults. Common post-traumatic nasal deformities that are amenable to re-operation are listed in **Box 2**.

Nasal Deviation/Asymmetry

Nasal deviation following blunt trauma is common. This injury typically occurs in response to a lateral blow to the nose affecting 1 or both of the nasal bones and/or the nasal septum. Either a portion of the nose or the entire nose will deviate from midline compared with a line drawn from the center of glabella to the center of cupids bow. Nasal osteotomies will almost certainly be needed to reset the nasal dorsum. Septoplasty with resec-tion or strut grafting will be required to straighten the lower third of the nose. Variably, spreader grafts, shield grafts, and batten grafts can be used to address vault collapse, nasal tip problems, and alar asymmetries, respectively.

Saddle Nose Deformities

The saddle nose deformity is one of the more unwelcome complications in maxillofacial trauma surgery. Severe nasal bone fracture, under-reduction and fixation of naso-orbital-ethmoidal (NOE) fractures, and the loss of dorsal septal carti-lage can cause a gross deformity characterized by a scooped out appearance from the profile view and an excessive nasal width from the frontal view. In 1949, Seltzer classified the saddle nose deformity into 3 types.[29] In 2007, Daniel and Brenner[30] described a more detailed classification system (**Box 3**).

Type 0/1 deformities

These deformities are classified such that they still maintain structural integrity of the septum. The base of the septal wall has been lowered but still remains strong enough to build on. Treatment of these deformities has ranged from injectable filler materials, silicone, or expanded polytetrafluoro-ethylene allografts, to autogenous bone or carti-lage grafts, with the bone or cartilage grafts seeming to be an ideal choice because of increased stability and decreased rates of

---

Box 2
Common posttraumatic nasal deformities amenable to reoperation

- Nasal deviation/crooked nose
- Nasal valve collapse
- Saddle nose deformity
- Septal deviation

Box 3
Daniel's classification of saddle nose deformity

- Type 0: pseudosaddle
- Type I: minor; cosmetic concealment
- Type II: moderate; cartilage vault restoration
- Type III: major; composite reconstruction
- Type IV: severe; structural reconstruction
- Type V: catastrophic; nasal reconstruction

Data from Daniel R, Brenner K. Saddle nose deformity: a new classification and treatment. Facial Plast Surg Clin North Am 2006;14(4):301–12.

---

infection.[31] Donor sites for reconstruction include the nasal septum, costal cartilage, rib, or cranial bone, as well as various pedicled flaps from the alar cartilage and facial components.[32]

Type II to V deformities

These deformities involve more structural bony damage and greater loss of septal support. Reconstruction is complex and may even involve multistaged procedures. Options for reconstruc-tion involve the usage of interpositional grafting, spreader grafts, grafting from septal cartilage, costal cartilage, calvarium, iliac crest, and, in more severe cases, possible forehead flaps, free-tissue transfer, or the use of nasal prosthetics.[33]

NOE FRACTURES

Naso-orbital-ethmoid complex fractures are historically known for their difficulty in treatment and diagnosis. The anatomy of the NOE complex tends to be detailed and small disruptions can lead to grossly apparent deformities. In a series by Ellis,[34] more than half of their patients with NOE-type fractures had other associated facial injuries. NOE injuries primarily result in aesthetic deformities. However, functional problems can occur with damage to the nasal airway, sinus drainage system, and the lacrimal system.[35] Repair of NOE fractures should be performed within the first weeks of injury to avoid soft tissue complications caused by scaring. Complications associated with NOE fractures include orbital damage, nasolacrimal injury, enophthalmos, residual telecanthus, saddle nose deformities, horizontal shortening of palpebral fissures, anosmia, and residual nasal deformity.[36]

Relevant Anatomy

The NOE complex is the superior aspect of the midface and allows communication and articula-tion of anterior skull base structures with the facial skeleton. The delicate bony structure of the ethmoid bone and lacrimal bones predispose this area to comminution of the anatomic architecture and disruption of complex soft tissue structures. The complex is composed of the nasal process of the frontal bone, nasal bones, the frontal processes of the maxilla, lacrimal bones, the ethmoids, the sphenoid posteriorly, and nasal septum. The importance of the medial canthal tendon (MCT) has been well described in the literature.[37] The MCT surrounds the lacrimal sac medially and blends with the contents of the eyelid laterally. Thus, disruption of this tendon leads to loss of eyelid support and blunting of the medial canthal angle. Normal intercanthal distances for white men range from 33 to 34 mm and 32 to 34 mm for white women. Intercanthal distances of 35 mm can be suggestive of an NOE-type fracture, whereas distances of 40 mm and more are diagnostic in the setting of trauma.[38]

Classification of NOE Fractures

Markowtiz and colleagues[37] described the classification of the NOE fracture based on the fracture pattern of the central bone and its relation to the MCT. This classification has allowed clinicians to discuss and plan the reconstruction of NOE fractures according to easily classifiable and relevant anatomic issues. Type I fractures are characterized by a large, intact, central bony fragment with full attachment of the MCT. Type II injuries involve comminution of the lacrimomaxillary region, but the MCT is still fully attached to a central bony segment. Type III fractures involve extensive comminution with the MCT either attached to a small bony segment or avulsed (**Fig. 10**).[38]

Work-up

Complications associated with NOE complex injuries are mostly aesthetic. However, occasionally patients may complain of functional deficits including ocular dysfunction, epiphora, or dacrocystitis, and nasal obstruction. A comprehensive physical examination of the complex should be performed including a complete ophthalmologic examination with proper examination of extraocular muscle function and visual fields as well as careful assessment of the nasal structures. The function of the lacrimal system should also be verified by history or examination.

Imaging studies should include axial, coronal, and sagittal CT scans in 1-mm cuts. Orbital volumes should be assessed for significant changes. The frontal process of the maxilla should be carefully evaluated, because this is the primary attachment of the MCT. In many cases, these patients will have had previous treatments at other institutions and operative records and imaging can be obtained to detail what forms of fixation and/or alloplasts have been used in primary or secondary treatment attempts (**Fig. 11**). It can also useful to

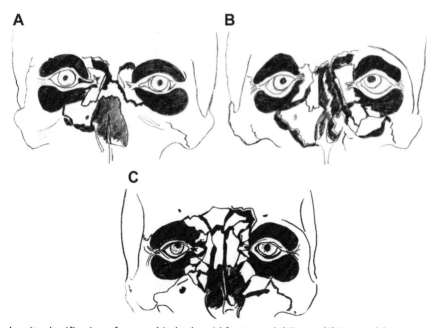

Fig. 10. Markowitz classification of naso-orbital-ethmoid fractures. (*A*) Type I. (*B*) Type II. (*C*) Type III. (*From* Reddy LV, Pagnotto M. Midface fractures. In: Fonseca RJ, Marciani R, Turvey T, editors. Oral and maxillofacial surgery. 2nd edition. St Louis (MO): Saunders Elsevier; 2009. p. 245 (v2); with permission.)

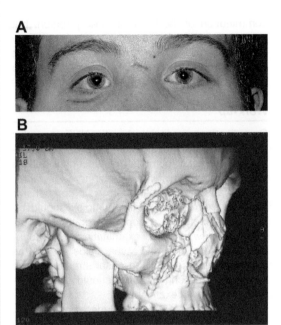

Fig. 11. (*A*) Patient with a right-sided orbitozygomatic and naso-orbito-ethmoid fracture treated at another institution. Patient has a postoperative telecanthus as well as vertical dystopia. (*B*) CT three-dimensional reconstruction of the same patient showing incomplete fixation of the right orbitozygomatic fracture and an untreated type I naso-orbitozygomatic fractures.

obtain images from the initial traumatic event. These images may give clues to the treating surgeon about the degree of anatomic distortion the patient initially suffered as well as how far they have come from their initial repair. As detailed earlier, the use of CT-assisted preoperative and intraoperative guidance can also help guide the reconstruction of enophthalmos correction from NOE fractures. In addition, a premorbid photograph should be obtained.

Surgical Techniques

Before the 1960s, closed reduction of NOE fractures was the treatment modality of choice. In 1964, Mustarde and Digman illustrated the importance of open reduction and internal fixation of NOE fractures with transnasal wiring.[39] It is now the gold standard to perform an open reduction with internal fixation in the form of micro- or miniplates, orbital mesh, and transnasal wiring for treatment of NOE fractures.

NOE fractures are notorious for their difficulty in primary reconstruction, and can be even more challenging in revision surgery. Ideal aesthetic outcomes are best achieved during the initial repair, and secondary procedures may be limited

by scar tissue and lack of primary bony support.[34] The former can be particularly vexing when attempting to reestablish medial canthal angle morphology and the spatial position of the canthus itself.

The operative techniques used for revision surgery of NOE complex fractures are similar to those of the primary surgery. Proper access should be achieved to expose the entire medial orbital wall. This exposure may necessitate the use of a coronal incision, although some achieve good results with the use of Lynch incisions. If the orbital floor needs to be accessed, then a lower-eye lid incision should also be used. Transconjunctival incisions may limit the medial extent of the dissection, but can be extended into transcaruncular incisions. Alternatively, a subciliary or lower lid incision can be used to allow more exposure to the entire medial orbital rim. The dissection of the medial orbital wall should be posterior enough for proper graft placement if enophthalmos is associated with an uncorrected medial orbital wall fracture.

The MCT should be located by the use of external landmarks and internal attachments. At the time of revision surgery, the insertion of the MCT might be located in an aberrant position. If difficulties locating the MCT are encountered, a skin incision can be made medial to the cantus to find the anterior portion of the tendon. The tendon can than be identified and secured for later canthopexy, if needed.

Osteotomies can be performed if necessary and correct anatomic reduction of the medial orbital rim can be established with transnasal wiring or plate fixation. Careful attention must be directed to the placement of the wiring. A hole must be drilled posterior to the lacrimal fossa to prevent lateral splaying of the posterior segment and residual telecanthus. If medial orbital wall reconstruction is needed, the surgeon's preference of grafting or reconstruction material should be used. The advantage of using titanium orbital plates/mesh includes the availability of holes in the mesh that can be used to secure transnasal wires in the absence of adequate bone. They are also of the right thickness for the delicate lamina papyracea and orbital floors, and can be visualized in postoperative radiographs. Autogenous bone grafts can make any future revision procedures easier because of the lack of tissue in-growth or inflammatory processes associated with alloplastic materials.[40] Canthopexy should be performed if the MCT is avulsed either from the primary injury or iatrogenically from soft tissue dissection. Positioning of the MCT should be slightly superior and posterior to its normal anatomic attachment

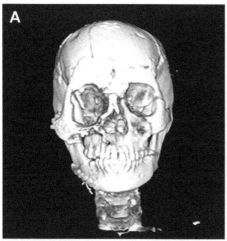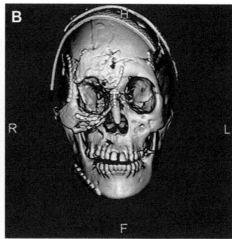

Fig. 12. Patient was assaulted with a hammer and initially treated by another surgeon. (*A*) A malpositioned zygoma and orbital floor as well as splayed frontal processes of the maxilla. (*B*) A repositioned zygoma and dorsal nasal grafting. Medial canthal repositioning was done and enophthalmos correction was performed with porous polyethylene. A medical model was used for planning. The patient still requires further maxillary reconstruction and orbital work.

to accommodate sag or relapse. Many have advocated the use of lead or silastic bolsters with a transcutaneous wiring technique. This method helps to support the repair and redrape soft tissue, in addition to reducing the bone and securing the wire effectively. When used, these bolsters are left in place for 7 to 10 days.

Primary dorsal grafting should always be considered because severe NOE fractures, by nature, will weaken the nasal septum and nasal bones, which are often comminuted beyond the ability to be fixated (**Fig. 12**). Markowitz and colleagues[37] used dorsal grafts in 42% of their NOE fractures, and a similar percentage of primary bone grafting was also shown by Gruss and colleagues[35] in his series.[41] In the setting of secondary surgery, the need for a dorsal graft will be indicated by a saddle nose deformity. The dorsal graft can be overprojected to camouflage any residual telecanthus, because an overprojected nasal dorsum is generally more aesthetically pleasing than one that is underprojected.

SUMMARY

In conclusion, reoperative midface surgery can be challenging. Although well-established surgical principles are still the basis of surgical approaches and techniques, the advent of new materials and technologies brings about opportunities to achieve the best possible outcomes with bony reconstruction and more precise results. Soft tissue deformities continue to be some of the

most challenging, especially as they relate to the orbit, but continually evolving techniques offer improved results for volume corrections to treat enophthalmos and diplopia. Conventional orthognathic and reconstructive rhinoplasty techniques can also be applied to great effect and with satisfying results to treat posttraumatic malocclusions and nasal deformities.

REFERENCES

1. Reddy L, Pagnotto M. Midface fractures. In: Marciani R, editor. 2nd edition, In: Oral and maxillofacial surgery, vol. 2. St Louis (MO): Saunders Elsevier; 2009. p. 239–55.
2. Sicher H, Tandler J. Anatomie fur Zahnarzte. Vienna (Austria): Springer; 1928.
3. Gassner R, Tuli T, Hachl O, et al. Cranio-maxillofacial trauma: a 10 year review of 9,543 cases with 21,067 injuries. J Craniomaxillofac Surg 2003;31(1):51–61.
4. Le Fort R. Études expérimentales sur les fractures de la mâchoire supérieure. Rev Chir 1901;23: 208–27.
5. Manson P, Hoopes JE, Su CT. Structural pillars of the facial skeleton: an approach to the management of Le Fort fractures. Plast Reconstr Surg 1980;66(1): 54–62.
6. Ferraro JW, Berggren RB. Treatment of complex facial fractures. J Trauma 1973;13(9):783–7.
7. Steidler NE, Cook RM, Reade PC. Residual complications in patients with major middle third facial fractures. Int J Oral Surg 1980;9(4):259–66.

8. Morgan BDG, Madan DK, Bergerot JPC. Fractures of the middle third of the face: a review of 300 cases. Br J Plast Surg 1972;25(2):147–51.

9. Baumann A, Ewers R. Midfacial degloving: an alternative approach for traumatic corrections in the midface. Int J Oral Maxillofac Surg 2001;30(4):272–7.

10. Gruss J, Phillips J. Rigid fixation of the Le Fort maxillary fractures. In: Yaremchuk MJ, Gruss JS, Manson PN, editors. Rigid fixation of the craniomaxillofacial skeleton. Boston: Butterworth-Heinemann; 1992. p. 283–301.

11. Covington DS, Wainwright DJ, Teichgraeber JF, et al. Changing patterns in the epidemiology and treatment of zygoma fractures: a 10-year review. J Trauma 1994;37(2):243–8.

12. Ellis E 3rd, el-Attar A, Moos KF. An analysis of 2,067 cases of zygomatico-orbital fracture. J Oral Maxillofac Surg 1985;43(6):417–28.

13. Souyris F, Klersy F, Jammet P, et al. Malar bone fractures and their sequelae. A statistical study of 1.393 cases covering a period of 20 years. J Craniomaxillofac Surg 1989;17(2):64–8.

14. Kelley P, Crawford M, Higuera S, et al. Two hundred ninety-four consecutive facial fractures in an urban trauma center: lessons learned. Plast Reconstr Surg 2005;3:42e–9e.

15. Kurita M, Okazaki M, Ozaki M, et al. Patient satisfaction after open reduction and internal fixation of zygomatic bone fractures. J Craniofac Surg 2010; 21(1):45–9.

16. Kaastad E, Freng A. Zygomatic-maxillary fractures. J Craniomaxillofac Surg 1989;17(5):210–4.

17. Migliori ME, Gladstone GJ. Determination of the normal range of exophthalmometric values of black and white adults. Am J Ophthalmol 1984;98(4): 438–42.

18. Manson PN, Clifford CM, Su CT, et al. Mechanisms of global support and posttraumatic enophthalmos: I. The anatomy of the ligament and its relation to intramuscular cone orbital fat. Plast Reconstr Surg 1986;77(2):193–202.

19. Manson PN, Grivas A, Rosenbaum A, et al. Studies on the enophthalmos: II. The measurement of orbital injuries and their treatment by quantitative computed tomography. Plast Reconstr Surg 1986; 77(2):203–14.

20. Clauser L, Galie M, Pagliaro F, et al. Posttraumatic enophthalmos: etiology, principles of reconstruction, and correction. J Craniofac Surg 2008;19(2):351–9.

21. Bell RB, Markiewicz M. Computer-assisted planning, stereolithographic modeling, and intraoperative navigation for complex orbital reconstruction: a descriptive study in a preliminary cohort. J Oral Maxillofac Surg 2009;67(12):2559–70.

22. Fuller SC, Strong EB. Computer applications in facial plastic and reconstructive surgery. Curr Opin Otolaryngol Head Neck Surg 2007;15(4):233–7.

23. Gellrich NC, Schramm A, Hammer B, et al. Computer-assisted secondary reconstruction of unilateral posttraumatic orbital deformity. Plast Reconstr Surg 2002;110(6):1417–29.

24. Kokemueller H, Tavassol F, Ruecker M, et al. Complex midfacial reconstruction: a combined technique of computer-assisted surgery and microvascular tissue transfer. J Oral Maxillofac Surg 2008; 66(11):2398–406.

25. Tessier P, Rougier J, Hervouet F, et al. Sequelae of orbital trauma. Plastic surgery of the orbit and eyelids. [transl by Wolfe SA]. New York: Masson; 1981. p. 99.

26. Haug RH, Prather JL. The closed reduction of nasal fractures: an evaluation of 2 techniques. J Oral Maxillofac Surg 1991;49(12):1288–92.

27. Rohrich RJ, Adams WP. Nasal fracture management: minimizing secondary nasal deformities. Plast Reconstr Surg 2000;106(2):266–73.

28. Verwoerd CD. Present day treatment of nasal fractures: closed versus open reduction. Facial Plast Surg 1992;8(4):220–3.

29. Dyer WK, Beaty MM, Prabhat A. Architectural deficiencies of the nose: treatment of the saddle nose and short nose deformities. Otolaryngol Clin North Am 1999;32(1):89–112.

30. Daniel R, Brenner K. Saddle nose deformity: a new classification and treatment. Facial Plast Surg Clin North Am 2006;14(4):301–12.

31. Türegün M, Sengezer M, Guler M. Reconstruction of saddle nose deformities using porous polyethylene implant. Aesthetic Plast Surg 1998;22(1): 38–41.

32. Kalogjera L, Bedekovic V, Baudoin, et al. Modified alar swing procedure in saddle nose correction. Aesthetic Plast Surg 2003;27(3):209–12.

33. Pribitkin EA, Ezzat WH. Classification and treatment of the saddle nose deformity. Otolaryngol Clin North Am 2009;42(3):437–61.

34. Ellis E III. Sequencing treatment for naso-orbito-ethmoid fractures. J Oral Maxillofac Surg 1993; 5(5):543–58.

35. Gruss J, Hurwitz J, Nik N, et al. The pattern and incidence of nasolacrimal injury in the naso-orbital-ethmoid fracture. Br J Plast Surg 1985;38(1): 116–21.

36. Buehler JA, Tannyhill RJ. Complications in the treatment of midfacial fractures. Oral Maxillofac Surg Clin North Am 2003;15(2):195–212.

37. Markowitz BL, Manson PN, Sargent L, et al. Management of the medial canthal tendon in nasoethmoid orbital fractures: the importance of the central fragment in classification and treatment. Plast Reconstr Surg 1991;87(5):843–53.

38. Paskert JP, Mason PN, Iliff NT. Nasoethmoidal and orbital fractures. Clin Plast Surg 1988;15(2): 209–23.

39. Papadopoulos H, Salib NK. Management of naso-orbital-ethmoidal fractures. Oral Maxillofac Surg Clin North Am 2009;21(2):221–5.

40. Wolfe SA, Ghurani R, Podda S, et al. An examination of posttraumatic, postsurgical orbital deformities: conclusions drawn for improvement of primary treatment. Plast Reconstr Surg 2008;122(6):1870–81.

41. Gruss JS. Naso-ethmoid-orbital fractures: classification and role of primary bone grafting. Plast Reconstr Surg 1985;75(3):303–17.

Reoperative Mandibular Trauma: Management of Posttraumatic Mandibular Deformities

Luis G. Vega, DDS

KEYWORDS

- Reoperation • Mandible fractures
- Posttraumatic deformities • Nonunion • Malunion
- Malocclusion

Mandibular fractures are one the most common maxillofacial injuries. Their management has been traditionally regarded as one of the cornerstones of oral and maxillofacial surgery. Despite many technological and technical advances, to consistently return patients to their preinjury state remains one of the main challenges in the management of these injuries. As a result, an unavoidable number of patients develop unsatisfactory results. Diagnostic errors, poor surgical technique, healing disorders, or complications may lead to the establishment of posttraumatic mandibular deformities. Nonunion, malunion/malocclusion, or facial asymmetry can be found early during the healing process or as long-term sequelae after the initial mandibular fracture repair. Although occasionally these problems can be solved in a nonsurgical manner, reoperations play an important role in the management of these untoward outcomes.

PATIENT EVALUATION
History

As in primary surgery, the value of a thorough history and physical examination cannot be over-emphasized. The patient's chief complaint, perceptions, expectations, and cooperation are essential to the surgeon's evaluation of the degree to which the existing result can be improved by reoperation. All preoperative, intraoperative, and postoperative data from previous surgical and nonsurgical treatments related to the mandibular trauma should be assessed. Special attention is required in those cases in which additional maxillary fractures were present because of the possibility of these injuries to contribute to the posttraumatic mandibular deformity. Reviewing the preinjury history allows the clinician to uncover preinjury problems or previous therapies, such as untreated dentoskeletal deformities, temporamandibular joint (TMJ) dysfunction, orthodontic therapy, or orthognathic surgery. These findings might better explain the previous poor result and might merit a change in the surgical treatment plan. Dental models and photographs from these previous therapies are always of great value for diagnosis and treatment planning. Additional considerations should be given to patients with a history of immunosuppression or polysubstance abuse because of their higher propensity to develop complications.

Examination

Problem-oriented physical examination is centered on evaluating facial height, width, and symmetry. Palpation of the mandible is necessary to assess for any bony deformities and mandibular and/or dental mobility. Intraoral examination

Division of Oral and Maxillofacial Surgery, Department of Surgery, University of Florida, Health Science Center at Jacksonville, 653-1 West 8th Street, Jacksonville, FL 32209, USA
E-mail address: luis.vega@jax.ufl.edu

Oral Maxillofacial Surg Clin N Am 23 (2011) 47–61
doi:10.1016/j.coms.2010.12.003

includes occlusion, dental decay, oral hygiene, and oral mucosa integrity. Determination of the degree of TMJ dysfunction requires quantification of the mandibular range of motion. Facial and trigeminal nerve evaluation should also be documented.

For better understanding of the traumatic forces, extent of the original injury, and initial state of the repair, radiographic examination should include imaging from any of the previous phases of treatment. If warranted, new plain films and computed tomographic (CT) scans with or without 3-dimensional reconstructions should be obtained. Stereolithographic models also aid the clinician to better understand the deformity and establish a treatment plan. Newer technologies such as computer-assisted surgical simulation and craniomaxillofacial navigation have been used for the assessment and correction of complex facial trauma cases.[1,2]

Occlusion is better evaluated by obtaining dental models. As discussed by Yang and colleagues elsewhere in this issue, the goal of secondary reconstruction in maxillomandibular trauma is not necessarily the reestablishment of the preinjury occlusion but rather a more ideal/functional relationship. Thus, consideration should be given for presurgical orthodontic or prosthodontic evaluation. When surgery is indicated, dental model surgery allows splint fabrication for intraoperative establishment of the occlusal relationship, as in orthognathic surgery.

ANALYSIS OF THE UNSATISFACTORY INITIAL RESULT

One of the most important aspects in treatment planning for reoperation is the establishment of the possible causes that contribute to the development of the posttraumatic mandibular deformity (**Box 1**). Knowledge of these factors allows the clinician to plan accordingly to avoid them, as just simply repeating the same surgical procedure most likely would lead to the same untoward result.

Box 1
Causes of posttraumatic mandibular deformities

- Diagnostic errors
- Poor surgical technique
    Inadequate fracture reduction
    Inadequate fracture fixation
- Infection
- Healing disorders

Diagnostic Errors

Failure to recognize, either clinically or radiographically, the morphology of the fracture or the presence of multiple mandibular fractures may lead to the selection of the wrong surgical approach and ultimately the wrong method of fixation. An example can be found in cases in which the clinician fails to identify fragments or microfractures adjacent to the main fracture (**Fig. 1**). Although good occlusion can be achieved at the immediate postoperative period, these fragments may become unstable and potentially lead to infection or nonunion. It is also important for the clinician to be familiar with certain clinical situations that are prone to posttraumatic deformities, such as multiple unilateral mandibular fractures, mandibular fractures in combination with segmental maxillary fractures, or severely atrophic mandibular fractures.

Poor Surgical Technique

Whether the mandible is treated using closed or open techniques, poor surgical technique is usually related to inadequate establishment of the occlusion or inadequate fracture reduction and/or fixation (**Fig. 2**).

Inadequate establishment of occlusion
Establishing the correct occlusion and maxillomandibular fixation (MMF) is the initial step toward achieving fracture stability. Failure to attain adequate occlusion is related to missing or decayed teeth, multiple fractures, tight MMF that creates buccal tipping, loose MMF that produces an open bite, or inadequately reduced fractures. In addition, poorly adapted plates may displace the occlusion because of their tendency to draw the fracture to the plate.

Inadequate fracture reduction
Good visualization of the mandibular fracture is vital for accurate bone alignment and stabilization.

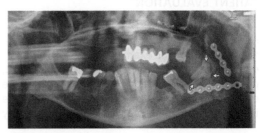

Fig. 1. Diagnostic errors. Panoramic radiograph of a comminuted left mandibular angle/ramus fractures. Clinician failed to identify the presence of comminution and wrong fixation was selected. The patient subsequently developed an infection caused by fracture instability.

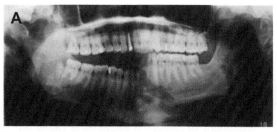
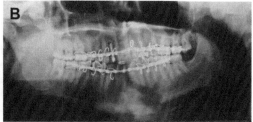

Fig. 2. Inadequate reduction caused by poor selection of surgical technique. (*A*) Panoramic radiograph of a severely displaced left mandibular body and mildly displaced right mandibular angle fractures. (*B*) Postoperative panoramic radiograph showing poor reduction of the left mandibular body fracture. The patient was later taken to the operating room for an open reduction and internal fixation.

A good example is a symphyseal fracture that appears well reduced at the level of the buccal cortex but the lingual cortex was not visualized or properly reduced. Poor reduction usually is associated with insufficient anatomic references such as inadequate dentition, multiple mandible fractures, dentoalveolar fractures, and segmental maxillary fractures. Moreover, inadequate reduction of the mandibular segments may diminish the area of osseous contact, making mobility of the fracture fragments more likely. In the presence of multiple fractures, inadequate reduction and stabilization of one of the fractures may hinder the reduction and stabilization of the other. Therefore, both fractures should be reduced before application of the fixation. Segments that are not properly reduced may lead to nonunion, malunion/malocclusion, or facial asymmetry.

Inadequate fracture fixation

Fracture stability is key for bone healing. The surgeon's knowledge of the biomechanical principles of fracture repair is paramount to institute the necessary fixation. Common infringements of rigid fixation principles include, for example, a plate that is too small, 1 plate instead of 2, placement of a screw into the line of fracture, too few screws per side of fracture, and inadequate plate bending (**Fig. 3**).[3] In addition, the clinician must remember that proper rigid fixation techniques call for good

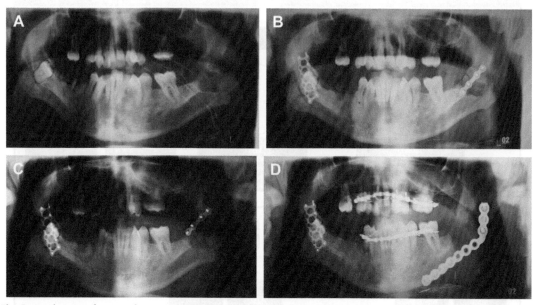

Fig. 3. Inadequate fracture fixation. A 46-year-old man with bilateral mandibular angle fractures that developed an infection on the left side before presentation to our institution. (*A*) Panoramic radiograph after incision, drainage, and extraction of tooth #17. (*B*) Postoperative radiograph after open reduction and internal fixation of both fractures. (*C*) Two-week follow-up panoramic radiograph of left failed fixation. Later surgery demonstrated the buccal plate holding the fixation fractured because of poor bone quality. (*D*) Panoramic radiograph after reoperation showing the placement of a larger reconstruction-type fixation plate.

irrigation while drilling to avoid bone overheating that could potentially lead to bone necrosis and hardware failure. Alpert[4] suggested that inadequacy of rigid internal fixation in concept and execution is the most common cause of failure and subsequent infection in postoperative mandibular fracture repair. Failed or failing rigid internal fixation cannot be repaired with antibiotics or MMF. It is basic that a foreign body that must be debrided from the fracture site.

Infection

Infections are the most common complication after repair of mandibular fractures. The rate of infection varies depending on the fracture location and type of surgical procedure performed. Postoperative infections are part of a vicious cycle that produces intricate relationships between etiologic factors and the formation of posttraumatic mandibular deformities. For example, a tooth in the line of a fracture leads to bacterial contamination of the fracture site, producing an infection that consequently may generate osteolysis around the screws, leading to fixation failure and ultimately a nonunion. Therefore, the causes of postoperative infections are multifactorial, and causes such as instability, failed hardware, teeth in the line of fracture, medically compromised patients, delay of treatment, and noncompliant patients have been described in the literature.[5] Controversy still exists with the treatment of teeth in the line of fracture,[6] delay of treatment,[7] and prophylactic antibiotic coverage.[8] In a recent systematic review, Kyzas[8] suggests that the evidence to support the prophylactic use of antibiotics in the treatment of mandible fractures is rather limited and of doubtful quality. A general algorithm for the management of an infected mandibular fracture after rigid fixation can be seen in **Fig. 4**.

Osteomyelitis may result if delayed or inadequate treatment of postoperative infections is rendered. Posttraumatic mandibular osteomyelitis occurs in 1% to 6% of cases and is more common with chronic disease.[9] Surgical treatments include debridement, sequestrectomy, mandibular resection, and immobilization of the fragments.[10]

Healing Impairment

The role of systemic disease and polysubstance abuse during treatment planning for reoperation cannot be underestimated. Several systemic diseases or abnormalities have been linked with healing impairment, including diabetes, anemia, human immunodeficiency virus (HIV) infection,

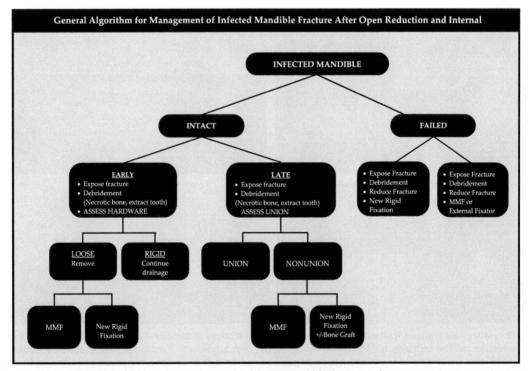

Fig. 4. General algorithm for the management of infected mandible fracture after open reduction and internal fixation. (*Modified from* Alpert B. Management of the complications of mandibular fracture treatment. Operat Tech Plast Reconstr Surg 1998;5(4):325–33; with permission.)

hyperparathyroidism, hyperthyroidism, osteomalacia, osteopetrosis, chronic renal disease, osteogenesis imperfecta, Paget disease, vitamin B or C deficiencies, and chronic steroid or bisphosphonate use.[9]

In a retrospective study, Senel and colleagues[11] found an increased risk for postoperative infection in HIV-positive patients and diabetic patients after mandibular fracture repair. Similarly, Benson and colleagues[5] associated treatment failure with immunosuppression after immediate bone grafting of clinically infected mandibular fractures. Increased risk of complications in patients who abused alcohol and drugs has also been identified in the literature.[11–14] Although the reason for this increase is also multifactorial, it has been suggested that nutritional deficiencies, changes in general health, life style, and personal/oral hygiene, and overall compliance are contributing factors.[13]

REOPERATION IN POSTTRAUMATIC MANDIBULAR DEFORMITIES

Posttraumatic mandibular deformities that may require reoperation for their correction include nonunion, malunion/malocclusion, and facial asymmetry. These deformities may be present alone or in combination, and one deformity could be the cause of the other (eg, malunion producing facial asymmetry).

NONUNION

A nonunion is a fracture with arrested healing that requires further surgical therapy to achieve union.[9] Haug and Schwimmer[12] considered a nonunion any mandibular fracture that exhibited mobility after 4 weeks without treatment or after 8 weeks with surgical management. The incidence of nonunion in mandibular fractures has been reported to be 0.1% to 9%, but rates vary considerably when evaluating specific fixation techniques.[3,15] Causes are multifactorial; however, several contributing factors have been described in the literature, such as soft tissue infection, osteomyelitis, fracture mobility, inaccurate reduction, delay in treatment, teeth in the line of fracture, alcohol and drug abuse, inexperienced surgeon, and poor patient compliance.[12,15,16] According to De Souza and colleagues,[17] early motion after fixation is the main contributor to nonunion. A considerable number of nonunions are secondary to infection. Ellis and Walker[18] suggested that the hypoxic environment of the scar tissue after a postoperative infection induces the lack of osseous tissue

formation in mandibular nonunions. Large fracture gaps or comminuted fractures may also lead to nonunions because of soft tissue entrapment and poor bone contact. Severely atrophic mandibular fractures are also particularly susceptible to develop nonunion because insufficient bone contact between fracture segments is present and mandibular mobility is more likely to occur.

Diagnosis of mandibular nonunion is usually made by clinical examination after identifying persistent mandibular mobility or tenderness at the fracture site. Irregular radiolucency with mottled fracture ends and/or hardware loosening are radiographic findings that also support the diagnosis. When closed reduction techniques are used, the diagnosis of nonunion comes after the release of the MMF.

Surgical Considerations

Mandibular nonunions are best approached by an extraoral approach. Ample and direct visualization of the fracture site allows for better debridement of the area of any fibrous tissue, necrotic bone, or failed hardware. Ideally, bone debridement requires the presence of bleeding bone. Once adequate occlusion and MMF are achieved, the fracture is reduced and a properly anchored reconstruction-type plate with screws is placed away from the fracture (3–4 screws at each side of the fracture). Recommendations of placing the screws no closer than 7 to 10 mm have been described in the literature, with the rationale that, although the bone may appear normal, there is less mineral content several millimeters from the fracture.[3,19] In younger patients or in well-vascularized areas, union generally occurs if the bone gap is small. If inadequate bone contact exists, autogenous bone grafting needs to be performed to reestablish the continuity of the mandible (**Fig. 5**).

MALUNIONS/MALOCCLUSIONS

Malunions can occur with any form of treatment of mandibular fractures. They occur when segments heal in an improper alignment. Malocclusions are the most common sign and symptom of malunions.[3] Malunions typically follow inadequate establishment of occlusion, lack of accurate anatomic reduction, and poor adaptation of the fixation plate. Rigid internal fixation is more often associated with malunion and malocclusion than closed techniques. The rigidity obtained prevents correction of technical errors without reoperation.[9] If minor occlusal disparities are

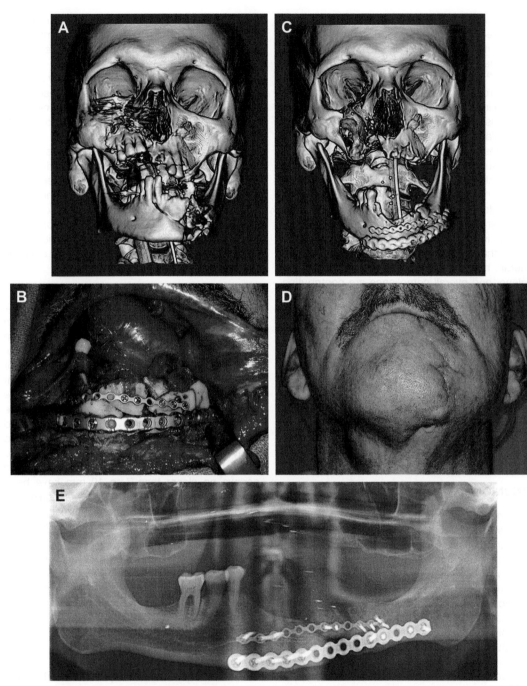

Fig. 5. Mandibular nonunion. A 55-year-old man with a gunshot wound to the face that developed a mandibular nonunion. Reoperation was performed 5 months after the primary surgery. (*A*) Three-dimensional CT reconstruction of the original injury. (*B*) Intraoperative view of the primary mandibular repair. (*C*) Immediate postoperative 3-dimensional (3D) CT reconstruction. (*D*) Draining purulent fistula in the right chin 4 months after the original surgery. (*E*) Panoramic radiograph showing a persistent radiolucency at the fracture site. (*F*) Intraoperative view of the mandibular nonunion after debridement. (*G*) Intraoperative view of the autogenous bone graft. (*H*) Immediate post-reoperative axial CT scan of the bone graft area. (*I*) Immediate post-reoperative 3D CT reconstruction. Maxillary reconstruction was achieved by placing zygoma implants.

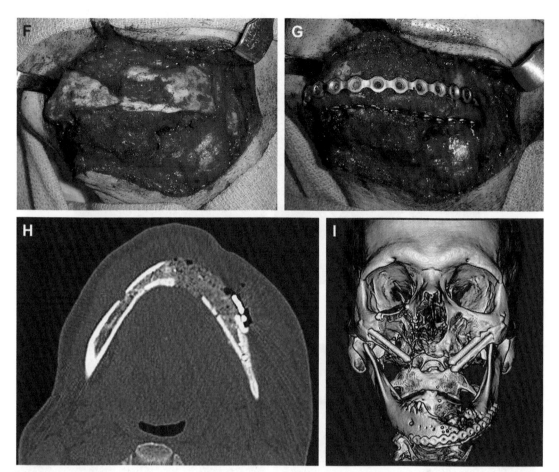

Fig. 5. (*continued*)

Surgical Considerations

When malocclusion is recognized early, it must be corrected or malunion will result. The mandible is approached in the same way as in the original repair. Hardware is removed, and proper occlusion is obtained via MMF. Fracture is properly reduced if needed, and a new fixation is applied. The revised occlusion is verified by releasing the MMF.

Surgical management of late malunions often includes osteotomies for the proper reestablishment of the mandibular anatomy and occlusion. Dental models are obtained to study the occlusion. Model surgery is performed, and the placement of the osteotomies is determined. Typically the osteotomies are at the previous fracture sites, but sagittal split or vertical ramus osteotomies can be used. A surgical splint is constructed to help establish the occlusal relationship. The surgical approach depends on the osteotomies to be

found, orthodontic therapy or occlusal adjustments can be instituted.

performed. Once the mandible is cut, the occlusion is set with the help of the surgical splint. MMF is obtained, and a new rigid fixation is applied. Occlusion is rechecked after releasing the MMF. Rarely the gap between the osteotomies require a bone graft (**Figs. 6** and **7**).

Malunions/maloccusions and condylar fractures

Controversy exists with regard to the best management of condylar fractures.[20] However, a vast majority of these fractures are treated closed, and they usually develop a malunion. Condylar malunion is not synonymous to malocclusion.[21] Ellis and Walker[18] suggested that the most important factor is not whether the patient was treated open or closed but the quality of functional rehabilitation of the mandible. Most of the patients have the biologic ability to adapt to their injury in a harmonius way.[22]

No treatment or unsuccessful treatment are the 2 main reasons of posttraumatic malocclusions secondary to condylar fractures. Minor malocclusion

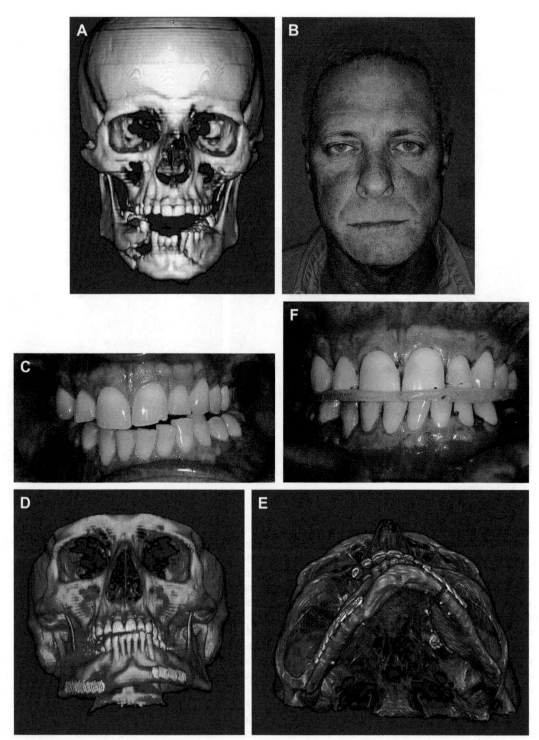

Fig. 6. Mandibular malunion/malocclusion. A 50-year-old man after work-related accident. He sustained bilateral mandibular body fractures that were repaired with open reduction and internal fixation. He presented to our institution after repair complaining of malocclusion. Reoperation was done 12 months after the original surgery. (*A*) Three-dimensional CT reconstruction of the original injury. (*B*) Preoperative photograph. (*C*) Preoperative photograph of the occlusion. (*D*, *E*) Three-dimensional CT reconstructions obtained to preoperatively study the shape of the mandible and the status of the original repair. Model surgery was performed, and a surgical splint was then fabricated. (*F*) Intraoperative view of the surgical splint and predetermined occlusion. (*G*) Intraoperative view of the right mandibular body osteotomy. (*H*) Intraoperative view of the left mandibular body osteotomy. Note the mental nerve lateralization. (*I*) Panoramic radiograph after reoperation. (*J*) Postoperative photograph 6 months after surgery. (*K*) Postoperative occlusion.

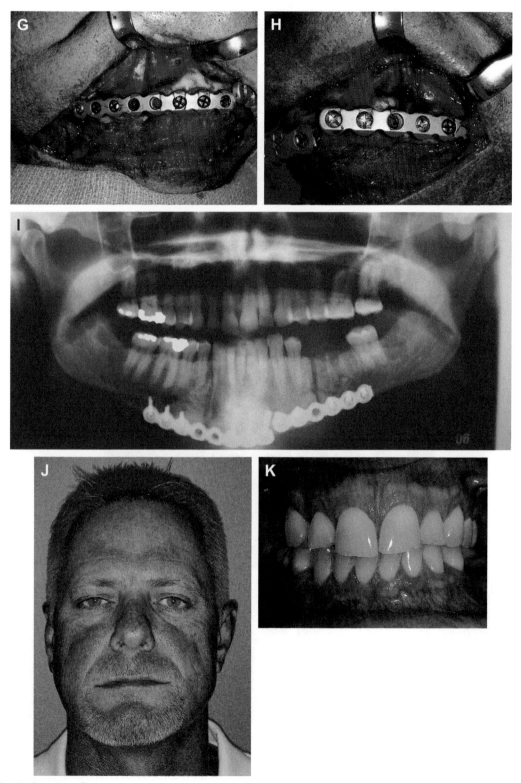

Fig. 6. (*continued*)

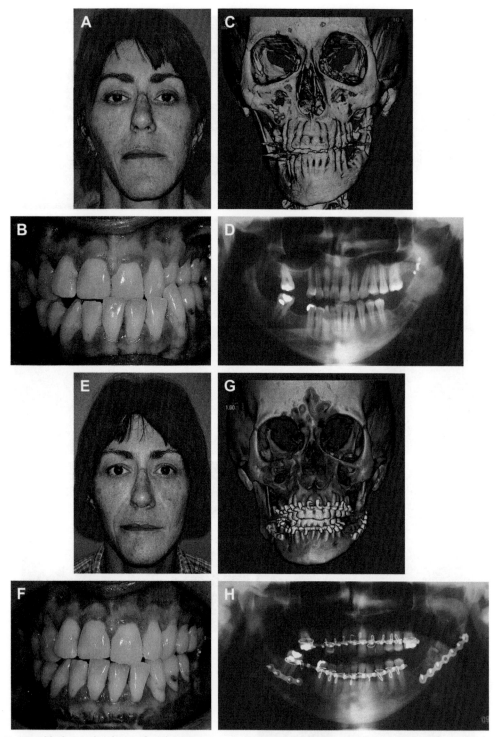

Fig. 7. Mandibular malocclusion/facial asymmetry. A 42-year-old woman who had a fall. She sustained a left mandibular angle fracture that was originally treated with closed reduction. Because of seizures, the MMF had to be released within days of the original surgery, and subsequently she was treated with an open reduction and internal fixation. She presented to our institution 2 years after the original surgery complaining of malocclusion and facial asymmetry. (*A*) Preoperative photograph. (*B*) Preoperative occlusion. (*C*) Three-dimensional CT reconstructions obtained to study the status of the original repair. (*D*) Preoperative panoramic radiograph. Patient underwent an extraoral vertical osteotomy in the area of the original fracture (*left*) and a sagittal osteotomy in the contralateral side (*right*). (*E*) Postoperative photograph. (*F*) Postoperative occlusion. (*G*) Postreoperative 3-dimensional CT reconstruction. (*H*) Panoramic radiograph after reoperation.

can be treated with orthodontics, prosthetics reconstruction, or occlusal adjustments.

Surgical Considerations

The degree of mandibular ramus deformity is the most important aspect to consider when planning

for reoperation of posttraumatic malocclusion after condylar fracture repair.[18] If the remaining mandibular ramus is short and multifragmented and the patient requires large movements to obtain proper occlusion, TMJ reconstruction may be the preferred method. A good example is a patient who presents with severe condylar

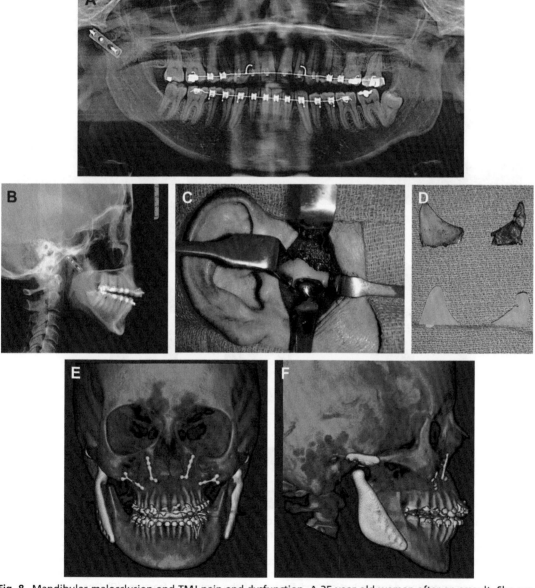

Fig. 8. Mandibular malocclusion and TMJ pain and dysfunction. A 35-year-old woman after an assault. She sustained a left subcondylar fracture that was originally treated with an open reduction and internal fixation. Patient presented to our institution 3 years after the original surgery, complaining of malocclusion and bilateral TMJ pain and dysfunction. (*A*) Preoperative radiograph showing severe resorption of the right condyle; note also degenerative changes on the left condyle. (*B*) Preoperative cephalometric radiograph showing the dentoskeletal deformity. Patient underwent a bilateral total TMJ replacement and a Le Fort I osteotomy. (*C*) Intraoperative view of the alloplastic total TMJ replacement. (*D*) Left condyle and coronoid. Comparison between planned and actual specimens. Note the severe resorption of the condyle. (*E, F*) Postoperative 3-dimensional CT reconstructions.

58

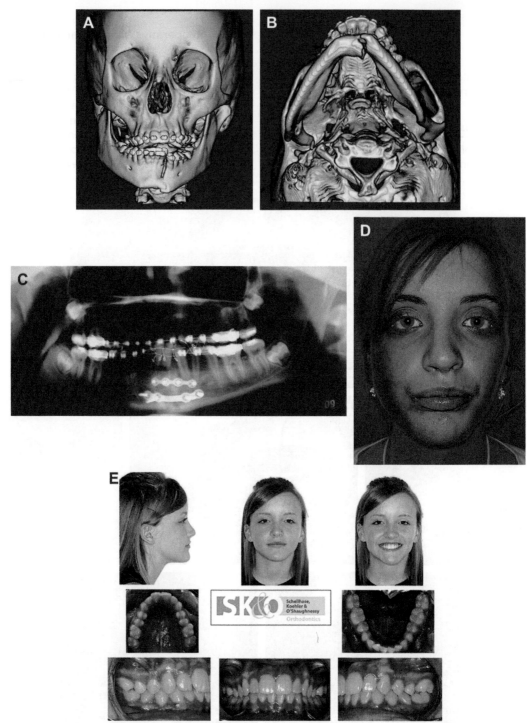

Fig. 9. Facial asymmetry. A 16-year-old girl after a motor vehicle collision. She sustained a mandibular symphysis and right condylar fractures. Patient's symphysis was treated with an open reduction and internal fixation, and the right condyle with a closed reduction. One month after the surgery, the patient complained of facial asymmetry with persistent right facial swelling but no malocclusion. (*A, B*) Three-dimensional CT reconstructions of the original injury. Note the displacement of the lingual cortices in the symphysis area. (*C*) Postoperative panoramic radiograph demonstrating good reduction and fixation of the symphysis fracture. (*D*) One-month follow-up photograph showing facial asymmetry and right "swelling that never goes away." (*E*) Preinjury orthodontic records used to plan her reoperation (*Courtesy of* Dr Karen Koehler, Jacksonville, FL). (*F, G*) Follow-up 3-dimensional (3D) CT reconstructions to study the cause of the facial asymmetry. Note the facial widening and the poor reduction of the lingual cortices at the symphysis area. (*H, I*) Post-reoperative 3D CT reconstructions. Lingual cortices were reduced by applying pressure on both mandibular rami until the buccal cortices began to separate. Note the decrease of the intergonial distance. The condylar fracture was treated closed. (*J*) Panoramic radiograph 1 year after reoperation. (*K*) Photograph 18 months after reoperation with good facial symmetry.

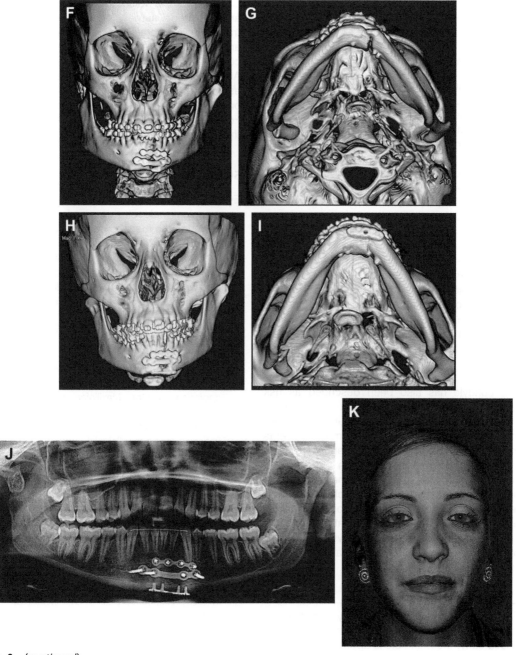

Fig. 9. (*continued*)

resorption after an unsuccessful open reduction and internal fixation (**Fig. 8**). Additional aspects to be considered are unilateral versus bilateral condylar fractures, time between injury and treatment of the malocclusion, and availability of a stable dentition.

Successful treatment of malocclusions can be achieved with functional therapy up to 3 months.[18]

In cases of long-standing malocclusions with stable temporomandibular articulations, orthognathic surgery has been advocated.[18,21,23–25] For unilateral condylar fractures, sagittal split, or vertical ramus, osteotomies have been used on the side of the fracture. Bilateral osteotomies may be used for more predictable results if only 1 condyle was affected.[18,21,24] Bilateral condylar fractures have the tendency to develop anterior open bites that can be treated with a Le Fort I or mandibular osteotomies.

FACIAL ASYMMETRY

Facial asymmetry can be found early during the healing period secondary to inadequate reduction (Fig. 9) or as long-term sequelae after malunions or, less commonly, nonunions. During the early phases of healing, clinical diagnosis is difficult because of postoperative swelling, but if suspected, imaging such as anteroposterior cephalometric radiography or CT scan can confirm the diagnosis. The clinician should be cognizant of several clinical scenarios that have the potential of developing facial asymmetries. Good examples are inadequate reduction with a combination of mandibular symphysis and subcondylar fractures. In these cases, overtightening the MMF causes rotation of segments, with loss of lingual contacts and flaring of the inferior border of the mandible. Furthermore, if a segmental maxillary fracture is also encountered, the ability to reestablish an arch form is lost and facial widening or asymmetry may result. The presence of multiple unilateral mandibular fractures such as mandibular angle and condyle has also been described as risk factors.[26] Additionally severe comminution of the mandibular body resulting in an inability to obtain intimate bony contact of all the small fragments may produce a bowing of the inferior border so that the injured side is lower than the uninjured side.[27] In rare cases, facial asymmetry is caused by the loss of posterior height, such as in severe resorption or malposition of the condyle after an open approach. Usually these patients present complaining of TMJ pain and dysfunction and often require autogenous or alloplastic total TMJ replacements.

Surgical Considerations

Facial asymmetry is treated similarly as malunions/malocclusions. If the facial asymmetry is diagnosed early, the mandible is approached through the original repair. Hardware is removed, the fracture is properly reduced, and a new fixation is placed. If the facial asymmetry is due to a symphysis fracture, Ellis and Tharanon[28] recommend pressing medially the mandibular rami until the buccal cortices begin to separate, indicating that the lingual cortices are in contact and proper reduction has been achieved.

Established facial asymmetries are treated similar to orthognathic surgery. Facial, dental, and radiographic analyses are performed. Determination of the osteotomies and splint fabrication is based on the results of the previous analyses and the model surgery. Surgical approach is intraoral or extraoral, depending on the location and type of the osteotomy to be used. Before cutting the mandible, all hardware are removed. After the mandible has been cut, occlusion is established and a new fixation is applied. If the original injury included a maxillary fracture, a Le Fort I osteotomy might be necessary to correct the deformity.

SUMMARY

Even with best efforts, unsatisfactory results such as nonunion, malocclusion, and facial asymmetry occur during the management of mandibular fractures. A clear understanding of the nature of these posttraumatic mandibular deformities helps to avoid them. Furthermore, the clinician should be familiar with the reoperative techniques used for the management of these deformities.

REFERENCES

1. Xia JJ, Gateno J, Teichgraeber JF. A new paradigm for complex midface reconstruction: a reversed approach. J Oral Maxillofac Surg 2009;67(3): 693–703.
2. Bell RB. Computer planning and intraoperative navigation in cranio-maxillofacial surgery. Oral Maxillofac Surg Clin North Am 2010;22(1):135–56.
3. Ellis E. Complications of rigid internal fixation for mandibular fractures. J Craniomaxillofac Trauma 1996;2(2):32–9.
4. Alpert B. Management of the complications of mandibular fracture treatment. Operat Tech Plast Reconstr Surg 1998;5(4):325–33.
5. Benson PD, Marshall MK, Engelstad ME, et al. The use of immediate bone grafting in reconstruction of clinically infected mandibular fractures: bone grafts in the presence of pus. J Oral Maxillofac Surg 2006;64(1):122–6.
6. Spinatto G, Alberto P. Teeth in the line of mandibular fractures. Atlas Oral Maxillofac Surg Clin North Am 2009;17(1):15–8.
7. Lucca M, Shastri K, McKenzie W, et al. Comparison of treatment outcomes associated with early versus late treatment of mandible fractures: a retrospective chart review and analysis. J Oral Maxillofac Surg 2010;68(10):2484–8.
8. Kyzas PA. Use of antibiotics in the treatment of mandible fractures: a systematic review. J Oral Maxillofac Surg 2010. [Epub ahead of print]. DOI:10.1016/j.joms.2010.02.059.
9. Koury M. Complications of mandibular fractures. In: Kaban L, Pogrel A, Perrott D, editors. Complications

in oral and maxillofacial surgery. 1st edition. Philadelphia: WB Saunders; 1997. p. 121–45.

10. Coviello V, Stevens MR. Contemporary concepts in the treatment of chronic osteomyelitis. Oral Maxillofac Surg Clin North Am 2007;19(4):523–34.

11. Senel FC, Jessen GS, Melo MD, et al. Infection following treatment of mandible fractures: the role of immunosuppression and polysubstance abuse. Oral Surg Oral Med Oral Pathol Oral Radiol Endod 2007;103(1):38–42.

12. Haug RH, Schwimmer A. Fibrous union of the mandible: a review of 27 patients. J Oral Maxillofac Surg 1994;52(8):832–9.

13. Passeri LA, Ellis E, Sinn DP. Relationship of substance abuse to complications with mandibular fractures. J Oral Maxillofac Surg 1993;51(1):22–5.

14. Serena-Gómez E, Passeri LA. Complications of mandible fractures related to substance abuse. J Oral Maxillofac Surg 2008;66(10):2028–34.

15. Mathog RH, Toma V, Clayman L, et al. Nonunion of the mandible: an analysis of contributing factors. J Oral Maxillofac Surg 2000;58(7):746–52 [discussion: 752–3].

16. Furr AM, Schweinfurth JM, May WL. Factors associated with long-term complications after repair of mandibular fractures. Laryngoscope 2006;116(3): 427–30.

17. De Souza M, Oeltjen JC, Panthaki ZJ, et al. Posttraumatic mandibular deformities. J Craniofac Surg 2007;18(4):912–6.

18. Ellis E, Walker R. Treatment of malocclusion and TMJ dysfunction secondary to condylar fractures. Craniomaxillofacial Trauma Reconstruction 2009; 2(1):1–18.

19. Mehra P, Van Heukelom E, Cottrell DA. Rigid internal fixation of infected mandibular fractures. J Oral Maxillofac Surg 2009;67(5):1046–51.

20. Laskin DM. Management of condylar process fractures. Oral Maxillofac Surg Clin North Am 2009; 21(2):193–6.

21. Becking AG, Zijderveld SA, Tuinzing DB. Management of posttraumatic malocclusion caused by condylar process fractures. J Oral Maxillofac Surg 1998;56(12):1370–4 [discussion: 1374–5].

22. Ellis E, Throckmorton G. Treatment of mandibular condylar process fractures: biological considerations. J Oral Maxillofac Surg 2005;63(1):115–34.

23. Spitzer WJ, Vanderborght G, Dumbach J. Surgical management of mandibular malposition after malunited condylar fractures in adults. J Craniomaxillofac Surg 1997;25(2):91–6.

24. Rubens BC, Stoelinga PJ, Weaver TJ, et al. Management of malunited mandibular condylar fractures. Int J Oral Maxillofac Surg 1990;19(1):22–5.

25. Laine P, Kontio R, Salo A, et al. Secondary correction of malocclusion after treatment of maxillofacial trauma. J Oral Maxillofac Surg 2004; 62(10):1312–20.

26. Cillo JE, Ellis E. Treatment of patients with double unilateral fractures of the mandible. J Oral Maxillofac Surg 2007;65(8):1461–9.

27. Ellis E, Muniz O, Anand K. Treatment considerations for comminuted mandibular fractures. J Oral Maxillofac Surg 2003;61(8):861–70.

28. Ellis E, Tharanon W. Facial width problems associated with rigid fixation of mandibular fractures: case reports. J Oral Maxillofac Surg 1992;50(1): 87–94.

Reoperative Soft Tissue Trauma

Tirbod Fattahi, MD, DDS

KEYWORDS

- Soft tissue trauma • Wound healing • Z-plasty
- Dermabrasion

There are more than 300 million people living in the United States.[1] Although the life span of the average American continues to increase, trauma remains the leading cause of death in the first 4 decades of life and is surpassed only by cancer and atherosclerotic disease as the overall leading causes of death.[2] There are more than 60 million injuries each year in the United States, with the annual medical cost exceeding $400 billion.[3] Many of these injuries involve the facial region, including soft tissue trauma. Because the face is considered the most conspicuous and significant portion of a person's identity, the importance of proper soft tissue management cannot be overemphasized. Clearly, any discussion of reoperative surgery must emphasize and highlight the necessary vigilance and attention to details required at the initial time of repair; this is no different for the face or any other part of the body. However, there are times when, irrespective of excellent initial management, revisions or reoperations become necessary. This scenario is certainly the case in major avulsive soft tissue trauma and after major oncologic resections (**Fig. 1**). In these situations, it is imperative to explain the extent of the injury to the patients and their families, emphasizing the importance of proper follow-up and the clinician's desire for continuity of care through the healing period. This article highlights the available modalities used in the management of unsightly scars or those scars whose location and appearance compromise function.

WOUND HEALING

Although it is beyond the scope of this article to discuss the initial management of facial soft tissue injuries, a brief overview of wound healing is necessary to understand the biology of wounds and the implications of the timing of secondary revision. Wound healing begins shortly after the initial traumatic event.[4] Hemostasis and formation of a clot followed by an inflammatory phase are the hallmarks of the initial few hours of wound healing. Derangements in hemostasis and excessive inflammation can certainly have a deleterious effect on the final aesthetic outcome of the scar. Cellular proliferation occurs in the next 2 to 5 days, marked by neovascularization as well as recruitment of mesenchymal cells and new keratinocytes. After the first week, the final phase of healing begins, which includes the formation of a scar followed by remodeling. Remodeling may take up to several months to complete. The greatest percentage of wound strength is generated in this phase, and as such, if an imbalance in cellular remodeling occurs, unwanted outcomes, such as a hypertrophic scar or keloid, may occur.[5]

Another factor that may influence the need for reoperation of a soft tissue injury is the manner in which the wound is managed (by the patient and the clinician) after the initial repair. Again, recalling the events at the cellular level is helpful. At the author's institution, all facial wounds are seen within 5 days for suture removal. Leaving sutures in for a longer period may leave "track" marks. Liberal use of adhesive bandages, such as

Division of Oral and Maxillofacial Surgery, University of Florida Health Science Center, Jacksonville, 653–1 West 8th Street, Jacksonville, FL 32209, USA
E-mail address: Tirbod.Fattahi@Jax.Ufl.Edu

Oral Maxillofacial Surg Clin N Am 23 (2011) 63–71
doi:10.1016/j.coms.2010.10.002
1042-3699/11/$ — see front matter © 2011 Elsevier Inc. All rights reserved.

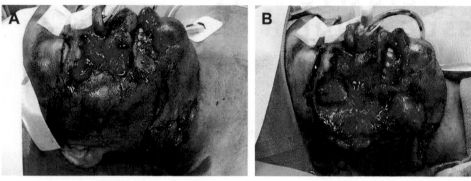

Fig. 1. Massive soft tissue trauma (*A, B*) often requires secondary revision.

Steri-strips (3M Company, Maplewood, MN, USA), obviates the sutures from remaining in place for a long time. After suture removal, the patient is asked to gently cleanse the laceration with a mild soap (eg, baby shampoo), dry the wound, and maintain a thin layer of antibiotic ointment on it until there is complete epithelialization (**Fig. 2**). This process typically occurs in the first 10 to 14 days. Sun protection is an important factor in the management of wounds. All patients are instructed to use an appropriate level of sunblock while the wound is remodeling. Sunblock should not be applied on a wound that has not completely epithelialized because it may irritate the wound. Ultraviolet rays (A and B) have been shown to cause photoaging and sunburn; they can also irritate the epidermis and dermis. Because a facial laceration usually extends well beyond the skin into the subcutaneous tissues, the epidermis and dermis are already injured; further sun damage only exacerbates the cellular response and the degree of inflammation. Along with sun protection, patients are instructed to massage the wound (after initial healing). Medicaments such as lotions, oils, and vitamins may assist, although scientific data regarding their efficacy are lacking.[6,7] However, silicone cream or sheets do have a significant role in the management of wounds. Although the exact mechanism of action remains unknown, it is thought that silicone may upregulate the action of collagenase (enhance collagen breakdown and reduce scarring) and decrease the production of transforming growth factor β_2, a proinflammatory mediator.[8–10] Silicone sheets and creams are routinely dispensed to the patients to augment the aesthetic outcomes of facial lacerations. There are multiple factors that must be kept in mind regarding the timing of scar revision. For example, wound healing occurs significantly quicker in a child than in an adult because of the abundance of collagen and elastin fibers. Therefore, it is acceptable to revise a scar in a child sooner (2–3 months)

than in an adult (4–6 months). Another consideration should involve the location of a scar and its effect on function (such as a periorbital laceration impeding eyelid closure). Loss or limitation of function is an indication of earlier scar revision, irrespective of age. Psychosocial considerations should also be included in the decision making regarding scar revision. Unattractive and unsightly scars can have an enormous emotional and psychological effect on the patient's life and quality of living. Sensitivity and understanding on the part of the clinician regarding this issue is desired.

SCAR ANALYSIS

Before reoperation of soft tissue injuries of the face, the clinician should evaluate the patient for several factors.[11] These factors are:

- Type and size of scar
  Flat versus raised, atrophic versus normal volume, keloid (beyond the margins of the initial wound)
- Location of scar in relation to skin tension lines and facial units
- Fitzpatrick classification of the patient
- Age of the patient
- Compromise in function.

Type and Size of Scar

Different types of scars may require different treatments. For example, a wide scar, irrespective of being flat, raised, or atrophic, may need reexcision and closure (**Fig. 3**). Types of closure may involve Z-plasty, W-plasty, geometric broken line closure, or a straight closure. The different types of closures are discussed later in this article. Hypertrophic and keloid scars need excision and other modalities, such as intralesional steroids and silicone sheets. In the author's experience, large hypertrophic scars and keloids do not respond

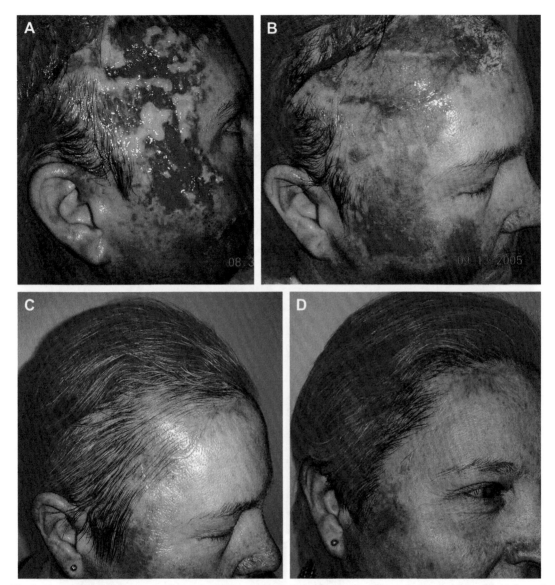

Fig. 2. Example of proper wound care by patient. (*A*) At 3 days after significant facial abrasion. (*B*) At 1 week after injury. (*C*) At 3 months after injury. (*D*) At 7 months after injury.

well to only excision or intralesional steroid injections; therapy must be directed toward a multimodal treatment. On the other hand, atrophic or volume-depleted scars require filling. This filling could encompass autogenous materials, such as fascia and fat, or synthetic dermal fillers.

Location of Scar in Relation to Skin Tension Lines and Facial Units

Resting skin tension lines have been described for more than 100 years.[12,13] Further enhancement of this concept led to the development of facial units and subunits.[14,15] Incisions made along the resting

tension lines tend to be less obvious.[16] It has been stated that no 2 zebras have identical stripe patterns. This dissimilarity may not be discernable to the eye at first glance because the general pattern of stripes and colors run in a specific direction. Similarly, the appearance of scars parallel to the skin lines may not be discernible at first glance, unlike those that are perpendicular. Regarding facial units and subunits, one of the well-respected concepts in oncologic skin resection is to remove the entire unit or subunit, even if the excision is slightly larger than needed. The benefit of this principle is in the secondary reconstruction of the said defect. If the resection and

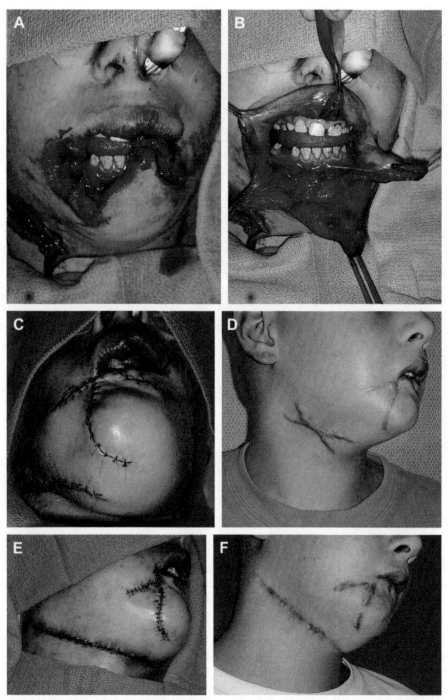

Fig. 3. Wide scar requiring excision before laser resurfacing. (*A, B*) Initial appearance after dog bite. (*C*) Immediately after repair. (*D*) Appearance at 4 months; notice raised and wide appearance. (*E*) Scar excision. (*F*) At 1 month after scar excision; the patient is ready for laser resurfacing.

reconstruction encompass an entire unit and subunit, the final outcome tends to blend in with the surrounding tissues and therefore is less conspicuous.

Fitzpatrick Classification of the Patient

Fitzpatrick[17] developed the skin sun reactivity classification in 1975. This useful classification assists in determining the degree of skin reaction to sun exposure as well as possible treatment modalities. The original use of this classification system was for skin rejuvenation, not facial trauma; however, knowing how a patient's skin may react to sunlight undoubtedly helps in choosing the correct treatment modality for scar revision.[18] Patients with high Fitzpatrick classification tend to experience postinflammatory dyspigmentation, encompassing both hyper- and hypopigmentation after soft tissue injury. Hyperpigmentation tends to be transient, but hypopigmentation tends to be permanent and is much more difficult to address. For this reason, a patient classified as Fitzpatrick type I or type II may respond well to a laser resurfacing procedure, whereas a patient classified as Fitzpatrick type IV or type V may need more conservative treatments such as superficial chemical peels and scar excision.[19,20]

Patient's Age

The old adage of waiting up to a year to perform scar revision is probably invalid. There is no scientific explanation for this practice.[21,22] A scar that is limiting function at 3 months or one that is perpendicular to a skin resting line at 3 months continues to limit function and be perpendicular to skin resting lines at 12 months. Some investigators argue that children, because of their rapid healing ability and higher concentration of collagen and elastin, should undergo scar revision after puberty. Psychosocial issues and limitation of function (eg, inability to close eyes) should supersede this principle.

Generally, scar revision can be done as early as few weeks if there is a functional impairment. In the absence of functional impairment, most scar revisions can be done between 4 and 6 months in adults. Revision can certainly be delayed up to 9 to 12 months assuming that further scar contracture and remodeling is occurring. The timing of scar revision is only one of many factors that

must be considered when contemplating reoperation.

Compromise in Function

Scars that interfere with normal facial functions, such as eyelid closure, lip competence, and lacrimal and salivary functions, must be addressed first (**Fig. 4**). Delay in secondary revision in these scenarios may increase morbidity and compromise other vital functions (lagophthalmos causing dry eyes leading to blurred vision).

TREATMENT OPTIONS

Most soft tissue reoperations include W- or Z-plasty, dermabrasion, laser resurfacing, and fat grafting. It is important to remember that other conservative options, such as silicone cream or sheets, steroid injections, Botox, and dermal fillers are acceptable, but this article emphasizes on the aforementioned more invasive or surgical modalities.

W-Plasty

The major indication for W-plasty is a long scar that is not orientated perpendicular to the skin tension lines.[23] The main advantage of W-plasty is that it does not increase the overall length of the scar, unlike Z-plasty. The scar is outlined circumferentially with multiple opposing W's, each with a limb no longer than approximately 5 mm. Once the scar is excised, the 2 flaps are brought together to create a series of small W's. Rearrangement of the scar from a wide and linear appearance into smaller geometric shapes improves the appearance of the scar (**Fig. 5**).

Z-Plasty

Z-plasty essentially involves the transposition of 2 triangular flaps to reorientate a scar. It is ideal for scars that cause functional impairment or are perpendicular to the resting skin lines because it changes the direction of the scar band

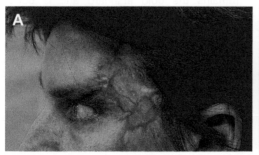
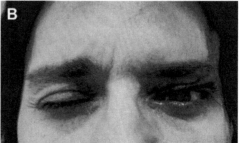

Fig. 4. Patient treated at another institution with a partial thickness skin graft to lateral orbit region causing scar contracture and inability to close eyelid (*A, B*).

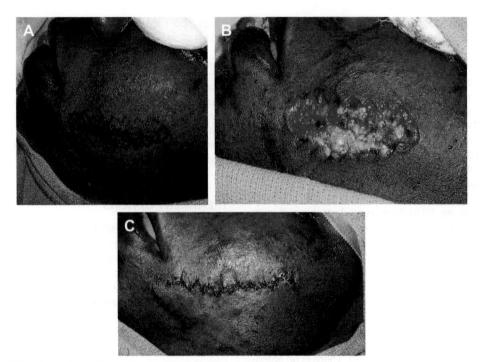

Fig. 5. W-plasty performed to address long scar along left cheek (*A–C*).

completely.[24–26] The central component of the Z must encompass the scar, and the other 2 limbs are designed so that the final flaps are as parallel to the resting skin lines as possible (**Fig. 6**). The angles between the 2 flaps can be 30°, 45°, or 60°. An angle of 30° increases the overall length of the scar by 25%, 45° by 50%, and 60° by 75%. Multiple Z-plasties can be performed simultaneously, although there is a significant increase in the overall length of the scar. It is also imperative to remember that irrespective of the method of skin rearrangement, further treatment modalities, such as dermabrasion and laser resurfacing, can certainly be done at another time to further enhance the final results.

Dermabrasion

Dermabrasion involves sanding of the scar using a high-speed rotary device. Dermabrasion is performed down to the level of the papillary dermis, which is easily recognized in the healthy skin by looking for pinpoint bleeders. When dermabrading a raised scar, pinpoint bleeding occurs almost instantaneously; therefore, care must be taken when performing this procedure. Dermabrasion is a wonderful tool in treating raised scars as well as atrophic or pitted scars (acne pits) (**Fig. 7**). By blending in the periphery of the dermabraded scar into the surrounding healthy tissues, a more

uniform and cosmetic outcome can be achieved. Also, because dermabrasion causes an insult to the papillary dermis, there is scientific evidence to demonstrate neocollagen formation as well as reorientation of the collagen fibers, which can further enhance the appearance of the scar.[27,28] Dermabrasion in dark-skinned individuals (Fitzpatrick IV and above) can cause significant dyspigmentation that may be permanent. If other options are not indicated, a test area (behind the ears) can be dermabraded to judge the skin reaction.

Laser Resurfacing

Perhaps the most powerful tool in scar modification in the appropriate patient is laser resurfacing (**Fig. 8**).[29] Carbon dioxide ultrapulse laser remains the gold standard and is constantly compared with other nonablative lasers, such as the YAG laser. Laser resurfacing effectively removes the entire epidermis and upper dermis and can stimulate significant neocollagen formation. Laser resurfacing is indicated in flat scars; hypertrophic scars are better treated using dermabrasion. The 2 modalities can be easily used simultaneously; after dermabrading a raised scar, the entire facial unit can be treated with laser (**Fig. 9**).[30] If the patient has generalized photodamage and melasma, then consideration should be given to resurface the entire face.

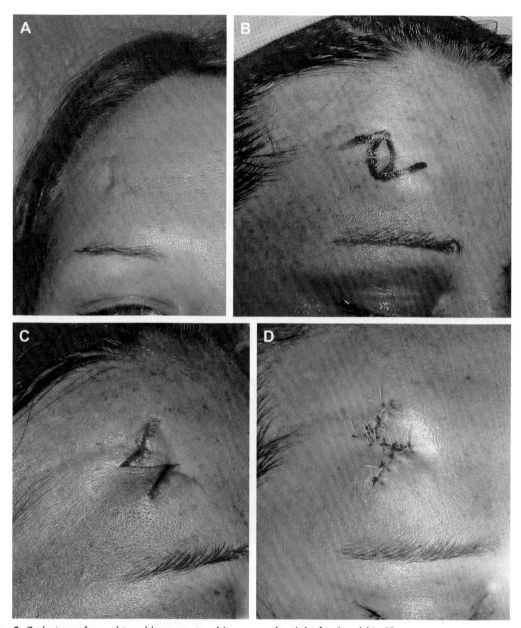

Fig. 6. Z-plasty performed to address an atrophic scar on the right forehead (*A–D*).

Full-face laser resurfacing does require pretreatment of skin with retinoids and bleaching creams to provide a balanced result. Similar to dermabrasion, laser resurfacing should not be done in dark-skinned individuals.[31]

Fat Grafting

Scars that are volume deficient and depressed can be easily augmented with fat transfer. An important consideration regarding autogenous fat transfer includes the need for overaugmentation because up to 40% of the transferred fat atrophies. Fat grafting can include dermal-fascia-fat grafting or liposuction and lipoinjection. Harvest of the dermal-fascia-fat requires another donor site incision, although it can easily be hidden on the inferior aspect of the umbilicus. Liposuction can be done on the lower abdomen and lateral thighs. Although some investigators advocate

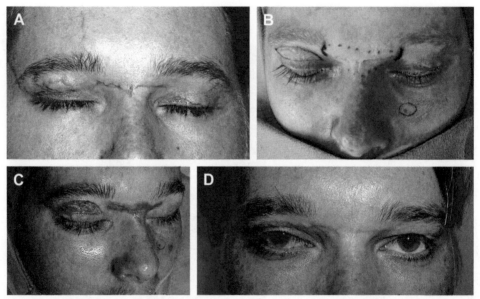

Fig. 7. Dermabrasion of the forehead area after soft tissue injury. The right upper eyelid scar is addressed through reexcision. (*A*) Appearance at 3 months after initial injury. (*B*, *C*) Intraoperative images during dermabrasion. (*D*) Appearance at 4 months after dermabrasion and scar revision.

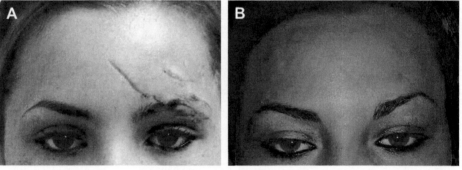

Fig. 8. Laser resurfacing of facial scars. (*A*) Appearance at 4 months after initial repair. (*B*) At 5 months after carbon dioxide laser resurfacing of forehead and upper eyelids.

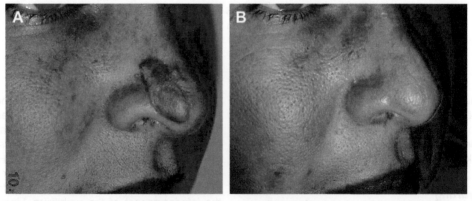

Fig. 9. Dermabrasion combined with carbon dioxide laser resurfacing after hypertrophic scarring after a fullthickness skin graft to right nose after a dog bite. (*A*) Appearance at 6 months after full-thickness skin graft. (*B*) Final appearance 4 months after simultaneous dermabrasion and laser resurfacing.

centrifuging of the harvested fat, this is usually not necessary for small scar revisions that require volume enhancement.[32,33]

SUMMARY

Soft tissue reoperation should be an integral part of the initial management of patients with soft tissue injuries. There are multiple modalities available to carry out scar revisions. A clear understanding of the wounding and healing process is important to determine the proper timing and the indicated surgical procedure for the individual patient.

REFERENCES

1. US Census Bureau. Available at: http://www.census. gov. Accessed September, 2010.
2. Advanced trauma life support. Chicago (IL): American College of Surgeons; 2000.
3. US Department of Health and Human Services. Available at: http://www.hhs.gov. Accessed September, 2010.
4. Broughton G, Janis JE, Attinger CE. The basic science of wound healing. Plast Reconstr Surg 2006;117:12S–34S.
5. Gorti G, Ronson S, Koch RJ. Wound healing. Facial Plast Surg Clin North Am 2002;10:119–27.
6. Khoosal D, Goldman RD. Vitamin E for treating children scars. Does it help reduce scarring? Can Fam Physician 2006;52:855–6.
7. Baumann LS, Spencer J. The effects of topical vitamin E on the cosmetic appearance of scars. Dermatol Surg 1999;25(4):311–5.
8. Agarwal US, Jain D, Gulati R, et al. Silicone gel sheet dressings for prevention of post-minigraft cobblestoning in vitiligo. Dermatol Surg 1999;25:102–4.
9. Ahn ST, Monafo WW, Mustoe TA. Topical silicone gel for the prevention and treatment of hypertrophic scars. Arch Surg 1991;126:499–504.
10. Ahn ST, Monafo WW, Mustoe TA. Topical silicone gel: a new treatment for hypertrophic scars. Surgery 1989;106:781–6.
11. Mustoe TA, Cooter RD, Gold MH, et al. International clinical recommendations on scar management. Plast Reconstr Surg 2002;110:560–71.
12. Gibson T. Karl Langer (1819–1887) and his lines [editorial]. Br J Plast Surg 1978;31:1–2.
13. Wilhelmi BJ, Blackwell SJ, Philips LG. Langer's lines: to use or not to use. Plast Reconstr Surg 1999;104: 208–14.
14. Gonzales-Ulloa M. Restoration of the face covering by means of selected skin in regional aesthetic units. Br J Plast Surg 1956;9:212.
15. Bush J, Ferguson MW, Mason T, et al. The dynamic rotation of Langer's lines on facial expression. J Plast Reconstr Aesthet Surg 2007;60(4):393–9.
16. Fattahi T. An overview of facial aesthetic units. J Oral Maxillofac Surg 2003;61(10):1207–11.
17. Fitzpatrick TB. [Soleil et peau]. J Med Esthet 1975;2: 33034 [in French].
18. Roberts WE. Skin type classification systems old and new. Dermatol Clin 2009;27(4):529–33.
19. Sriprachya-anunt S, Marchell NL, Fitzpatrick RE, et al. Facial resurfacing in patients with Fitzpatrick skin type IV. Lasers Surg Med 2002;30(2):86–92.
20. Taylor S, Grimes P, Lim J, et al. Postinflammatory hyperpigmentation. J Cutan Med Surg 2009;13(4): 183–91.
21. Lee KK, Mehrany K, Swanson NA. Surgical revision. Dermatol Clin 2005;23(1):141–50.
22. Grotting J. Scar and scar revision. Reoperative aesthetic and reconstructive plastic surgery. St Louis (MO): Quality Medical Publishing, Inc; 2007.
23. Isken T, Izmirli H, Onyedi M. A useful tool for design of the W-plasty in the excision of irregular lesions. Dermatol Surg 2009;35(12):2053–5.
24. Burke M. Z-plasty. How, when and why. Aust Fam Physician 1997;26(9):1027–9.
25. Furnas DW. The four fundamental functions of the Z-plasty. Arch Surg 1968;96:458–63.
26. Rohrich RJ, Zbar RI. A simplified algorithm for the use of Z-plasty. Plast Reconstr Surg 1999;103:1513–7.
27. Harmon CB, Zelickson BD, Roenigk RK, et al. Dermabrasive scar revision. Immunohistochemical and ultrastructure evaluation. Dermatol Surg 1995;21:503–8.
28. Robinson JK. Improvement of the appearance of full-thickness skin grafts with dermabrasion. Arch Dermatol 1987;123:1340–5.
29. Stratigos AJ, Dover JS. Overview of lasers and their properties. Dermatol Ther 2000;13:2–16.
30. Fezza JP. Laserbrasion: the combination of carbon dioxide laser and dermasanding. Plast Reconstr Surg 2005;118:1217–21.
31. Alster TS, Khoury RR. Treatment of laser complications. Facial Plast Surg 2009;25:316–23.
32. Carraway JH. Volume correction for nasojugal groove with blepharoplasty. Aesthet Surg J 2010; 30:101–9.
33. Carraway JH, Mellor CG. Syringe aspiration and fat concentration: a simple technique for autologous fat injection. Ann Plast Surg 1990;24:293–6.

Reoperative Orthognathic Surgery

Johan P. Reyneke, BChD, MChD, FCMFOS (SA), PhD[a,b,c,d,e,*]

KEYWORDS

• Reoperation • Complications • Orthognathic surgery

Favorable treatment outcomes in orthognathic surgical treatment can be achieved if the criteria of a comprehensive diagnosis, accurate treatment planning, and a sound surgical technique are closely adhered to. However, a small percentage of cases may require a second corrective surgery. Complications requiring reoperation are usually experienced by all clinicians eventually. Management of the complications by reoperation is usually more difficult than the primary surgery, and is often cumbersome. The best chance of achieving a pleasing surgical result is always by succeeding with the first operation.

The key to obtaining a successful secondary corrective procedure is to understand and appreciate the nature of the complication and the possible reasons for the complication to have occurred. This will enable a comprehensive treatment plan to be developed to manage the problem.

A second surgical procedure or reoperation is required when the surgical treatment goals have not been achieved and the results obtained are not acceptable from a functional and/or esthetic point of view. From an ethical point of view, it is essential to inform the patient once the complication has been identified. It is not a pleasant task for a clinician to inform a patient that a second surgical procedure is required to address an untoward result. The nature of the problem, the possible reasons for it to have occurred, and the proposed method of managing the problem should be explained to the patient in a compassionate way. In confirming the necessity of the second surgical procedure to the patient, it should

be stressed that alternative, conservative means of fixing or attempting to fix the problem by orthodontic means will compromise the result and lead to an unwanted outcome. However, some patients may refuse any further surgery and accept the compromised result. Factors that may motivate patients not to accept the reoperation may include the financial implications, work situation, studies, or loss of confidence in the surgeon. It is imperative that the possible consequences of choosing the nonsurgical option are thoroughly explained.

Operative complications requiring reoperation can be classified as (**Box 1**):

1. Intraoperative complications requiring an intraoperative correction
2. Immediate postoperative complications
3. Complications that develop some time after surgery
4. Surgical technique for the correction of complications.

INTRAOPERATIVE COMPLICATIONS REQUIRING INTRAOPERATIVE CORRECTIVE MEASURES

The best time to identify a surgical problem is at the time of surgery. Critical intraoperative evaluation of each surgical step is mandatory. Orthognathic surgery requires a sophisticated and accurate technique showing utmost respect for the hard and soft tissues involved in the treatment. The surgeon should have a specific routine for each orthognathic surgical procedure, with a clear

---

[a] Department of Maxillofacial and Oral Surgery, University of the Witwatersrand, Johannesburg, South Africa
[b] Department of Oral and Maxillofacial Surgery, University of Oklahoma, Oklahoma City, OK, USA
[c] Department of Oral and Maxillofacial Surgery, University of Florida, Gainesville, FL, USA
[d] Department of Oral and Maxillofacial Surgery, University of Monterrey, Monterrey, Mexico
[e] Private practice, Sunninghill Hospital, Johannesburg, South Africa
* Center for Orthognathic Surgery & Implantology, Sunninghill Hospital, Suite 25 West Wing, Cnr Nanyuki and Witkoppen Roads, Sunninghill Park, 2157, South Africa.
E-mail address: drjprey@global.co.za

Oral Maxillofacial Surg Clin N Am 23 (2011) 73–92
doi:10.1016/j.coms.2010.10.001
1042-3699/11/$ — see front matter © 2011 Elsevier Inc. All rights reserved.

Box 1
Orthognathic surgery complications requiring reoperation

Intraoperative complications requiring corrective measures

1. Incorrect condylar positioning

    Central condylar sag

    Peripheral condylar sag type II

2. Shift of occlusion during placement of rigid fixation

Immediate postoperative complications requiring reoperation

1. Inaccurate surgical splint
2. Incorrect condylar positioning during surgery

    Central condylar sag

    Peripheral condylar sag type II

3. Failure of rigid fixation
4. Neuromuscular relapse

Late postoperative complications requiring reoperation

1. Unexpected posttreatment skeletal growth
2. Postoperative dental relapse
3. Postoperative skeletal relapse

    Condylar resorption

        Idiopathic condylar resorption

        Peripheral condylar sag type I

    Neuromuscular relapse

4. Unsatisfactory esthetic results

    Soft tissue esthetic problems

        Nasal esthetics

        Midface esthetics

        Lip esthetics

    Hard tissue esthetic problems

        Facial asymmetry

        Anteroposterior problems

        Vertical problems

Surgical technique for correction of complications

understanding of the sequence and implication of each step. For each step during the procedure there are certain tips simplifying the surgery, but also certain traps. Being aware of these tips and traps will enable the surgeon to constantly critically evaluate the surgical progress and allow the operation to be performed with confidence to achieve optimal results.

Incorrect Condylar Positioning During Surgery

Correct positioning of the condyles into the articular fossa is probably the single most important maneuver during orthognathic surgery. The advent of rigid fixation for the stabilization of osteotomized segments has placed a greater challenge on the correct positioning of the mandibular condyle in its fossa. However, there is no consensus as to what constitutes an ideal functional and stable relationship between the condyle, the disc, and the glenoid fossa.

Condylar sag produces repeatable patterns of malocclusion after removal of the maxillomandibular fixation (MMF), which can be used to diagnose the specific condition and to identify the offending side.[1] Reyneke and Ferretti[2] described the various types of condylar sag and the typical malocclusions associated with each type to assist in the intraoperative identification of condylar malpositioning. In some cases condylar sag may not be identified during surgery and the problem may only become evident at the first postoperative visit or even later.

Evaluation of the occlusion during surgery is done on release of MMF. The mandible is opened and closed, and the condyles gently translated out of the fossa by pulling the mandible anteriorly and moving it left and right. The procedure is repeated after a minute and then, with light digital pressure on the chin, the mandible is rotated until first occlusal contact occurs. The occlusion is then checked. The temptation to force the teeth into occlusion should be resisted. The occlusion is deemed to be correct when it corresponds with the planned occlusion.

Mandibular surgery

Central condylar sag Central condylar sag occurs when the condyle is positioned inferiorly in the glenoid fossa and makes no contact with any part of the fossa. After removal of the MMF and in the absence of intracapsular edema or hemarthrosis, the condyle will move superiorly, causing a malocclusion (**Fig. 1**). When bilateral condylar sag has occurred, the mandible will rotate clockwise and backward causing a class II occlusion with a slight anterior open bite. However, the dental midlines will be coincidental (**Fig. 2**). When condylar sag has occurred, only on 1 side, the occlusion will be class II, on the effected side and the lower dental midline will be displaced toward the offending side. In the presence of intracapsular edema or hemarthrosis, the condyle may be pushed downwards by hydraulic pressure in the joint capsule, making intraoperative diagnosis of central sag difficult.[2]

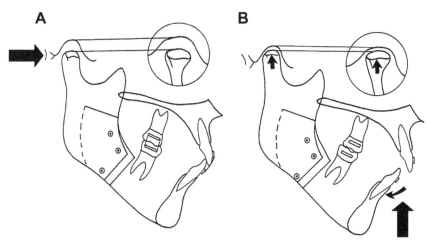

Fig. 1. (*A*) The teeth are held in the planned occlusion by MMF and the mandibular bone segments are held together by rigid fixation. The condyle is displaced inferiorly (*arrow*) in the glenoid fossa with no contact with bone. (*B*) After the removal of the MMF, the condyle(s) moves superiorly (*top arrows*) into the glenoid fossa with immediate dental relapse (*lower arrows*).

Treatment The MMF should first be replaced with the teeth in the planned occlusion and then the rigid fixation removed on the offending side(s). It is less cumbersome and less traumatic on the temporo-mandibular joints and soft tissues to remove the rigid fixation with the jaws stabilized by MMF. The condyles are now gently positioned into the glenoid fossa with a posterior vector of force using a condylar positioner and superior vector of force applied digitally at the mandibular angle.

Peripheral condylar sag type II Peripheral condylar sag type II occurs when the condyle is correctly positioned in the fossa while MMF is in position and the teeth are in occlusion. However, lateral flexural stress is placed on the proximal segment by the application of unfavorable forces on the bone segments during placement of rigid fixation (application of a bone clamp or lag screws) (**Fig. 3**). When peripheral condylar sag type II has occurred bilaterally, the bite will be open on both

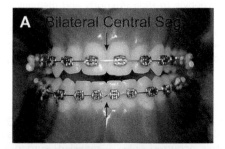

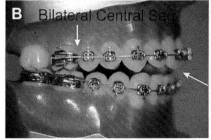
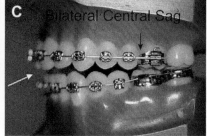

Fig. 2. The occlusion after central condylar sag. (*A*) Frontal view of the occlusion: the dental midlines are correct and the bite open anteriorly (*arrows*). (*B, C*) Lateral views of the occlusion: in a class II molar (*top arrows*) and canine relationship and increased overbite (*bottom arrows*).

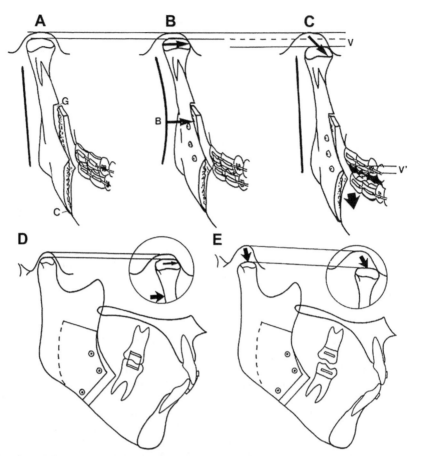

Fig. 3. Peripheral condylar sag type II. A frontolateral view of the glenoid fossa, condyle, the distal and proximal bone segments, and posterior occlusion. (*A*) Note the bone defect G, and the area of bone contact between the segments C. (*B*) Rigid fixation forces the segments together and places a torque force on the proximal segment (*bottom arrow*) and condyle (*top arrow*) causing a bowing effect B. (*C*) Once the MMF is removed, the tension on the ramus is released causing the condyle to slide inferiorly and medially (*top arrow*) on the medial wall of the fossa and a posterior open bite will occur (*bottom arrow*). The change in the condylar position V is equal to the posterior open bite V'. (*D*) A lateral view of the condyle, glenoid fossa, and the distal and proximal segments. The condyle seems to be correctly positioned in the fossa, however is forced medially (*arrows*); once the MMF is released (*E*), the condyle slides downwards (*arrows*) causing a posterior open bite and an edge-to-edge incisor relationship.

sides posteriorly and the incisor teeth will have an edge-to-edge relationship with the dental midlines coincidental. If peripheral sag has occurred only on 1 side, the bite will be open posteriorly on the offending side, the incisors will be edge to edge on the same side, whereas the lower dental midline will be displaced to the side opposite to the offending side (**Fig. 4**).[2]

Treatment The condylar positioning maneuver should now be repeated as described earlier. Special care should be taken during placement of rigid fixation not to force the bone segments together by clamping or lag screws. The occlusion is again checked on release of MMF.

Maxillary surgery
Central condylar sag may also occur after Le Fort I maxillary surgery. After intraoperative removal of MMF, the occlusion is checked in a similar fashion to that described earlier. During the surgical repositioning of the maxilla (with MMF in place), the condyles may be distracted from the glenoid fossa as a result of bony interference at the posterior maxilla. When the teeth are placed in the planned occlusion and MMF applied, the mandible will rotate with the posterior teeth as fulcrum, distracting the condyles inferiorly. Once the MMF is removed, the condyles will return to their normal position, resulting in a class II anterior open bite (**Fig. 5**).[3]

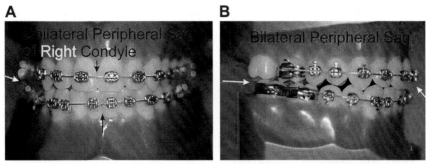

Fig. 4. Unilateral peripheral condylar sag type II of the right condyle. (*A*) Frontal view of occlusion: the mandibular midline is displaced toward the left (*black arrows*). The bite opens on the right (*white arrow*). (*B*) Right side of the occlusion: an edge-to-edge incisor (*right arrow*), tendency to a class III molar and canine dental relationship, and posterior open bite (*left arrow*).

Treatment The rigid fixation should be removed and the MMF left in place to maintain the teeth in the planned occlusion. The maxillomandibular complex should now be rotated closed carefully until first bone contact is observed. The surgeon should be able to detect the area of bony interference at the posterior maxilla. Using a pear-shaped bur, the bone interference can be removed, preferably from the inferior part (tuberosity region) of the maxilla (see **Fig. 5**). The process is continued until no resistance is felt and reference marks coincide with the anterior bone contact. Ensure intraoral reference marks are not lost by removing too much bone or bone in the wrong areas. This would jeopardize the planned vertical position of the maxilla. Once satisfied that all the

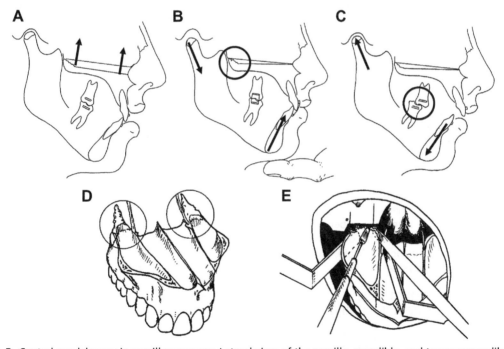

Fig. 5. Central condylar sag in maxillary surgery. Lateral view of the maxilla, mandible, and temporomandibular joint. (*A*) Surgery for superior repositioning of the maxilla is planned (*arrows*). (*B*) Inadequate bone has been removed at the posterior maxilla (*circle*). The bone interference at the posterior maxilla prevents rotation of the maxillomandibular complex around a point at the condyle. To achieve bone contact at the anterior maxilla, the maxillomandibular complex is rotated (*bottom arrow*) around the bone interference (*circle*), whereas the condyle moves inferiorly (*top arrow*) in the fossa. (*C*) Once the MMF is release, the condyles moves superiorly into the glenoid fossa (*top arrow*), the mandible rotates backward (*bottom arrow*) in a clockwise direction, with the posterior molars as fulcrum (*circle*). An anterior open bite and class II dental relationship will result. (*D*) Common areas for bone interference are at the junction between the pterygoid plates and the tuberosities of the maxilla (*circles*). (*E*) The bone interferences should carefully be removed using a large bur.

bony interferences have been removed, the rigid fixation is replaced. Do not use the same screw holes because this would repeat the error. The MMF is removed and the occlusion checked. Do not accept an incorrect occlusion at this point because it will not improve the next day!

Shift of the Occlusion During Placement of Fixation

Mandibular surgery

Inadequate MMF and excessive forces used during the placement of rigid fixation may cause the occlusion to shift. This complication is more likely to occur when a surgical splint is not used. The change from the planned occlusion is observed before MMF removal when the occlusion is checked and should be differentiated from condylar sag.

Treatment Remove the rigid fixation and replace the MMF with the teeth in the planned occlusion. The rigid fixation can now be replaced taking care not to apply any lateral forces on the bone. Avoid using the same screw holes. Keep in mind that self-tapping screws only require a rotational force and no pushing forces.

Maxillary surgery

The maxilla may be displaced, leading to a shift in the occlusion by excessive forces during placement of rigid fixation. Inaccurate bending of bone plates may either displace the maxilla (or segments) or place tension on the bone that will only become evident after removal of MMF or the surgical splint. Differentiate the problem from condylar malpositioning.

Treatment Remove the rigid fixation and MMF. Reposition the teeth into the planned occlusion and reapply MMF. Check the accuracy of the bone plates and, if necessary, rebend the plates to fit snugly on the bone. The bone screws can now be carefully replaced. Avoid the previous holes drilled into the bone.

IMMEDIATE POSTOPERATIVE COMPLICATIONS REQUIRING REOPERATION

Certain complications may occur during the healing phase in the first few weeks after surgery and may require reoperation.

Malocclusion as a Result of an Inaccurate Surgical Splint

At the first postoperative visit, usually 1 week after surgery, the occlusion should be carefully examined to detect any obvious malocclusion or centric relation occlusal discrepancies. It is the author's policy not to use a final surgical splint, because it is not possible to accurately evaluate the occlusion intraoperatively as well as immediately after surgery with a surgical splint in place. Any occlusal or skeletal discrepancy caused by an inaccurate splint will only become evident once the splint has been removed. In a small percentage of patients, small occlusal discrepancies caused by a poorly fabricated and inaccurate surgical splint may be managed orthodontically. However, unplanned additional orthodontic treatment will add to the treatment time. Once the surgical splint has been removed, the occlusion should be carefully evaluated and, if any discrepancy is identified, the clinician should differentiate between a small dental discrepancy and skeletal discrepancies. If small dental discrepancies are detected, the orthodontist should see the patient as soon as possible. The orthodontist should then establish whether the discrepancy can be managed by orthodontic means alone. The implications should be discussed with the patient. An inaccurate surgical splint may lead to inaccurate surgical repositioning of the jaw(s) or dentoalveolar segments. In these cases, the malalignment should be corrected surgically.

Incorrect Condylar Positioning During Surgery

An incorrect position of the condyle may only become apparent after surgery.

Central condylar sag

Indiscriminate and rough surgical technique may cause intraoperative intracapsular edema or hemarthrosis in the temporomandibular joint.[2–4] With time, the condyle(s) seat into the glenoid fossa(e) a few days after surgery, leading to postoperative malocclusion. Strong interdental elastics placed at the time of surgery may also disguise central condylar sag. The problem is then only identified once the elastics are removed at the first postoperative visit. The author is not in favor of the placement of strong interdental elastics after surgery, and recommends light 100-g (3.5 oz), 6-mm (0.25-inch) elastics bilaterally in the canine area. If a malocclusion that indicates central condylar sag is noticed at this stage, the patient should be informed about the surgeon's concerns and the best mode of correction explained. The diagnosis can be confirmed by a lateral cephalometric radiograph (**Fig. 6**). Elastic therapy at this stage will be futile. Strong class II elastics to advance the mandible, and vertical elastics to close the open bite, will again distract the condyles out of the fossae and extrude the incisor teeth.

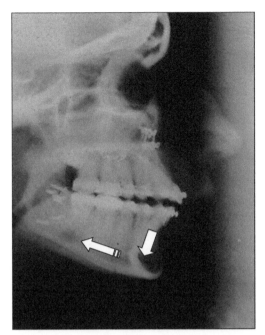

Fig. 6. A class II and anterior open bite as a result of central condylar sag is shown on the postoperative lateral cephalometric radiograph. The lower incisors moves downward (*right arrow*) and the mandible backward (*left arrow*) as a result of the condyles settling superiorly into the glenoid fossa.

Treatment It is ideal for both patient and surgeon to have the problem corrected as soon as possible after it is identified. Orthognathic records, photographs of the occlusion, and radiographs should again be obtained. It is impractical and unnecessary to have dental models redone. It is hoped that the original dental casts will still be available as a reference. Under general anesthesia, the teeth are positioned into the planned occlusion and secured by MMF. The osteotomy site(s) are exposed and a mental note is made of the initial amount of mandibular movement by comparing the vertical osteotomy lines between the segments. The rigid fixation is removed and the bone segments gently separated using a periosteal elevator. If the correction is performed within the first 2 to 4 weeks after the primary surgery, the segments will separate easily. However, separation after a longer period of time may require an osteotome. Ensure that the proximal segment can be moved posteriorly without interference, and carefully position the condyle into the glenoid fossa as discussed earlier. Note the amount of mandibular movement again at the vertical osteotomy lines. It should be different to before separation. No difference will indicate that the condylar repositioning was not successful. The MMF is now removed and the occlusion carefully checked.

Peripheral condylar sag type II

The mechanism of the development of condylar sag type II has been discussed earlier, but the problem might not be diagnosed intraoperatively. The malocclusion may only become apparent a few days or even weeks after surgery.

Treatment Small discrepancies can be corrected by orthodontic means alone; however, attempts to correct larger occlusal discrepancies with interocclusal elastics will increase the load on the condyle(s), which may result in condylar resorption. Large discrepancies should be corrected by reoperation.

Failure of Rigid Fixation

Mandibular surgery

The advent of rigid fixation has had a major influence on not only patients undergoing orthognathic surgery but also the surgeons performing the surgery. With the use of rigid fixation, patients recover more safely and more comfortably, and the treatment results are more stable.[5] It is also less cumbersome for the surgeon who previously had to rely on suspension wires and MMF. However, rigid fixation may fail. Failure of fixation usually becomes evident within the first week after surgery when a change in the occlusion is noticed. The typical occlusal changes associated with bilateral failure of fixation are: (1) development of an anterior open bite, (2) the mandible moves forward with the molars into a class III relation, (3) the incisors develop an anterior cross bite, and (4) when the patient occludes, an early posterior dental contact followed by movement of the anterior mandible is usually noticed. By placing an index finger intraorally (offending side) on the external oblique ridge and a thumb on the lower tooth surfaces, mobility between the segments will be evident. In cases in which the fixation failed on 1 side only the signs listed earlier will occur on the offending side. Extraorally, the antegonial notch will be accentuated because of counterclockwise rotation of the proximal segment. The rotation of the proximal segment can also be identified on a panoramic radiograph (**Fig. 7**).

Treatment In cases in which the intersegmental mobility is slight and the occlusal discrepancy small, the segments can by immobilized by means of MMF or tight interarch elastics for 2 to 4 weeks.

If intersegmental mobility and occlusal discrepancy are severe, the only method of correction is to replace the fixation surgically. For these cases, correction should take place as soon as possible. The sagittal split is repeated after removal of fixation, as previously described. Identify the reason

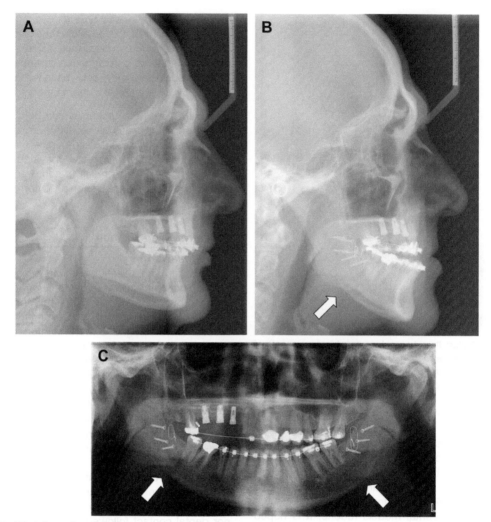

Fig. 7. (*A*) A lateral cephalometric radiograph of a patient with a class II malocclusion requiring mandibular advancement. (*B*) A postoperative radiograph of the patient in (*A*). A class III anterior open bite has developed as a result of failure of the rigid fixation (*arrow*). (*C*) A postoperative panoramic radiograph of the patient in (*A*) showing the rotation of the proximal segments (*arrows*).

for failure to prevent a repetition of the problem. Failure of bicortical fixation may be caused by: (1) inadequate length of the screws, (2) inadequate number of screws, (3) poor configuration of the screws (if a bone plate is used the plate may be too short with inadequate screws), and (4) following an unfavorable split, the bone contact may be inadequate. Ensure correct replacement of the fixation and check the occlusion.

Maxillary surgery
Mobility of the maxilla is usually evident at the first postoperative evaluation. A change from the planned occlusion is seen and, when the patient occludes, mobility of the maxilla or maxillary segment will be observed.

Treatment Unilateral segmental or slight maxillary mobility can be treated by the placement of MMF or tight interarch elastics for 2 to 4 weeks and ensuring that the patient remains on a soft diet. Severe bilateral mobility should be corrected by reoperation and repeat of rigid fixation.

Chin surgery
The chin segment is usually fixated by means of tricortical screws or bone plates after repositioning. Inadequate fixation will lead to mobility of the segment as a result of forces from the suprahyoid muscles. A sudden postoperative change in chin esthetics, loss of labiomental fold, shortening of the chin-throat length, and pain are typical signs of failure of internal fixation. This

complication can be diagnosed on a lateral cephalometric radiograph.

Treatment Expose the mental area through the intraoral incision. Remove the fixation (screws or bone plates) and identify the reason for failure. Place the chin segment in the planned position and replace adequate rigid fixation.

Neuromuscular Relapse

Mandibular surgery

Mandibular relapse after bilateral sagittal split osteotomy has been the topic of study for many years and was until recently considered one of the common complications associated with this procedure.[6–8] However, with the introduction of internal rigid fixation, more predictable results have been achieved.[5] Various treatment methods have been implemented to prevent skeletal relapse, such as overcorrection, suprahyoid muscle detachment, medial pterygoid and stylomandibular ligament detachment, prolonged MMF, and a variety of methods of fixation.[9] Reports in the literature identify 3 main soft tissue factors that may influence the skeletal stability after surgery: (1) neuromuscular adaptation, (2) stretching of soft tissue, and (3) alteration of the muscle orientation.[8] These factors are important when large skeletal movements are performed, inadequate muscle stripping has been done, or as a result of poor proximal segment control.

Treatment Any attempt to control the potential relapse with tight elastics or MMF carries a poor prognosis. The skeletal changes should not be followed by orthodontic compromise. Although a short-term improvement may be achieved by orthodontic tooth movement, the result is seldom stable in the long-term. In most cases, reoperation is required after careful assessment of the cause of relapse. Surgical correction should address the problem areas. First establish possible reasons for poor neuromuscular adaptation, for example: (1) failure to strip muscles from repositioned bone causing muscle interference at the time of first surgery. During reoperation, special care should be given to adequate stripping of muscles to ensure free repositioning of the jaws. (2) Large skeletal movements leading to stretching of the musculature. The surgical design may have to be altered to prevent large repositioning of the jaws (ie, bimaxillary surgery instead of single-jaw surgery).

Maxillary surgery

The 2 most unstable orthognathic surgical procedures are:

1. Maxillary expansion.[8,10] Stretching of the soft tissue of the hard palate plays a major role in stability after segmental expansion of the maxilla. The firm palatal soft tissue tends to resist expansional forces during surgery. In addition, postoperative scarring of the palatal soft tissue may be an important factor causing transverse relapse in the long-term.

2. Surgical advancement of the maxilla and/or expansion in patients with cleft lip and palate. Patients with cleft lip and palate have often had several surgical procedures for the correction of the lip and hard and soft tissue defects at a younger age. Each procedure will have caused scaring of the soft tissues. Correction of the occlusion by means of a Le Fort I maxillary osteotomy is usually one of the last corrective procedures to be performed. The fibrous tissue will not only resist maxillary advancement and/or expansion during surgery but will significantly reduce postoperative stability.

Treatment Adequate subperiosteal dissection or even incision of the palatal soft tissue is recommended to release the tension for cases requiring large expansion. However, maintaining adequate blood supply to the segments is mandatory, especially in patients with cleft palate. Ensure that the nasal mucosa is intact when incising the palatal mucosa. Postoperative control by means of a surgical splint followed by orthodontic control of the transverse dimension is mandatory for stability. These principles should be adhered to when a second procedure is performed. Transverse palatal distraction (surgically assisted expansion) may also be considered when a second procedure is indicated.[11,12]

LATE POSTOPERATIVE COMPLICATIONS REQUIRING REOPERATION
Unexpected Postoperative Growth

Late relapse after healing can be the result of several factors, including postoperative growth, orthodontic relapse, or condylar remodeling or relapse. Late postoperative growth is a risk often associated with mandibular setback procedures, especially in male patients, who may show continued facial growth well into their 20s.[13]

An intimate knowledge of the embryophysiology and growth of the cranium and maxillofacial skeleton will greatly assist both the orthodontist and the surgeon in harnessing the growth spurts in an attempt to simplify treatments.[14] The orthodontist can apply orthopedic and orthodontic forces during these active growth phases. However, once growth is deemed to be complete, correction

82 Reyneke

of dentofacial anomalies will be largely surgical in nature. There is a danger that, if surgery is performed before skeletal maturity has been obtained, continued facial growth will necessitate reoperation. It is mandatory that the family of the patient and other attending physicians be made aware of the possibility of a second corrective procedure once skeletal maturity has been obtained.

There are circumstances when surgery is recommended for patients with an immature skeleton.[15] For patients with poor self-image, especially in young developing girls, or patients with severe functional problems, the advantages of early surgical intervention may outweigh the risks of waiting. Growing patients undergoing surgery should be aware of the possibility that a second corrective procedure may be required at a later stage (**Fig. 8**).

The exact point at which facial growth is complete is impossible to determine. A combination of indicators, such as the hand/wrist radiograph (to determine the epiphyseal closure), serial cephalometric radiographs (6 months apart), or skeletal scintigraphy (technetium 99m), are useful tools, but are not a guarantee that no further growth can occur.

There is a distinction between prolonged excessive mandibular growth and early cessation of maxillary growth. The clinician should be aware that, if the problem is in the maxilla, surgery for the correction of maxillary anteroposterior deficiency can be performed earlier. A class III malocclusion will be the result of one of the following skeletal malrelationships: (1) anteroposterior mandibular excess (mandibular prognathism), (2) anteroposterior maxillary deficiency, (3) vertical maxillary deficiency, and (4) a combination of

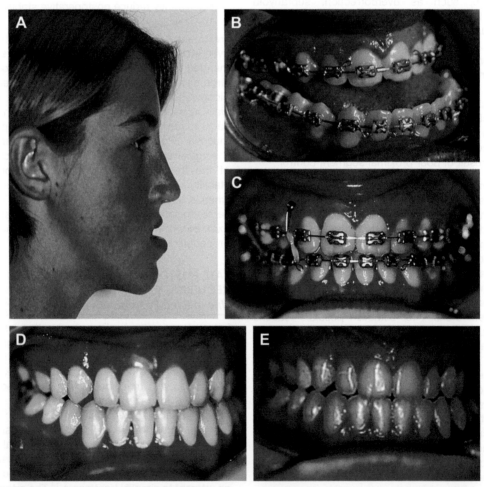

Fig. 8. (*A*) A lateral view of a 13-year-old patient with a severe class III occlusion as a result of maxillary anteroposterior deficiency and mandibular anteroposterior excess. (*B*) The presurgical class III occlusion, (*C*) the immediate postoperative occlusion, (*D*) the slight occlusal relapse as result of postoperative mandibular growth 18 months after surgery, and (*E*) the occlusion 3 years after surgery.

these. Orthognathic surgical correction of class III malocclusion is dependant on the cessation of mandibular growth. Mandibular growth in adolescent patients requiring orthognathic surgery should be monitored because experience has shown that prognathic mandibles tend to continue growth longer than normal mandibles, especially in men. Surgical correction of cases in which an apparently normal mandible is present and the problem has been diagnosed as being primarily in the maxilla can be performed earlier than in their mandibular counterparts once the mandible has ceased growing.

Unexpected late facial growth may take place several months or even years after treatment. This may pose a dilemma to the orthodontist as to whether relapse should be treated orthodontically or surgically, and whether mandibular growth has ceased.

A change in occlusion some time after completion of orthognathic surgical treatment may be caused by dental relapse, skeletal relapse, and late skeletal growth. The diagnosis should be based on clinical and radiographic findings.

Treatment

Patients should be debanded and placed in retention. Serial cephalometric radiographs should be used to monitor and confirm cessation of growth before any corrective procedure is contemplated.

Once the surgeon is comfortable that facial growth has stabilized, the patient should be rebanded and any minor orthodontic preparation in terms of arch alignment and compatibility should be addressed.

At surgery, the rigid fixation is removed and the sagittal split osteotomy repeated. The bicortical screws are often well integrated into the bone and may be difficult to remove. It is common for the screw heads to be damaged or broken, and it is recommended that no further attempts to remove the screws are made and that the screws are cut using a diamond fissure bur.

Postoperative Dental Relapse

A change in postoperative occlusion may be the result of dental relapse. Clinicians should carefully differentiate between dental and skeletal relapse. Dental relapse should be corrected orthodontically.

Postoperative Skeletal Relapse

Condylar resorption

The first sign of relapse is usually a change in the occlusion. This can occur as result of skeletal changes from the planned results after initial treatment.[16]

Remodeling of the mandibular condyles has been noted after both orthodontic treatment alone or in combination with orthognathic surgery. This remodeling is in response to altered muscle dynamics of masticatory forces on the condylar head or alternatively as a result of forceful seating of the condyle in the glenoid fossa during the placement of rigid fixation in mandibular surgical procedures. The remodeling may continue for several years after treatment. In extreme cases, it may lead to resorption of the condyle causing a shortening of the mandibular ramus, and may lead to a class II anterior open bite malocclusion (**Fig. 9**). When considering the correction of an anterior open bite caused by bilateral condylar resorption, the clinician should differentiate between myogenic condylar resorption, idiopathic condylar resorption, degenerative joint disease, and destructive rheumatic joint diseases such a rheumatoid or psoriatic joint disease.

Idiopathic condylar resorption Idiopathic condylar resorption is believed to be related to chronic excessive loading of the mandibular condyle. It may occur in isolation or after mandibular surgery.[17] This condition requires reoperation.

The features of condylar resorption are as follows: (1) it usually occurs in women between the ages of 15 and 30 years (predominantly in their teens), (2) it affects both condyles and the pattern is usually symmetric, (3) it is self-limiting, (4) resorption is progressive and leads to a gradual loss of the ramus height, (5) patients develop a class II anterior open bite, (6) it is usually painless, (7) joint noise may be present, and (8) resorption may progress to the level of the sigmoid notch.

Treatment There are 2 important principles in the correction of this deformity:

1. Ensure that the resorption process is inactive. A technetium 99m bone scan will assist in establishing the bone activity in the condyle. The occlusion should be stable for a minimum of 1 year.
2. Treat the deformity in such a way that the condyles are not loaded, for example by avoiding lengthening the posterior height of the mandible, large mandibular advancements, and being gentle during condylar positioning.

Posttreatment stability of the occlusion in these patients treated by means of orthognathic surgery may be unpredictable. Further consideration may be given to superior distraction osteogenesis of the condylar stump or replacement of the mandibular condyle by a total-joint temporomandibular

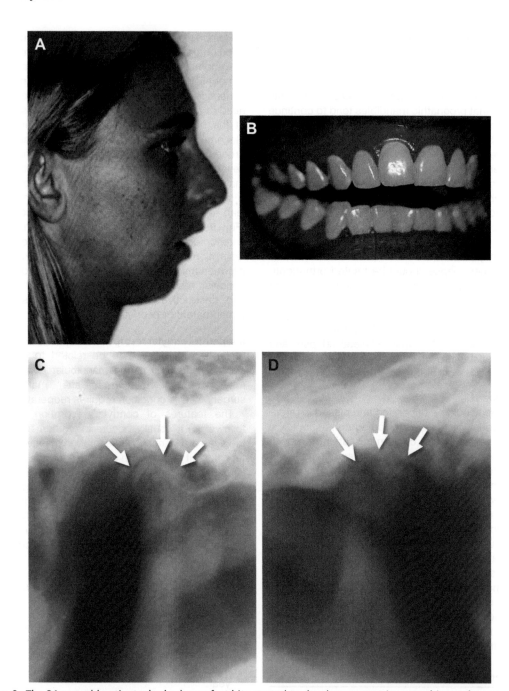

Fig. 9. The 24-year-old patient who had a perfect bite started to develop an anterior open bite at the age of 18 years, 3 years after orthodontic treatment. (*A*) Profile view showing the increased lower facial height as a result of clockwise rotation of the mandible. (*B*) The severe class II anterior open bite as result of bilateral shortening of the condyles. (*C*, *D*) Tomograms of the right and left condyles showing the severe shortening of the condyles as a result of resorbtion (*arrows*).

joint prosthesis in patients with severe functional and esthetic deformities.[18,19]

Peripheral condylar sag type I Peripheral condylar sag type I occurs when lateral forces are applied to the mandibular condyle during placement of rigid

fixation, causing the condyles to slide inferiorly but to maintain contact with the glenoid fossa laterally (**Fig. 10**).[1] The bone contact between the condyle and the fossa provides stability to the occlusion, and the problem can therefore not be identified at the time of surgery. It is more likely

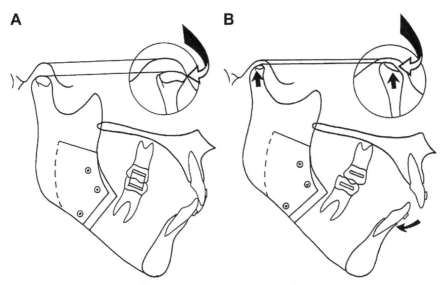

Fig. 10. Peripheral condylar sag type I. (*A*) The condyle is forced medially and slides inferiorly on the medial wall of the fossa during placement of rigid fixation. The problem cannot be identified because the condyle-fossa contact provides physical support to the occlusion after removal of MMF. (*B*) Condylar resorption in the contact area will lead to superior movement of the condyle, which will later cause posterior relapse of the mandible.

to occur in cases in which bicortical screw fixation is used, because there is often a tendency for the surgeon to attempt better bone contact between the proximal and distal segments by forcing them closer together. These patients often experience immediate postoperative pain over the temporomandibular joint area on the offending side(s).

This problem only becomes apparent several weeks or months after surgery when resorption of the lateral poles (the contact areas) of the condyle occurs (see **Fig. 10**). This resorption will cause the condyle to slide superiorly into the fossa, causing the mandible to relapse posteriorly (on the offending side). Modern imaging techniques, such as cone beam scanning, may allow the identification of the condylar resorption, especially on the anteroposterior views in which lateral resorption will be evident. The resorption occurs more on the lateral pole and less on the superior aspect of the condylar surface. Presumably, once the load on the condyle is removed, the resorption process should cease. It is therefore recommended that the problem be corrected as soon as a diagnosis is made.

Treatment The complication should not be corrected by orthodontic treatment. The sagittal split osteotomy is repeated on the offending side after removal of the rigid fixation. Special care is taken not to apply any lateral force to the proximal segment either with a bone clamp or lag screws that may force the segments together. Any gap

between the bony segments should be maintained during placement of the rigid fixation and, where required, the defect should be grafted. Remove the MMF and check the occlusion.

Neuromuscular relapse

Mandibular surgery Relapse as a result of neuromuscular influences in response to the repositioning of the jaws may only become apparent weeks, or even months, after surgery. Inadequate stripping of muscle attachments to the mandible may cause stretching of the muscles or the muscles themselves may interfere with surgical repositioning (medial pterygoid and stylomandibular ligament attachments on the medial aspect of the mandibular angle).[20] Incorrect positioning of the proximal mandibular segment (clockwise or counterclockwise rotation) will change the orientation of the masseter muscle fibers, which may lead to skeletal relapse and malocclusion. A clockwise rotation of the proximal segment usually occurs with mandibular setback procedures, whereas counterclockwise rotations will occur more often with mandibular advancement procedures.

Treatment Inadequate stripping of muscles and ligamentous attachments may stretch the muscles and ligamentous attachment to the mandible. These patients may need reoperation to correct the occlusion through correct positioning of the proximal segment and adequate stripping of muscular and ligamentous attachments.

Maxillary surgery

Transverse relapse The surgeon should ensure that the posterior teeth have not been orthodontically expanded beyond the bony base before surgery in an attempt to close an anterior open bite by means of orthodontics. Transverse relapse requiring reoperation often only becomes apparent several weeks or months after surgery. Transverse relapse may present with lateral crossbites, an edge-to-edge incisor relationship that may further deteriorate to an anterior open bite (**Fig. 11**). Postoperative orthodontic control is mandatory after surgical expansion of the maxilla by means of a continuous arch wire, through the bite elastics or a palatal bar.

Anteroposterior relapse When maxillary anteroposterior relapse occur an edge-to-edge or class III dental relationship with anterior and/or lateral cross bites will develop.[21] Nonunion of the maxilla may occur after large maxillary advancement procedures and will have a strong tendency to relapse. It is advisable to ensure adequate bone

contact and improved stability by the placement of bone grafts into bone defects and by using adequate rigid fixation. Patients not adhering to the prescribed soft diet after surgery may also be at risk to develop nonunion of the maxilla after surgery.

Vertical relapse Maxillary downgraft procedures are considered to be among the most unstable of all orthognathic procedures.[8] The loss of surgically created maxillary height after maxillary downgrafting procedures is believed to occur as a result of the action of the muscles of mastication (especially temporalis and masseter) and encroachment of the freeway space. The amount of vertical increase of the maxilla, and also the type of interpositional bone grafting material, may influence the postoperative stability; however, the use of rigid fixation has improved long-term stability.[22]

Treatment

Transverse relapse Establish whether relapse is caused by skeletal or dental change. Postoperative

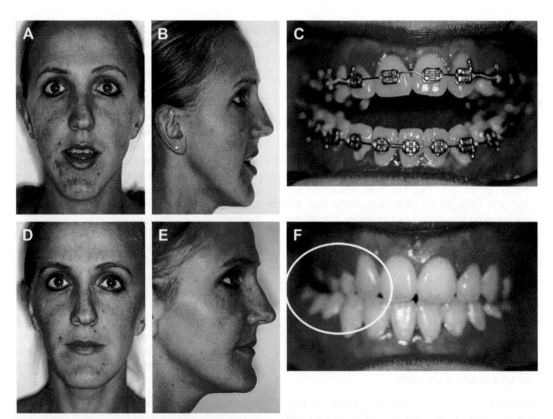

Fig. 11. The treatment of the patient with a severe class III anterior open bite malocclusion consisted of superior repositioning and expansion of the maxilla by means of a 3-piece Le Fort I maxillary osteotomy and setback of the mandible by means of a bilateral sagittal split mandibular ramus osteotomy. (*A*) Frontal view, (*B*) profile view, and (*C*) preoperative occlusion. Posttreatment: (*D*) frontal view, (*E*) profile view, and (*F*) occlusion. The postoperative transverse relapse and development of an edge-to-edge incisor relationship, especially on the right (*circle*) are evident.

transverse dental relapse may often occur after excessive presurgical orthodontic expansion. The posterior teeth should be orthodontically uprighted and placed in the middle trough of bone before corrective surgery. It is also recommended that a surgical splint be worn for at least 6 weeks after surgery, and orthodontic control of the transverse expansion should start immediately after splint removal.

Anteroposterior relapse Large maxillary surgical advancement will often have a tendency to relapse because of muscular stretching. In patients with cleft lip and palate, fibrous tissues after primary cleft repair will resist jaw repositioning and will be a factor causing relapse. During reoperation the surgeon should ensure adequate mobilization of the maxilla, and adequate internal rigid fixation and bone grafting should further enhance stability.

Vertical relapse Severe vertical relapse of the maxilla will also have anteroposterior implications. Loss of maxillary height will allow the mandible to autorotate into a class III occlusion.

Reoperation should be approached with caution, paying careful attention to the possible causes of the initial relapse and their future prevention. These causes can be addressed through the use of additional and more rigid internal fixation, the use of a different interpositional grafting material, and possibly considering a decrease in the amount of vertical downgrafting planned. Limiting the vertical increase of the maxilla will reduce the autorotation of the mandible, which in turn may necessitate an additional anteroposterior occlusal correction by maxillary advancement or mandibular setback. To allow consolidation of the maxilla in its new position, a prolonged period of soft diet may also be beneficial.

Unsatisfactory Esthetic Results

Patients having orthognathic surgery should be warned that initial esthetic results should not be evaluated within the first 4 to 6 weeks after their operation. Although most of the postoperative swelling subsides within the first 2 weeks, soft tissue settling, function, and animation of the mimic muscles will usually take substantially longer. Final evaluation of the esthetic result should therefore only be made 6 to 8 months after surgery, after removal of the orthodontic bands. However, certain esthetic problems do become apparent soon after surgery. As with most other complications requiring reoperation, esthetic problems should ideally be avoided. However, despite accurate planning and meticulous surgery

with the best intentions, they sometimes do occur. Although some of these problems may be diagnosed early in the healing phase, they can only be critically evaluated and should be corrected only when all the swelling has disappeared.

Soft tissue esthetics

Nasal esthetics During maxillary superior repositioning or advancement procedures, inadequate control of the nasal septum during a Le Fort I maxillary osteotomy will result in buckling of the nasal septum and asymmetry of the columella (**Fig. 12**).[23]

Widening of the alar bases and tipping up of the nasal tip may occur because of inadequate contouring of the piriform rims and anterior nasal floor during maxillary superior repositioning and/or advancement. Creation of adequate nasal volume through contouring of the bone is critical to avoid this complication (**Fig. 13**).[23,24]

An excessively prominent anterior nasal spine (anterior and/or superior) will tend to tip the nasal tip upwards, cause asymmetry of the columella, and increase the nasolabial angle. Potential esthetic problems can be avoided by shortening the anterior nasal spine when indicated.

Treatment Unacceptable nasal esthetics should be corrected once the clinician is convinced that postoperative swelling has subsided. Corrections of the problems are as follows:

Trimming of the nasal septum and control of the septum by means of a suture placed through the septum and a hole made through the anterior nasal spine

Contouring of the piriform rim and use of a cinch suture to narrow the alar base

Trimming of the anterior nasal spine.

These procedures are usually performed through the Le Fort I incision, but can also be performed through a closed rhinoplasty incision.

Midface esthetics The accurate and careful reapproximation of the submucosal soft tissue including the mimic muscles after the Le Fort I maxillary osteotomy will avoid the development of chubby cherub cheeks and/or asymmetry between the left and right sides of the midface.

Treatment Once the soft tissues have healed and scar tissues have matured, correction through reoperation is not successful.

Lip esthetics Suturing of the soft tissues after completion of the osteotomies can be seen as

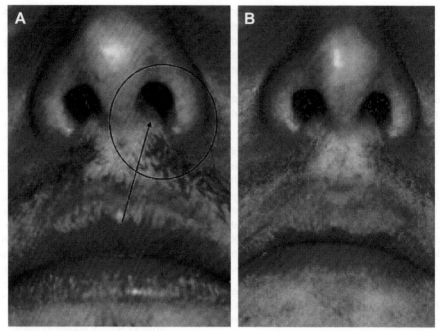

Fig. 12. (A) The nasal septum has buckled (*circle and arrow*) as a result of poor nasal septum control during superior repositioning of the maxilla. (B) The symmetry of the nasal columella is restored through a closed rhinoplasty approach.

the signature of the surgeon on his work and is equally as important and demanding as repositioning of the jaws. Varying degrees of esthetic changes may occur after maxillary surgery and inadequate soft tissue management. Lip thinning and/or shortening with reduced lip pout may be

prevented by V-Y mucosal suturing and accurate nasolabial reapproximation.[25–27]

Lip asymmetry Once the soft tissue swelling has subsided, asymmetry of the lip may become apparent. One side of the lip may appear thinner

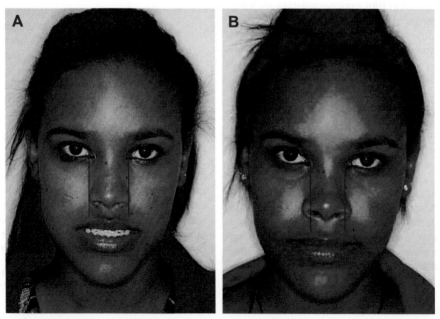

Fig. 13. (A) The alar width of the patient is normal before surgery. (B) A large maxillary advancement and inadequate control of the alar width of the nose lead to an unesthetic widening of the alar base after surgery.

and/or shorter than the opposite side as a result of unequal soft tissue suturing of the left and right sides of the upper lip. The philtrum of the upper lip may be asymmetric to the columella of the nose or dental midline as a result of asymmetric suturing of the submucosal soft tissues or malalignment of the mucosa of the lip. Always place the midline suture in line with the facial midline first and then suture the incision by starting laterally and working toward the midline. It is important to decide on the cause of the soft tissue asymmetry before resuturing.

Treatment

Upper lip A mucosal incision is performed as for a Le Fort I osteotomy, but only extended to the first bicuspid. Should the submucosal tissue require realignment, an incision is made down to the periosteum and the submucosal tissues elevated from the bone. The perioral muscles should be dissected from the mucosal layer and then resutured symmetrically. If a V-Y suture is required, it is placed first in the center of the lip and then aligned with the dental and facial midlines. The upper lip closure is then completed by suturing from lateral to medial.

Lower lip Excessive muscle stripping during subperiosteal dissection, failure to accurately reapproximate the mentalis muscles, and/or inaccurate mucosal suturing after genioplasty will result in poor lower lip and chin esthetics (**Fig. 14**). A mucosal incision is made followed by a subperiosteal dissection. The mentalis muscles are then carefully dissected from the mucosal layer and reapproximated followed by symmetric suturing of the mucosa. Place the midline suture first and carefully align it with the dental and facial midline.

Hard tissue esthetics

Facial asymmetry The accurate correction of a facial asymmetry is extremely challenging, and all patients undergoing such attempts at correction should be warned that no facial features are truly symmetric. Therefore, correction of an asymmetric face can never achieve symmetry.

Dental midlines Malalignment of the dental midlines with the opposite jaw or facial midline is of one of the most common surgical errors. When single jaw surgery is performed, the responsibility of ensuring that the midline of the unoperated jaw corresponds with the facial midline rests with the orthodontist because the operated jaw will be aligned with the prepared unoperated jaw at surgery. If the midline is then not coincidental, the postoperative orthodontic correction may be complicated or, often, not possible. This discrepancy may then require correction by reoperation. When double-jaw surgery is performed, dental midline alignment to the midline of the face is the responsibility of the surgeon. It is

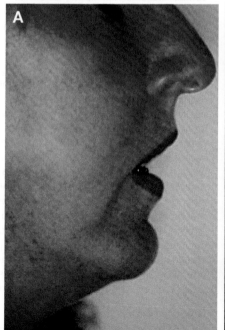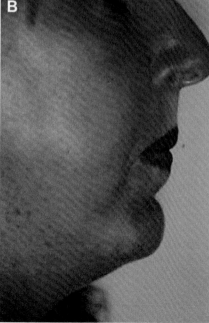

Fig. 14. (*A*) The postoperative result after genioplasty. Inadequate suturing of the mentalis muscles has resulted in shortening of the lower lip, exposure of the lower incisor teeth, poor chin shape, and unesthetic chin contour. (*B*) The severe lower lip strain in an attempt to create lip seal is evident.

particularly disappointing to realize on the day after surgery that the dental midline and facial midline do not coincide.

Correction of an occlusal plane cant Correction of a transverse occlusal plane cant is often an integral part of the overall correction of facial asymmetry. However, there is often a tendency to undercorrect this problem, limiting the surgical outcome. Reoperation is indicated when the transverse occlusal plane cant is significant after surgery.

Posterior facial asymmetry Posterior facial asymmetry may occur after surgical correction of mandibular asymmetry. Inadequate transverse control of the proximal mandibular segments after rotation of the distal segment may result in a unilateral prominence at the mandibular angle: the so-called swelling that never goes away. Once the swelling has subsided and the asymmetry is evident at the mandibular angle areas, the skeletal prominence should be evaluated by means of a *posteroanterior* cephalometric radiograph or computed tomography scan. Small skeletal discrepancies can be corrected by intraoral contouring of the bone, whereas larger asymmetric discrepancies require a repeat of the bilateral sagittal split osteotomies, taking special care to control the transverse positioning of the proximal segments.

Chin asymmetry The chin forms an important and conspicuous part of facial esthetics, and postoperative chin asymmetry will certainly be noticeable and a possible source of patient dissatisfaction. Correction of chin asymmetry is usually performed last during the surgical procedure and requires accurate presurgical assessment, planning, and surgical technique. Poor chin symmetry often stems from failure to address a cant at the lower border of the mandible in the mental area. Postoperative chin asymmetry should be corrected surgically.

Anteroposterior problems Unsatisfactory facial profile esthetics may result from incorrect orthodontic and/or surgical treatment planning, but may also result from inaccurate execution of the treatment plan. Critical evaluation of the postoperative facial esthetics should only take place once all the swelling has subsided. Patients with unrealistic expectations may voice their dissatisfaction with the surgical outcome (often immediately after surgery) and will need consultation and explanation. Reoperation in these instances will often be counterproductive. In some cases, the patient will have legitimate concerns regarding the esthetic outcome. At this stage, the surgeon would

also have noticed that the esthetic treatment objectives have not been achieved. The exact nature of the patients dissatisfaction should be established and the postoperative result carefully scrutinized. It is recommended that new orthognathic records be obtained, and the postoperative result evaluated and compared with the preoperative esthetic treatment objectives. Possible reasons for this complication should be identified and corrective measures instigated with the consent of the patient.

Vertical problems Overcorrection of vertical maxillary excess is possibly the most common postoperative esthetic complication when a Le Fort I maxillary osteotomy is performed. Excessive superior repositioning of the maxilla will leave the patient with an edentulous appearance and poor lip support that will worsen in time.

Treatment The corrective surgical measure will require a maxillary downgraft procedure.

SURGICAL TECHNIQUE

Before reoperating, the surgeon should have a clear idea of the reason(s) for the failure of the initial procedure, and the surgical treatment plan should focus on the specific correction of the problem.

Sagittal Split Ramus Osteotomy

Early correction
Reoperation of the mandible within the first 6 weeks after the primary surgery should not require cutting of the bony cortex by means of a bur or saw. After the removal of the internal rigid fixation through an extraoral or intraoral approach, as required, the proximal and distal segments should easily separate with an osteotome. Take care to identify and protect the inferior alveolar neurovascular bundle and ensure adequate mobility of the segments by restripping the pterygomasseteric sling, the medial pterygoid muscle, and the stylomandibular ligament. The teeth are then placed into the planned occlusion and immobilized by means of MMF. After the placement of the rigid internal fixation, the MMF is removed and the occlusion carefully tested. The second procedure should be performed with the primary cause for reoperation in mind, and special care should be taken to prevent a repeat of the problem.

Late correction
Reoperation several months after the primary surgery is more challenging. At this stage, bone healing has taken place and often osseointegration of the titanium fixation screws (and plates)

has occurred. It may not be possible to remove the screws, and the surgeon may be forced to cut through the screw using a diamond bur. Splitting the mandibular ramus will now require conventional surgical technique using a bur or saw to initiate the split, followed by separation of the bone segments using osteotomes. The procedure can now be completed as described earlier.

Le Fort I Maxillary Osteotomy

Early correction
Reoperation within the first 6 weeks after the initial surgery allows remobilization of the maxilla without much intervention. The internal rigid fixation plates and screws are identified and moved and the maxilla downfractured. The problem areas identified as the cause of the complication are addressed and the maxilla fixated in the adjusted position. Ensure that the original screw holes are avoided when replacing the fixation.

Late correction
Removal of rigid fixation from the maxilla several months after the initial orthognathic surgery is more difficult and cumbersome. At this stage, the plates and screws are often partially covered by bone and care should be taken not to fracture the thin maxillary bone during removal. Damage to the bone at the previous fixation sites may compromise the positioning and/or stability of the refixation hardware, which may adversely affect the final outcome.

Genioplasty

Early correction
Once the bone and internal rigid fixation are exposed, the cause for reoperation is identified and corrected. Replace the fixation avoiding the screw holes of the previous fixation.

Late correction
Removal of the rigid fixation is often not possible if the genioplasty procedure was performed a long time previously. Bone integration with titanium fixation or bone covering the screws and/or plates will force the surgeon to cut through the plates or screws using a diamond bur.

SUMMARY

Orthognathic surgery provides the orthodontist and surgeon with an effective and dynamic means to correct dentofacial deformities whether they are developmental, posttraumatic, or congenital in nature. Complications may occur at any stage, or multiple stages, of care, from the initial diagnosis to the treatment planning, orthodontic treatment,

surgery, and postoperative orthodontic care. The treatment team should continually strive for greater acuity with every step of the treatment to provide safer and more effective care to patients. Seemingly small technical issues in the operating room can significantly affect the outcome and may result in reoperation.

REFERENCES

1. Arnett GW, Tamborello JA, Rathbone JA. Temporomandibular joint ramifications of orthognathic surgery. In: Bell WH, editor. Modern practice in orthognathic and reconstructive surgery. 1st edition. Philadelphia: WB Saunders; 1992. p. 523–33.
2. Reyneke JP, Ferretti C. Intraoperative diagnosis of condylar sag after bilateral sagittal ramus split osteotomy. Br J Oral Maxillofac Surg 2002;40(4): 285–92.
3. Reyneke JP. Intraoperative diagnosis of condylar sag after Le Fort I osteotomy (chapter 5). In: Reyneke JP, editor. Essentials of orthognathic surgery. 1st edition. Chicago: Quintessence; 2003. p. 304–7.
4. Stroster TG, Pangrazio-Kulberch V. Assessment of condylar position following bilateral sagittal split ramus osteotomy with wire fixation or rigid fixation. Int J Adult Orthodon Orthognath Surg 1994;9:55–63.
5. Watzke IM, Turvey TA, Phillips C, et al. Stability of mandibular advancement after sagittal osteotomy with screw or wire fixation: a comparative study. J Oral Maxillofac Surg 1990;48:108–21.
6. Schendel SA, Epker BN. Results after mandibular advancement surgery: an analysis of 87 cases. J Oral Surg 1980;38:265–82.
7. Costa F, Robiony M, Politi M. Stability of sagittal split ramus osteotomy used to correct class III malocclusion: review of the literature. Int J Adult Orthodon Orthognath Surg 2001;16:121–9.
8. Proffit WR, Turvey TA, Phillips C. Orthognathic surgery: a hierarchy of stability. Int J Adult Orthodon Orthognath Surg 1996;11:19–204.
9. Van Sickels JE, Tiner BD, Keeling SD, et al. Condylar position with rigid fixation versus wire osteosynthesis of a sagittal split advancement. J Oral Maxillofac Surg 1999;57:31–4.
10. Jacobs JD, Bell WH, Williams CE, et al. Control of the transverse dimension with surgery and orthodontics. Am J Orthod 1980;77(3):284–306.
11. Koudstaal MJ, Poort LJ, van der Wal KGH, et al. Surgical assisted rapid maxillary expansion (SARME): a review the literature. Int J Oral Maxillofac Surg 2005;34:709–14.
12. Mommaerts MY. Transpalatal distraction as a method of maxillary expansion. Br J Oral Maxillofac Surg 1999;37:268–72.
13. Enlow GH, Facial growth. 3rd edition. Philadelphia: Saunders; 1990. p. 193–221. Chapter 6.

14. Turvey TA, Simmons K. Orthognathic surgery before completion of growth. In: Fonseca RJ, Betts NJ, Turvey TA, editors. Orthognathic surgery, vol. 2. 1st edition. Philadelphia: Saunders; 2000. p. 535–49. Chapter 26.

15. Reyneke JP. Mandibular anteroposterior excess (chapter 4). In: Reyneke JP, editor. Essentials of orthognathic surgery. 1st edition. Chicago: Quintessence; 2003. p. 171–5.

16. Huang YL, Pogrel MA, Kaban LB. Diagnosis and management of condylar resorption. J Oral Maxillofac Surg 1997;55:114–9.

17. Posnick JC, Fantuzzo JJ. Idiopathic condylar resorption. Current clinical perspectives. J Oral Maxillofac Surg 2007;65:1617–23.

18. Schendel SA, Tulasne J, Linck DW. Idiopathic condylar resorption and micrognathia: the case for distraction osteogenesis. J Oral Maxillofac Surg 2007;65:1610–6.

19. Reyneke JP. The bilateral sagittal split mandibular ramus osteotomy-surgical manual. 2nd edition. Jacksonville (FL): Biomet Micro Fixation; 2006.

20. Reyneke JP, Ferretti C. Anterior open bite correction by Le Fort I or bilateral sagittal split osteotomy. Oral Maxillofac Surg Clin North Am 2007;19(3):321–38.

21. Dowling PA, Espeland L, Sandvic L, et al. Le Fort I maxillary advancement: 3-year stability and risk factors for relapse. Am J Orthod Dentofacial Orthop 2005;128:560–7.

22. Wardrop RW, Wolford LM. Maxillary stability following down-graft and/or advancement procedures with stabilization using rigid fixation and porous block hydroxyapatite implants. J Oral Maxillofac Surg 1989;47:336.

23. Reyneke JP. The Le Fort I maxillary osteotomy - surgical manual. Jacksonville (FL): Biomet Micro Fixation; 2006.

24. Jensen AC, Sinclair PM, Wolford LM. Soft tissue changes associated with double jaw surgery. Am J Orthod Dentofacial Orthop 1992;1101:266–75.

25. Timmes DP, Larsen AJ, Van Sickels JE. Labial morphology following Le Fort I osteotomy and V-Y closure. J Dent Res 1986;65:350–1.

26. Talebzadeh N, Pogrel MA. Upper lip length after V-Y versus continuous closure for Le Fort I maxillary osteotomy. Oral Surg Oral Med Oral Pathol Oral Radiol Endod 2000;90:144–6.

27. Reyneke JP. The sliding genioplasty - surgical manual. 2nd edition. Jacksonville (FL): Biomet Micro Fixation; 2007.

Avoiding Revision Rhinoplasty

Peter D. Waite, MPH, DDS, MD

KEYWORDS

• Reoperation • Revision • Rhinoplasty

Septorhinoplasty is one of the most difficult surgical procedures performed by maxillofacial surgeons. Functional and cosmetic perfection, in the mind of the patient, is difficult to achieve. A great deal of time must be spent explaining surgical goals, expected outcomes, risks, benefits, and alternatives with patients before surgery. Nasal surgery is extremely difficult for the surgeon to master, because of the complex three-dimensional anatomy and a relationship of hard and soft tissue, healing, scar contracture, surgical access, and manipulation. Therefore, it is also difficult for patients to understand and conceptualize the limitations of their own surgery. Most often, reoperation of the nose is because of patient dissatisfaction, resulting from poor diagnosis, poor explanation, poor planning, and poor execution by the surgeon. Inexperienced surgeons do not know what they can or cannot achieve and tend to oversell the procedure. It is only through poor results that surgeons gain experience. Revision rhinoplasty of the nose is reported to be 8% to 15%.[1] Reoperation should be performed to correct deformities that were not diagnosed or addressed in previous surgeries, such as those from poor planning and/or performance and poor surgical healing. Disturbance of the skin and subcutaneous tissues during primary surgery may lead to postoperative scarring and a late-onset deformity or asymmetry. Postoperative results take months to years before becoming fully apparent, and the novice surgeon is unable to reliably predict the outcome. There are multiple pitfalls that must be addressed and avoided by the nasal surgeon (**Box 1**).

Pitfalls in nasal surgery can easily result in complications. The experienced nasal surgeon learns to anticipate the pitfalls and navigate between the hazards. Most surgeons learn when to operate, but it takes time and complications to learn when to stop. Overoperation of the nose often results in a poor result. Nowhere is this more true than in cosmetic nasal surgery; the enemy of good is better. Michelangelo once said: "Trifles make perfection, but perfection is no trifle." The nasal surgeon must have a good idea of what to expect and how the healing process will change the configuration of the nose in the 12 months after the operation. The most common reason for reoperation of the nose is simply a failure to plan. No one plans to fail, they just fail to plan.

AVOIDING REVISION RHINOPLASTY
Lack of Planning and Individualizing the Operation

Poor planning or standardized procedures often result in unpredictable results or the observation that all results tend to look the same. The nose must be individualized to fit the face. A routine nasal surgery can never be performed on all people in the same way. It must be individualized for the patient. One must consider such things such as age, sex, height, and ethnicity. Nasal surgery must be functional and balance the facial harmony. For example, men can tolerate a stronger, broader dorsum, and, likewise, a tall woman might tolerate a longer, stronger dorsum than a shorter, petite woman (**Fig. 1**).

Poor Selection of Patients

The surgeon should develop clear inclusion and exclusion criteria. Psychologically unstable patients with unrealistic expectations should be excluded. The acceptable candidates for surgery are those with reasonable expectations, who

Department of Oral and Maxillofacial Surgery, University of Alabama School of Dentistry, University of Alabama at Birmingham, SDB 419, 1919 7th Avenue South, Birmingham, AL 35294-0007, USA
E-mail address: pwaite@uab.edu

Oral Maxillofacial Surg Clin N Am 23 (2011) 93–100
doi:10.1016/j.coms.2010.10.007
1042-3699/11/$ — see front matter. Published by Elsevier Inc.

Box 1
Pitfalls in nasal surgery leading to reoperation

- Inadequate diagnosis and treatment planning
- Improper patient selection
- Operating beyond one's surgical ability
- Poor septal management
- Too many, or incorrect, intranasal incisions
- Inappropriate dorsal hump reduction
- Aggressive septal resectioning/shortening
- Poor and/or excessive nasal narrowing
- Hazards of the nasal tip/base surgery

---

seem to understand the goals and objectives of the treatment plan. Identify limiting physical factors such as extensive septal deformities, thick sebaceous skin, flaccid nasal cartilages, excessive size, abnormal width and tip projection, extremely small nasal anatomy, infantile nose, and lack of nasal seal or alar base. These physical factors are often difficult to improve. It is best to identify 1 major deformity that can be easily and predictably corrected. Identify psychological factors such as poor motivation, unrealistic expectations, and vague goals. Patients who have had multiple cosmetic procedures and have expressed dissatisfaction will usually be dissatisfied again. Avoid anxious patients making hasty decisions. It

is usually best that patients seriously consider their operation and seek family support. Encourage patients to seek a second opinion because, if they return for surgery, this will only strengthen and embolden the surgeon/patient relationship. Avoid recent emotional crisis such as a divorce or physical facial injury. Look for the narcissistic, manipulative patient desiring facial perfection and/or the noncompliant personality. Careful patient selection will greatly diminish reoperation of the nose.

Operating Beyond One's Ability

There have been multiple surgical adages such as "To thyself be true," "Know your limitations," "Don't be too eager to operate," and, of course, "First, do no harm." Septorhinoplasty is a difficult operation and it takes years to develop deft, delicate, and accurate technique. Overoperation and aggressive surgery often result in asymmetric volume reduction of the tip, asymmetry, loss of tip support, excessive scarring, and cephalic alar retraction. Overaggressive surgery and technical errors can result from poor scars, especially in external rhinoplasty, perforations, cartilage displacement, incorrect suture placement, and supratip scarring (**Fig. 2**).

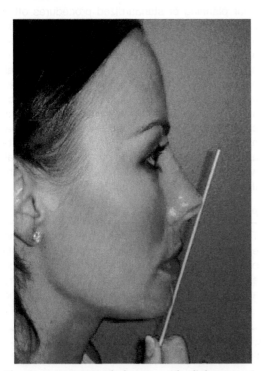

Fig. 1. Strong natural dorsum with slight supratip break and youthful nasolabial angle.

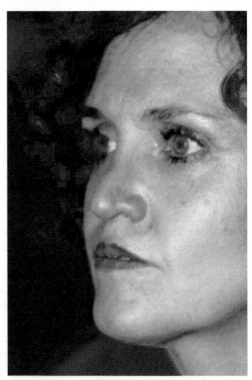

Fig. 2. Excessive cartilage resection resulting in alar retraction and tip ptosis.

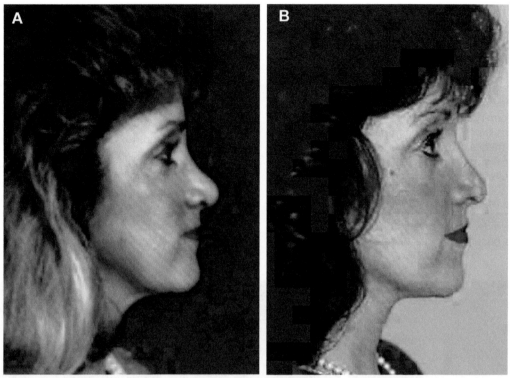

Fig. 3. (*A*) Poor tip support and pollybeak deformity with supratip scarring. (*B*) Revision surgery required tip rhinoplasty with columella strut and excision of supratip scar from an external technique.

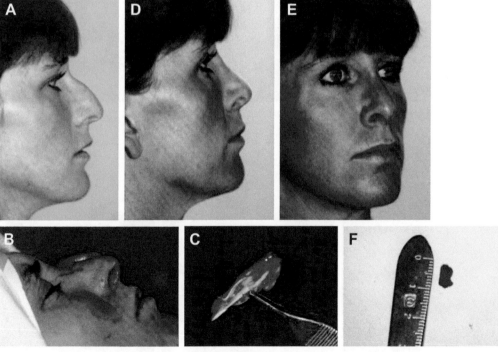

Fig. 4. (*A, B*) A large dorsal hump reduction by an internal rhinoplasty requires more intranasal incisions and greater risk for abnormal scarring and soft tissue retraction. (*C*) Two-thirds of the dorsal hump should be cartilage, but this will include septum and portions of the upper lateral cartilage. (*D–F*) An excellent result, but a small bone irregularity developed 1 year after surgery and was easily removed by reoperation.

Inappropriate Septal Caudal Shortening May Result in Malposition of the Columella

Aggressive dissection of the caudal edge of the septum will disrupt the medial footplates and fixation point of the medial crural cartilage. This disruption will result in tip ptosis, narrowing the nasal labial angle and possibly causing a pollybeak deformity. It is important to understand the cartilaginous tripod concept and preserve tip support of the medial crural footpads for support of the nasal tip.[2] Almost every surgical procedure in rhinoplasty results in compromising nasal tip support (**Fig. 3**).

Too Many Intranasal Incisions

The external rhinoplasty or open nose technique has become popular because it allows excellent access and vision for the novice and also limits the number of intranasal incisions. Limiting the intranasal incisions improves mucosal healing and prevents postsurgical scarring, but it also limits the potential violation of cartilaginous fixation points. The endonasal approach produces multiple different incisions with the potential of producing a stellate scar contraction, and this may retract or collapse the nasal valve area.[3] Excessive nasal scarring often leads to difficult reoperation and, therefore, the external nasal approach is ideal for reoperation procedures. Most surgeons today seem to prefer the external rhinoplasty technique.[4] It is clearly indicated for revision or reoperation of the nose, twisted tip deformities of the nose, and cleft nose deformities. If an isolated nasal deformity can be identified and a simple, single,

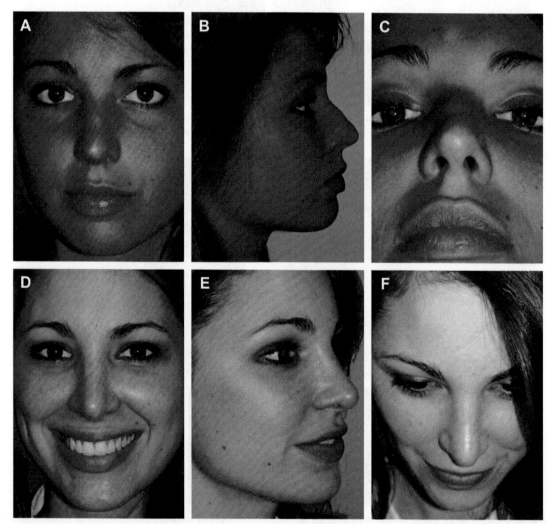

Fig. 5. (*A–C*) The initial nasal surgeon failed to remove the bony dorsum and left an open roof deformity. (*D–F*) Revision surgery was to finish the operation by reducing the dorsum, narrow the open roof, and maintain a supratip break.

intranasal incision made for access, the results are usually predictable. Such situations might include a small dorsal defect requiring an isolated rasp reduction or augmentation (**Fig. 4**).

Poor Hump Removal

Some of the patients who are most satisfied with their nasal reoperations have been those who simply had inadequate hump removal leaving a supratip fullness and/or pollybeak deformity (**Fig. 5**). The inexperienced surgeon often removes too much bone and not enough cartilage, thereby deepening the nasal frontal angle and leaving a pollybeak deformity. When reducing the dorsal hump, one should consider the thickness of the skin at the bony dorsum, the thin skin overlying rhinion, and the possibility of the tip settling, leaving a fullness in the supratip region. Therefore, a straight-line hump removal is usually not acceptable because the result is the depression at rhinion and a pollybeak deformity caused by loss of the supratip support. Excessive hump reduction can alter the nasal valve and compromise airflow.[5-7] It is wise to spend time counseling patients with

large nasal dorsa that it is best not to make an extreme change in the deformity but rather attempt a realistic improvement. A large dorsum is often not only bone and cartilage but thick, sebaceous skin.

Inadequate Septal Surgery

Cosmesis should never compromise airway function. Untreated asymptomatic septal deviations will often become apparent to the patient after nasal surgery, or the memory of the deviation will act as a rudder on a boat and deform the nose, creating an asymmetry. Inadequate septal surgery may result in nasal asymmetry, pollybeak deformity, and persistent septal deviations. Superior septal deviations are extremely difficult to correct and must be identified before surgery, with good patient explanation.[8] Dislocated caudal septums, either deflected at the time of the surgery or acquired, may be repaired and sutured to the anterior nasal spine. Patients with nasal deviations are frequently only part of a larger facial asymmetry and will benefit from maxillofacial surgery or repositioning the anterior nasal spine.

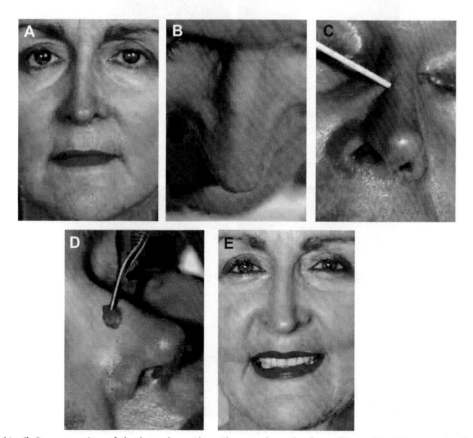

Fig. 6. (*A–C*) Over-resection of the lateral crural cartilage and nasal valve collapse. (*D, E*) Reoperation involved spreader grafting and additional auricular cartilage to correct the contour.

Incorrect Nasal Narrowing

In the past, overaggressive procedures narrowing the nose resulted in hideous deformities that are difficult to correct. It was believed that over-resection of the cartilages would result in a more elegant appearance. With time, these procedures have resulted in scar contracture, asymmetry, and nasal valve collapse (**Fig. 6**). Narrowing the nasal vault/bones often results in middle vault collapse. Disruption of the upper lateral cartilage to the nasal bones allows the upper lateral cartilage to collapse and fall in with inspiration.[3,5] Incorrect lateral nasal osteotomies compromise the bony cartilage support. However, failure to perform lateral nasal osteotomies will often result in an open roof deformity. Although seldom used, medial osteotomies should be short to avoid rocker deformities, and should follow the dorsum. Medial nasal osteotomies should be anticipated in patients with large nasal bones and/or previous nasal trauma. Lateral osteotomies are almost always indicated when the dorsum has been aggressively reduced. If the previous surgeon performs dorsal reduction but not lateral nasal osteotomies, this deformity can be easily corrected by simply completing the operation. Lateral osteotomies should begin at the junction of the inferior turbinate and begin low at the piriform aperture, extending upward quickly. A lateral osteotomy placed too low will often disrupt the inferior turbinate and lead to nasal obstruction and, if placed too high on the nasal dorsum, will be visible on the thinner skin.

Hazards of Nasal Tip/Base Surgery

Understanding the nasal base and the tripod concept is essential to performing septorhinoplasty. The tip of the nose is supported by a tripod.

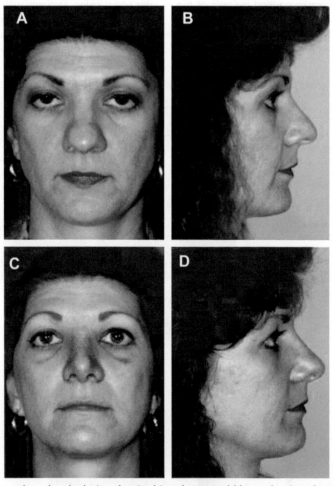

Fig. 7. (*A, B*) Failure to reduce the ala during the tip rhinoplasty would leave the tip volumetrically much smaller than the alar base, resulting in an unnatural result. (*C, D*) Result after alar base surgery performed as a second stage.

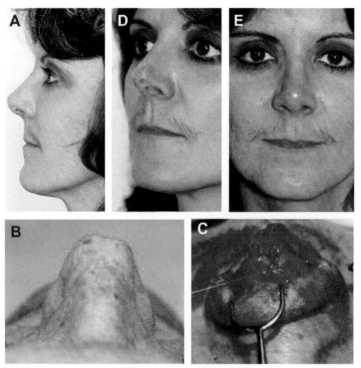

Fig. 8. (*A*, *B*) Surgical division of the cartilage at the dome will result in knuckles and bossa over time in the thin-skinned patient. The first surgeon did not carefully smooth and contour the medial crural cartilage. (*C*) Reoperation required tip rhinoplasty to reshape the cartilage tip. (*D*, *E*) Postoperative tip rhinoplasty.

The 2 lateral crural cartilages form 2 legs of the tripod and the 2 medial crural cartilages fixated to the caudal edge of the septum just above the anterior nasal spine form the central leg of the tripod. From the lateral view, the tip lobule should be equal in mass to the alar base. From the basal view, the tip is about one-third that of the nostril base. Tip surgery must be carefully planned and executed to produce symmetric results. Violation of the lateral cartilage in an asymmetric fashion will result in tip deviation. Aggressive volumetric reduction of the tip may give a refined, smaller tip, but one that is out of proportion with the alar base; the tell-tale sign of an unnatural rhinoplasty. In some cases it may be necessary to reduce the ala by a Weir resection (**Fig. 7**),[5] particularly in cleft patients. It is usually impossible to narrow the nose within the inner canthal dimension, although that is the esthetic norm. The most predictable tip rhinoplasty procedure is the complete strip, which is a partial resection of the cephalic edge of the lower lateral cartilage. This procedure allows a volumetric reduction of the tip, decreasing the bulbosity and adding to the more refined, chiseled appearance. Oversection of the lateral crura cartilage may, in the short-term, seem to give a more narrowed nasal tip but this will invariably result in

excessive alar retraction and a more pinched nasal appearance. Complete sectioning of the cartilage without careful resection of the sharp edges will sometimes result in knuckling and bossa. The sharp edges of the cartilage in time will wear through and make a skin prominence (**Fig. 8**).

SUMMARY

Reoperation of the nose is challenging and sometimes emotionally difficult for the surgeon and patient. There are multiple pitfalls to be avoided and it is always best to carefully diagnose and establish a surgical treatment plan. Even among the best of plans and surgical techniques, revision may be necessary. The patient and surgeon should understand the limitations of the surgical techniques and the individual anatomy.

REFERENCES

1. Becker DG, Bloom J. Five techniques that I cannot live without in revision rhinoplasty. Facial Plast Surg 2008;24:358–64.
2. Sandel HD IV, Perkins SW. Management of the short nose deformity in revision rhinoplasty. Facial Plast Surg 2008;24:310–26.

3. Fedok FG. Revision rhinoplasty using the endonasal approach. Facial Plast Surg 2008;24:293–309.

4. Paun SH, Nolst Trenite GJ. Revision rhinoplasty: an overview of deformities and techniques. Facial Plast Surg 2008;24:271–87.

5. Ballert JA, Park SS. Functional considerations in revision rhinoplasty. Facial Plast Surg 2008;24:348–57.

6. Sykes JM. Management of the middle nasal third in revision rhinoplasty. Facial Plast Surg 2008;24:339–47.

7. Cobo R. Correction of dorsal abnormalities. Facial Plast Surg 2008;24:327–38.

8. Sillers MJ, Cox AJ III, Kulbersh B. Revision septoplasty. Otolaryngol Clin N Am 2009;42:261–78.

Considerations in Revision Rhinoplasty: Lessons Learned

Tirbod Fattahi, MD, DDS

KEYWORDS

- Revision rhinoplasty • Open structure rhinoplasty
- Graft materials

In the preceding article (Dr Peter Waite, Avoiding Revision Rhinoplasty), readers were introduced to the author's suggestions regarding ways and techniques to avoid a revision rhinoplasty. It is imperative to point out that avoiding a reoperation is much more desired that redoing an operation. As has been said before, one has the greatest chance of surgical success the first time around. No one will argue that any secondary operation is typically more challenging than the primary event. Not only has the surgical field not been violated, but dissection during a primary operation is also significantly easier than dissection during a secondary operation. This article is intended to deal with the difficult subject matter of revision rhinoplasty. It is impractical to cover the entire gamut of revision rhinoplasty in a few pages; numerous multivolume textbooks have been written on this subject. Since there is consensus that rhinoplasty is one of the most difficult aesthetic surgery procedures with a high rate of revision (up to 21%),[1–4] one would make the inference that a revision rhinoplasty should also be one of the more difficult revision surgeries. The intent of this article is to share with the readers a few pearls and lessons learned dealing with revision rhinoplasty.

STEP 1—RECOGNITION

Most rhinoplasty patients are seen within a few days following the operation. Typically, the splint (external or internal) and sutures are removed, and the nasal cavity is cleansed. Pictures are taken, and the patient is given routine instructions about wound care and is asked to follow up. Although the nose is quite swollen at this point, gross issues are easily recognized even at this early stage. A major nasal complex deviation at this stage will not go away. The surgeon must recognize this right away; clearly, something has occurred that was not planned. While it might be prudent to wait a bit longer to let the swelling resolve before informing the patient (assuming the patient does not inform the clinician first), the surgeon must begin to plan for the inevitable: revision surgery.

On the other hand, minor issues may not become evident and their revision surgery not necessary until several months following the original surgery. There truly is no consensus as to the timing for a revision surgery. There are many factors involved. Timing for revision surgery will be discussed later in this article.

STEP 2—CONSULTATION

Perhaps the most important consideration in revision rhinoplasty is determining what the patient's concerns are and then verifying the validity of the complaint with a complete internal and external examination of the nose. The clinician must see what the patient sees; otherwise, a proper doctor—patient relationship may never begin. Clearly, there are instances where patient's expectations or complaints are less than reasonable or appropriate; these instances will not be discussed

Division of Oral and Maxillofacial Surgery, University of Florida Health Science Center, Jacksonville, 653-1 West 8th Street, Jacksonville, FL 32209, USA
E-mail address: Tirbod.Fattahi@Jax.Ufl.Edu

Oral Maxillofacial Surg Clin N Am 23 (2011) 101–108
doi:10.1016/j.coms.2010.10.008

here. Listening intently to the patient and determining the patient's chief complaint is paramount in revision rhinoplasty. More than likely, the patient is not fully content with his or her result. He or she may not be the happiest patient. Sensitivity on the part of the clinician in addressing the patient's concerns is required.

Once the patient's complaints have been determined, a full examination of the nose is performed. The author begins with the external examination. Quality and thickness of the skin must be recorded. Generally speaking, patients with thick, sebaceous skin such as those of Middle Eastern descent are much more challenging to revise.[5,6] Presence of abnormalities such as bossae, convexities or concavities along dorsal side walls, degree of projection and rotation of the nose, and dorsal profile must be addressed. Assuming that the patient had his or her initial surgery performed by another practitioner, it is very beneficial to obtain all previous treatment records. One must know how the nose was approached: endonasal versus an open technique. Another important consideration is the status of the septum; is it still there? Most revision rhinoplasty procedures require grafting. If the nasal septum is still present, then it can be used. One can determine the presence of the septum by gently pressing a cotton tip applicator along the quadrangular septum to verify its presence. Certainly, septal incisions such as hemi-transfixion incisions can be a clue that the septum has been manipulated. If previous records are available, it is prudent to ascertain whether the septum was scored to remove deviation or if it was harvested completely. If it was harvested, it would also be helpful to know how much was left behind in the L strut. Assessment of the inferior turbinates must also be done during the internal examination of the nose, since hypertrophic turbinates often can cause air flow restriction.

Another important consideration is whether the patient is experiencing nasal air flow obstruction and whether this was present before surgery. Midvault narrowing following a rhinoplasty can collapse the internal nasal valve leading to restriction of airflow. One of the worst complications following a rhinoplasty is development of a new nasal air flow obstruction. A thorough speculum-assisted examination of the nose should reveal areas where air flow can become restricted. Postoperative synechiae can cause airflow restriction; they are thankfully easily addressed by simple cautery or excision (**Fig. 1**). Although airflow manometry is an option in determining air flow obstruction, it is seldom used.[7]

During the consultation, a treatment plan should be formulated regarding the sequence of the

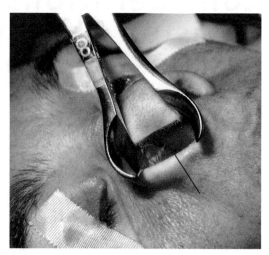

Fig. 1. Postoperative synechia in right nostril causing air flow obstruction (*arrow*).

revision surgery. Certainly, this treatment plan can be modified before surgery once all of the required information has been gathered. Nevertheless, Gunter rhinoplasty diagrams and software (Canfield Scientific Incorporated, Fairfield, NJ, USA) are extremely valuable in the treatment planning phase. Not only can a road map be created, but the author also routinely prints this diagram, uses it during surgery (along with patient's photos), and then stores it as a permanent part of the patient's medical records (**Fig. 2**).

STEP 3—TIMING

The old adage that one must wait an entire year to perform a revision rhinoplasty is without scientific merit. There is no physiologic explanation that somehow a twisted nose at 4 months after primary surgery will magically untwist itself by 12 months. If it looks bad at 4 months; it will look ugly at 12! Having said this, there is merit in waiting and patience when it comes to minor issues. A slight supratip fullness may respond well to massaging or steroid injections. A transcolumellar incision that appears somewhat red may respond favorably to wound care. Conversely, a tension nose with lack of proper projection a few weeks following surgery will more than likely become worse with time. Major postoperative issues such as new air flow obstruction, persistent dorsal hump, deviated nasal complex, widened dome, and lack of nasal tip support warrant a revision surgery within a few weeks to months. A clinician may opt to wait to get the patient mentally ready for another operation, but it is the opinion of the author that the aforementioned issues following a primary rhinoplasty should be addressed quickly.

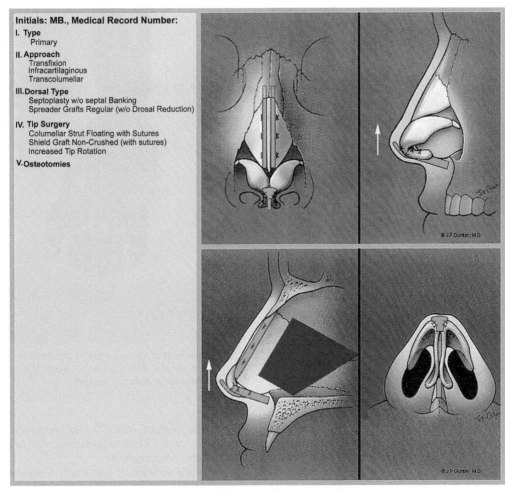

Initials: MB., Medical Record Number:

I. Type
   Primary

II. Approach
   Transfixion
   Infracartilaginous
   Transcolumellar

III. Dorsal Type
   Septoplasty w/o septal Banking
   Spreader Grafts Regular (w/o Drosal Reduction)

IV. Tip Surgery
   Columellar Strut Floating with Sutures
   Shield Graft Non-Crushed (with sutures)
   Increased Tip Rotation

V. Osteotomies

Fig. 2. Gunter rhinoplasty diagrams. (*Courtesy of* J.P. Gunter, MD.)

STEP 4—RESTRUCTURING THE NOSE

Revision nasal surgery is a difficult operation. Because of the scarring process following the primary operation, dissection is tedious, and landmarks are lost (**Fig. 3**).[8,9] Most experts will favor an open rhinoplasty technique in cases of major revision surgery. There is no question that the open technique will offer an extended view and access to nearly the entire nasal complex, thereby allowing precise maneuvers and placement of sutures and grafts (**Fig. 4**). Following primary rhinoplasty, the natural plane of dissection between the lower cartilages and overlying skin envelope is lost; therefore careful separation of the cartilages from the soft tissue is paramount to avoid inadvertent damage to the underlying cartilages. Open structure rhinoplasty is a term popularized by

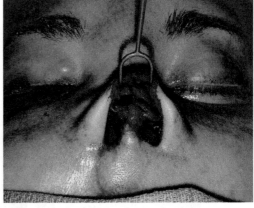

Fig. 3. Loss of normal surgical planes during revision surgery. Notice the amount of scarring between lower lateral cartilages and overlying soft tissue.

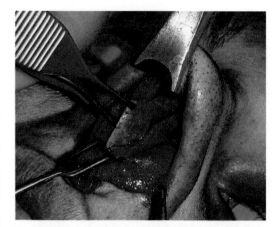

Fig. 4. Open structure rhinoplasty technique will provide an excellent view of the nasal complex.

Toriumi.[10,11] It not only describes the technique (open), but it emphasizes the concept of structuring and building a nose, a clear distinction from the old philosophy of overoperated and destructive rhinoplasty procedures of 20 years ago or so. Once the nasal complex has been degloved via an open technique, a clear view of the underlying anatomy becomes evident. The clinician can then address each component of the patient's complaints appropriately. Incremental dorsal reduction can be done under direct visualization. Placement of spreader grafts between the upper lateral cartilages (ULC) and dorsal septum can be performed if nasal air flow obstruction is due to a restricted internal nasal valve (**Fig. 5**). Tip plasty can be done through cephalic trim of the lateral crura to achieve tip rotation, along with transdomal suturing and placement of shield grafts. Cookie cutter graft templates and a hand press can be used for this purpose (**Fig. 6**). Most open rhinoplasty techniques will cause some degree of tip ptosis; to combat this, columellar

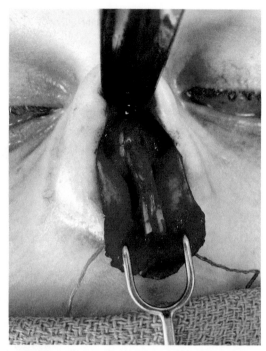

Fig. 5. Placement of spreader grafts to relieve air flow obstruction. Grafts are placed between the upper lateral cartilages and dorsal septum.

strut grafts must be used. This is especially true in revision surgery if lack of tip support and projection is noted preoperatively.

If the nose is twisted, one must determine its cause. As the old saying goes: "as the septum goes, so does the nose." If the septum is still present, it must be addressed to ensure that it is in fact in the midline and not twisted. If it is twisted, then it can be scored to straighten it, or more preferably, it can be harvested, an appropriate sized L strut left behind, and used as donor material for

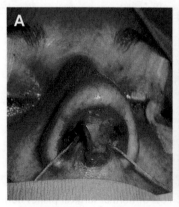
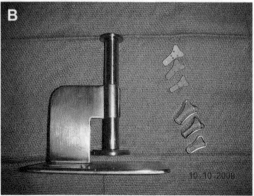

Fig. 6. Placement of shield graft. (*A*) Graft in place. (*B*) Cookie cutter and templates used in creating the shield graft.

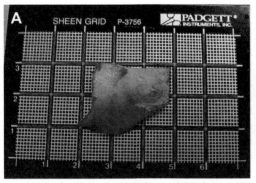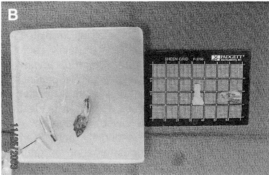

Fig. 7. (*A, B*) Harvested septum to be used for various grafts (shield graft, spreader grafts). Most revision rhinoplasty will not yield this amount of cartilage.

rebuilding the nose. Lateral and medial osteotomies also can be used to address a crooked nose, although again it is important to ensure that the septum is in the midline.

STEP 5—GRAFT-DEPLETED PATIENT

It is not uncommon to examine a patient for revision surgery and realize that the patient no longer has any nasal septum available for grafting.[12–15] This is a difficult situation, since most revision rhinoplasties require some level of augmentation

to correct what has been taken away. "Conserve and preserve; don't resect and regret!" (Peter Adamson, MD, personal communication, 2006). Unfortunately this statement is often times ignored during primary rhinoplasty and only comes to fruition during revision surgery when the clinician realizes that too much cartilage has been removed and the nasal complex lacks structural support (**Fig. 7**).

It is prudent to determine preoperatively if augmentation of the nose is needed. Septal cartilage remains the material of choice for secondary

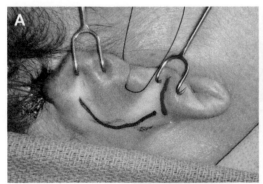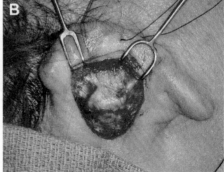

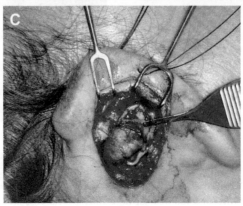

Fig. 8. Harvest of auricular cartilage form a posterior approach. (*A*) Outline. (*B*) Exposure. (*C*) Harvested cartilage.

revision. If absent, other options include harvesting of auricular cartilage, harvesting of rib grafts, cranial bone grafts, allografts such as irradiated rib cartilage, and alloplasts.[16–21] Certainly each option carries its own advantages and disadvantages that must be discussed with the patient. Auricular cartilage is easy to harvest with little morbidity, but it lack stiffness (**Fig. 8**). It is ideal for dorsal camouflage and lower cartilage onlay grafts. Autogenous costochondral grafts can certainly provide tremendous amount of graft material; however, there is potential for some morbidity associated with this procedure, and it may require hospitalization. Considering that most rhinoplasty procedures are done at a surgery center as outpatient procedures, harvesting a simultaneous rib graft might be a challenge. Nevertheless, in cases where complete restructuring of the nose is required (such as severe saddle nose deformity or cocaine nose), autogenous rib grafts are the materials of choice. Irradiated homologous costal cartilage grafts have been studied extensively and are an acceptable alternative to autogenous rib graft harvesting. Advantages include decreased operating time, lack of donor site and potential harvesting complications, and its availability. There is a slight risk of resorption over time, although the overall rate of complications is quite low. Cranial bone grafts can be used to provide support in severe saddle nose deformities, although their harvest may require an overnight stay in the hospital (**Fig. 9**). Alloplasts such as silastic or porous polyethylene have been used in nasal and facial augmentation surgery for quite a long time. While the overall success rate of facial implants is high, it is the

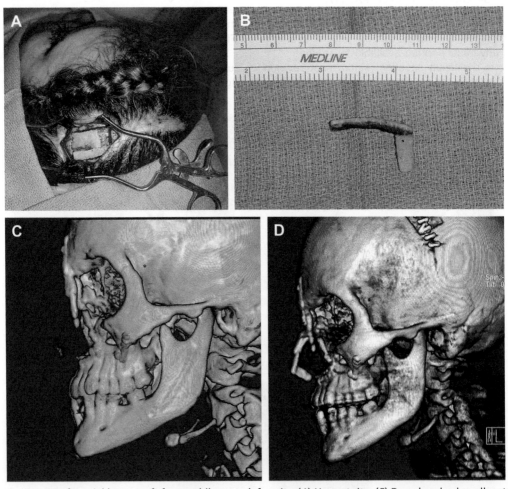

Fig. 9. Harvest of cranial bone graft for a saddle nose deformity. (*A*) Harvest site. (*B*) Dorsal and columellar struts created. (*C, D*) Pre- and postoperative three-dimensional computed tomography scan reconstruction.

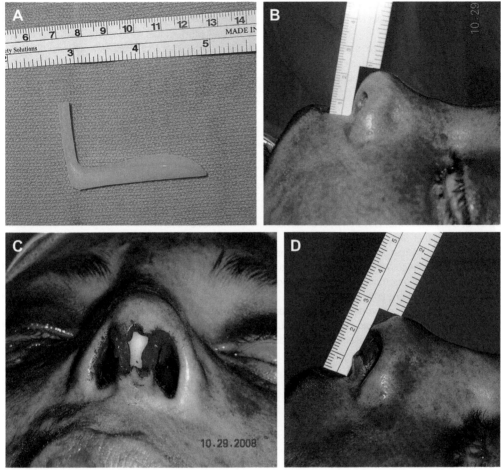

Fig. 10. Silicone dorsal–columellar implant. (*A*) Implant. (*B*) Preinsertion measurement of nasal projection. (*C*) Implant in place. (*D*) Postinsertion measurement of nasal projection.

opinion of the author to limit the use of alloplasts in patients who have thick nasal skin and who object to the use of autogenous or homologous rib grafts (**Fig. 10**). Patients with thin soft tissue envelopes may reject these materials over time and will often present with extrusion of the implant and foreign body reaction. While it is beyond the scope of this article to discuss every advantage or disadvantage of graft materials, it is important to include this discussion with the patient who desires revision rhinoplasty, since most revision rhinoplasties are in fact graft-depleted individuals.

SUMMARY

Revision rhinoplasty is a difficult operation. It poses a unique set of challenges to the clinician. However, it can also be a rewarding operation. Recognition of the patient's chief complaint and proper treatment planning, along with proper surgical execution, can certainly improve

outcomes. It is imperative to determine if the patient needs graft augmentation before revision, as most do, and most are in fact graft depleted.

REFERENCES

1. Warner J, Gutowski K, Shama L, et al. National inter-disciplinary rhinoplasty survey. Aesthet Surg J 2009; 29(4):295–301.
2. Parkes ML, Kanodia R, Machida BK. Revision rhinoplasty: an analysis of aesthetic deformities. Arch Otolaryngol Head Neck Surg 1992;118(7):695–701.
3. Kamer FM, McQuown SA. Revision rhinoplasty: analysis and treatment. Arch Otolaryngol Head Neck Surg 1988;114(3):257–66.
4. Wright MR. Management of patient dissatisfaction with results of cosmetic procedures. Arch Otolaryngol Head Neck Surg 1980;106(8):466–71.
5. Daniel RK. Middle Eastern rhinoplasty in the United States. Part II: revision rhinoplasty. Plast Reconstr Surg 2009;124(5):1640–8.

6. Azizzadeh B, Mashkevich G. Middle Eastern rhinoplasty. Facial Plast Surg Clin North Am 2010;18(1):201–6.
7. Fattahi T. Internal nasal valve: significance in nasal air flow. J Oral Maxillofac Surg 2008;66(9):1921–6.
8. Becker DG, Bloom J. Five techniques that I cannot live without in revision rhinoplasty. Facial Plast Surg 2008;24(3):358–64.
9. Thomson C, Mendelsohn M. Reducing the incidence of revision rhinoplasty. J Otolaryngol 2007;36(2):130–4.
10. Toriumi DM. Structural approach to primary rhinoplasty. Aesthet Surg J 2002;22(1):72–84.
11. Toriumi DM. Structure approach in rhinoplasty. Facial Plast Surg Clin North Am 2005;13(1):93–113.
12. Byrd HS, Constantian MB, Guyuron B, et al. Revision rhinoplasty. Aesthet Surg J 2007;27(2):175–87.
13. Constantian MB. Indications and use of composite grafts in 100 consecutive secondary and tertiary rhinoplasty patients: introduction of the axial orientation. Plast Reconstr Surg 2002;110(4):1116–33.
14. Constantian MB. Four common anatomic variants that predispose to unfavorable rhinoplasty results: a study based on 150 consecutive secondary rhinoplasties. Plast Reconstr Surg 2000;105(1):316–31.
15. Constantian MB. Rhinoplasty in the graft depleted patient. Oper Tech Plast Recontr Surg 1995;2:67–81.
16. Murrell GL. Auricular cartilage grafts and nasal surgery. Laryngoscope 2004;114(12):2092–102.
17. Marin VP, Landecker A, Gunter JP. Harvesting rib cartilage for secondary rhinoplasty. Plast Reconstr Surg 2008;121(4):1442–8.
18. Mernger DJ, Gilbert J, Trenite N. Irradiated homologous rib grafts in nasal reconstruction. Arch Facial Plast Surg 2010;12:114–8.
19. Kridel RW, Faramarz A, Liu E, et al. Long-term use and follow-up of irradiated homologous costal cartilage grafts in the nose. Arch Facial Plast Surg 2009;11:378–94.
20. Romo T 3rd, Sclafani AP, Sabini P. Reconstruction of the major saddle nose deformity using composite allo-implants. Facial Plast Surg 1998;14(2):151–7.
21. Romo T 3rd, Zoumalan RA. Porous polyethylene implants in rhinoplasty: surgical techniques and long-term outcomes. Oper Tech Otolaryngol 2007;18:284–90.

Reoperative Face and Neck Lifts

Jacob Haiavy, MD, DDS[a,b,]*

KEYWORDS

- Secondary facelift • Revisional facelift • Reoperative facelift
- Secondary neck lift • Revisional neck lift
- Reoperative neck lift • Platysmaplasty
- Secondary rhytidectomy

In the past decade cosmetic surgery has become more common and accepted in our society. Face and neck lift procedures can be routinely viewed on the Internet or television. With easy access to the information and reality shows demonstrating success stories, there has been an increase in demand for these procedures. This increase has given rise to a new generation of patients who have undergone a facelift or a neck lift procedure and, because of the continued effects of aging, request a secondary operation.

When performing a secondary facelift or neck lift, the surgeon needs to consider the effects of the primary procedure on the tissues. Even though there are a few techniques of performing a facelift or a neck lift, the factors that need to be considered when performing a secondary procedure are the same:

- Previous incision placement and resulting scars
- Amount of skin laxity
- Earlobe deformity
- Hair pattern changes
- Fat irregularities and deficiencies
- Fascial laxity leading to deep nasolabial folds and jowls
- Cervicomental angle obtusity
- Platysmal laxity and banding
- Presence of unusual rhytids.

Most patients requesting secondary facelifts or neck lifts have some form of laxity and want to maintain their facial appearance. In addition, most of the patients seeking secondary facelifts are older in age and often have other ailments concomitant with aging. Therefore, the preoperative assessment should include a thorough medical history and physical examination. This assessment should include a history of over-the-counter and herbal medicines, because many of the patients who seek secondary facelift or neck lift take herbal medicine with potential ill effects on surgery. For example, ginkgo biloba and testosterone can potentially induce hypertension.[1] Many of the herbal products are blood thinners and can affect the coagulation cascade, such as ginkgo biloba, garlic tablets, ginger, St John's wort, and ginseng. The author recommends that patients stop all herbal medicines for 2 weeks before and after surgery. When necessary, appropriate referrals to the primary care physician, cardiologist, or other specialist should be made to obtain a clearance and minimize risk of perioperative complications.

In general, the author's approach to a secondary procedure is the opportunistic approach and is tailored to the patient's needs and existing anatomy.[2] Each patient presents with different skin thickness and elasticity, variable amount of subcutaneous tissue, variable amount of laxity and thickness of their superficial fascia, and variable amount of scarring from their primary facelift or neck lift. When evaluating the patient, the surgeon should look for residual signs of aging that have not been addressed in the primary procedure. It is not uncommon to see a patient who has had a facelift seeking a secondary procedure and on examination most of the laxity is

[a] Inland Cosmetic Surgery, 8680 Monroe Court, Suite #200, Rancho Cucamonga, CA 91730, USA
[b] Department of Oral & Maxillofacial Surgery, Loma Linda University, 11234 Anderson Street, Loma Linda, CA 92354, USA
* Inland Cosmetic Surgery, 8680 Monroe Court, Suite #200, Rancho Cucamonga, CA 91730.
E-mail address: Jhaiavy@yahoo.com

Oral Maxillofacial Surg Clin N Am 23 (2011) 109–118
doi:10.1016/j.coms.2010.10.006
1042-3699/11/$ — see front matter © 2011 Elsevier Inc. All rights reserved.

concentrated in the upper face and periocular region, which was not addressed in the primary surgery (**Fig. 1**). During the secondary facelift, the surgeon can and should address those areas to achieve the best possible result.

Generally, most of the patients seeking a secondary procedure have their skin envelope tightened with the primary procedure, and therefore, little skin needs to be removed in the secondary procedure. On the other hand, their superficial musculoaponeurotic system (SMAS) and the muscles in the neck are commonly lax compared with the tightened skin envelope.[3,4] In recent years, the popularity of various forms of short-scar facelifts has given rise to an increasing number of patients with this presentation.

Because most of the primary facelifts performed do not involve an extensive sub-SMAS dissection, the secondary facelift will benefit from some form of SMAS undermining and tightening. The subcutaneous layer, which is the most common plane of dissection in a facelift, may be thinner after the trauma of the original procedure and facial fat atrophy,[5] creating a challenge in a thin patient. In those cases, it may be more prudent to perform an SMASectomy with plication rather than an SMAS elevation.

INCISIONS AND SCARS

Incision placement during the secondary procedure is largely dictated by the incision line that was made during the first operation. The author's preference is to make a tragal margin incision or a retrotragal incision because it is easier to hide the scar and the scar heals well. Before making the incision, careful assessment of the amount of skin laxity present should be made, and if enough laxity is present, a preauricular incision can be converted to a tragal or retrotragal incision during the reoperation (**Fig. 2**). On closure of the flap, there should be minimal tension on the tragus. To minimize tension, the skin flap is sutured above and below the tragus with 4-0 Monocryl sutures.

EARLOBE DEFORMITY

Another common stigmata of facelifts is the "bat ear" or "pixie ear" deformity (**Fig. 3**A). This deformity is a result of poor incision placement and excess skin removal caudal to the ear lobe during closure of the primary procedure. The closure of the earlobe cannot be under tension. The deeper structures of the jaw line and neck should be secured to a stable structure such as the postauricular fascia or the mastoid fascia, and the skin should be closed passively around the earlobe. To correct this deformity, the surgeon should incise the earlobe to a more rounded appearance and then inset the earlobe to its proper position, which is 10° to 20° posterior to the axis of the pinna (see **Fig. 3**B).[6] One should never attempt

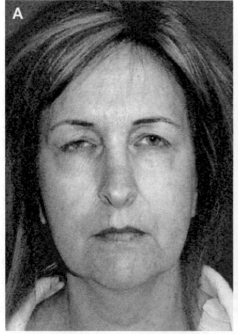
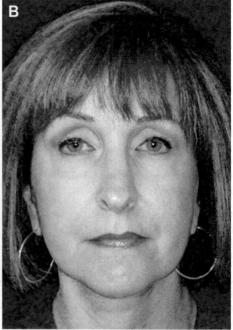

Fig. 1. (*A*) A 62-year-old woman 10 years after her primary facelift complaining of recurrent sagging in the face and jowls. (*B*) Same patient 3 months after facelift revision, endoscopic brow lift, and full-face CO$_2$ laser resurfacing.

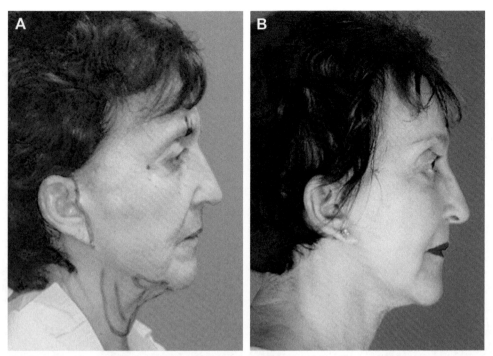

Fig. 2. (*A*) Preoperative markings of a 65-year-old woman 8 years after her primary facelift demonstrating a tragal margin incision. (*B*) Same patient 3 months after revisional facelift and neck lift with fat transfer to lower eyelids and a full-face trichloroacetic acid peel.

to hang the cheek on the earlobe during flap re-draping. Instead, the skin flap should be secured to the base of the ear lobe with a 3-0 Monocryl or 3-0 Vicryl suture. The skin of the earlobe is then closed with a 5-0 plain catgut suture under minimal tension (see **Fig. 3**C).

HAIR PATTERN CHANGES

One of the greatest challenges with incision placement in revisional facelift or neck lift is problems with hairline shifting and bold spots from the primary operation. Another common stigma of facelifts is distortion or the loss of sideburn and temporal hairline. This problem can occur when the cervicofacial flap is advanced too far in the cephalad direction, causing the hairline shift. For example, transposition of the sideburn above the helical rim can leave a bold spot above the ear. This problem is difficult to correct. It is occasionally possible to rotate the temporal hairline inferiorly and partially lower the sideburn. As is commonly the case, avoidance of this problem is the best course of action.

The author prefers to make the temporal incision in the hairline at the initial procedure and leave the sideburn or 1 cm of hair-bearing skin attached at the base of the helix. This method avoids improper transposition of hair in the temporal region. If skin

needs to be removed at that location, it is done in a conservative fashion, bearing in mind not to shift the temporal hairline. Another alternative for correction of this problem is to place the incision along the temporal hairline in the secondary procedure and avoid any additional hairline shifting at the time of flap advancement.[1]

In the postauricular region, there is a potential for visible scars when the incision in the primary procedure was made along the posterior scalp hairline. This scar can become wide and more visible when the neck tissues are suspended to the postauricular scalp skin as opposed to the deeper scalp structures. In the revisional procedure, the surgeon has the opportunity to remove some or the entire scar as long as enough laxity is present. It is the author's preference to make the new incision in the hairline cephalad to the old scar in a line that is perpendicular to the vector of pull. If the incision is made in a beveled manner and the dissection is made in a plane to avoid damage to the hair follicles, this incision heals so well that it is almost invisible a year later when the hairs have grown into the scar. When advancing the posterior cervical skin flap in a cephalic direction, the author places 1 or 2 deep permanent sutures (2-0 Ethibond or Nurolon [Ethicon, San Angelo, TX, USA]) that secure the deep portion of the skin flap to the deep posterior

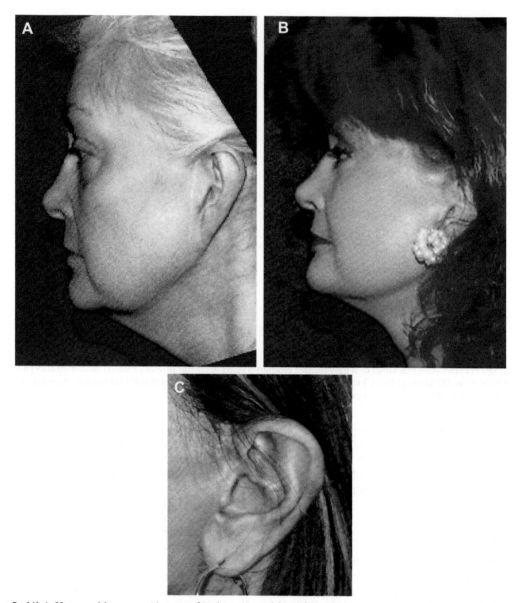

Fig. 3. (*A*) A 62-year-old woman 10 years after her primary facelift, with a visible preauricular scar and pixie ear deformity. (*B*) Same patient after secondary facelift with revision of preauricular scar, conversion to a tragal margin scar, and correction of pixie ear. (*C*) Close-up of a corrected earlobe with a previous pixie deformity.

scalp fascia and/or the periosteum (**Fig. 4**A). The excess skin and the old scar are then trimmed, and the incision is closed with staples passively under no tension. Care is taken to align the posterior hairline during closure (see **Fig. 4**B).

FAT IRREGULARITIES AND DEFICIENCIES

Because patients continue to age after their primary surgery, there is continued laxity of the skin and underlying tissues and facial fat atrophy. In addition, because patients are seeking these

procedures at an early age and have minimal neck laxity, surgeons have become more aggressive with cervical and facial fat removal. This situation had led to the problem of the patients presenting for a secondary procedure with an overskeletonized neck and submalar hollowing (**Fig. 5**A). This lack of subcutaneous fat makes it difficult to disguise the fascial and platysmal irregularities that may occur during surgical manipulation, especially on a thin patient. To correct this problem, in the secondary procedure instead of removing fat, the surgeon should attempt

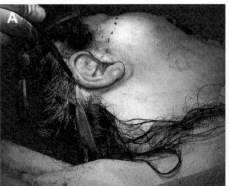
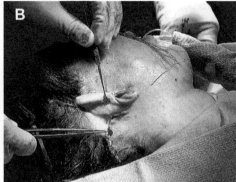

Fig. 4. (*A*) Advancement and fixation of posterior cervical skin flap. Note the alignment of hair. (*B*) Closure and alignment of temporal and posterior scalp hairline.

redraping the patient's existing fat from the jowls cephalically over the buccal recess. In the author's practice, it has been more common to perform fat grafting than fat removal procedures during facelift revisions. Fat grafting can correct the hollowing in the submalar, infraorbital, and perioral regions (see **Fig. 5**B). Patients need to understand that they may need multiple fat grafting sessions to achieve the optimal results. With the advancements in stem cell research and isolation of stem cell from adipose tissue, it may not be long before revisional surgery can be combined with one session of stem cell–enriched fat grafting to correct these problems.

FASCIAL LAXITY

Patients presenting for a secondary facelift or neck lift usually have minimal skin laxity, but more commonly they have some form of laxity in the deeper layers (SMAS and platysma muscle) that can lead to deepening of nasolabial folds, jowls, and platysmal banding. Usually, SMAS elevation is limited during the primary procedure. Therefore,

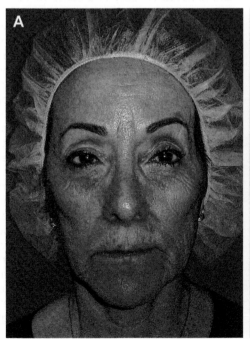
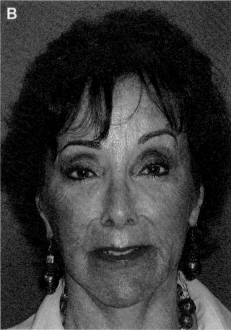

Fig. 5. (*A*) A 62-year-old woman demonstrating infraorbital, submalar, and cervical hollowing caused by fat atrophy after the primary procedure. (*B*) Same patient after reoperative facelift, endoscopic brow lift, and fat transfer to the eyes, cheeks, and lips, with full-face CO_2 laser resurfacing.

most patients benefit from reelevation and tightening of the deeper fascial layers (**Fig. 6**).[1,7]

The surgeon should be cautious because scarring form previous surgery can distort the anatomy. Fortunately, the scarring is mostly over the parotid gland, where the facial nerve branches are deep to the plane of dissection. It is also important not to carry the dissection too deep over the parotid, as damage to the gland can lead to a sialocele. Once the SMAS is freed past the parotid gland, the dissection becomes easier in the sub-SMAS areolar plane. It is important to understand the anatomy and relationship of the facial nerve to the SMAS and facial muscles (**Fig. 7**). The zygomaticus major and zygomaticus minor as well as orbicularis oculi and platysma muscles receive their innervations through their deep surface, whereas the buccinator, levator anguli oris, and mentalis muscles are innervated along their superficial surface.[6] Therefore, when the SMAS elevation is performed, as long as the dissection is carried out along the superficial surface of the facial muscles, injury to the facial nerve is not likely. Furthermore, as mentioned earlier, the author's approach is opportunistic, and the dissection is carried out medially only to the point needed to achieve adequate release and correction. This approach varies with each patient. If extensive scarring is present to the point where the relationship between the superficial and deep fascial layers is obscured, a simple SMAS plication is preferable (**Fig. 8**). Also, if the SMAS is found to be very thin and attenuated, it becomes difficult to perform a smooth elevation of that layer because it may tear. Therefore, a simple plication in this case may serve the patient and the surgeon better.

THE CERVICOMENTAL ANGLE AND PLATYSMA

The cervicomental angle has been studied extensively. For ideal aesthetics, it should be

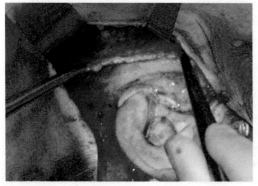

Fig. 6. Elevation of the deep layer and SMAS in a revisional facelift.

approximately 90°, but a wide range of normal neck morphology exists and the angle may vary from 105° to 120°.[8,9] The angle is usually more obtuse in women compared with men. A low and anteriorly positioned hyoid bone also leads to a more obtuse angle. This morphology can be camouflaged by placement of a chin implant to give the illusion of a more acute angle.[10] Because primary surgeries are being done at early ages, they usually involve removal of preplatysmal fat and tightening of cervical skin. With aging, the platysma muscle becomes more attenuated and the platysmal bands become more obvious. Another factor that can contribute to cervicomental obtusity is fat accumulation under the platysma. In a revisional surgery, it is more common to see this condition than the accumulation of preplatysmal fat if the patient has gained significant weight. Therefore, in the revisional facelift or neck lift, every effort should be made to preserve the fat on the cervical skin flap, especially if subplatysmal fat removal is planned. The author does not routinely perform submental liposuction when performing a revisional neck lift, especially if an extensive platysmaplasty is planned.

The author's approach to the neck is through the submental incision centrally and the postauricular incision laterally. Once adequately exposed, the amount of platysmal laxity is evaluated, and if necessary, excess muscle and fat are clamped and removed centrally in a conservative fashion to prevent undue tension on the suture plication. The subplatysmal fat is then exposed by elevation of the medial borders of the platysma from the mentum to the level of the cricoid cartilage. The excess fat is then removed under direct vision with the Bovie cautery and scissors. Careful hemostasis must be obtained. This fat contouring has to be precise, and care should be taken to avoid overresection of fat in the submental region. This overresection can lead to a hollowed out submental appearance that is difficult to correct. A greater amount of fat can be removed at the level of the hyoid, where it helps to deepen the cervicomental angle. In addition, releasing the muscle laterally by performing a myotomy either at the level of the hyoid or just caudal to the last muscle plication suture relieves some of the tension along the platysmal plication and allows the platysma to shift superiorly, creating a deeper cervicomental angle (**Fig. 9**). This back cut or myotomy of the platysma is parallel to the inferior border of the mandible and away from the submandibular gland, facial artery, facial vein, and the facial nerve. After adequate mobilization of the platysma, the edges of the muscle are grasped and overlapped in the midline. Platysmal plication is then performed

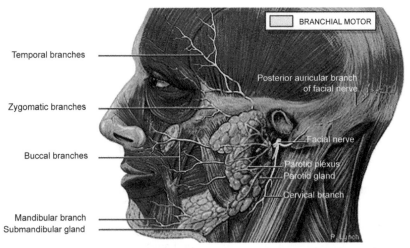

Fig. 7. Relationship of the facial nerve to the facial muscles. (*From* Yale Center for Advanced Instructional Media, copyright 1998. All rights reserved; with permission.)

with interrupted 3-0 Vicryl or 3-0 silk sutures from the mentum to at least the level of the hyoid bone. The author often continues this plication lower to the level of the thyroid cartilage, especially on a long-necked person with long bands. In very thin patients with little subcutaneous fat, it is important to bury the knots and be careful to create a smooth contour because the anatomy created with the muscle plication is immediately visible under the skin with little padding. The goal of muscle plication is to produce an even smooth platysma contour that tightly adheres to the underlying structures, producing a proper framework for redraping of the cervical skin.

On occasion, patients presenting for secondary facelift or neck lift have bulging of their submandibular gland. This presentation can be secondary to overaggressive liposuction during the primary procedure or just ptosis of the gland with attenuation of the deep fascia and gland capsule. Some patients may accept this side effect of the primary procedure as an explanation of normal anatomy. During the secondary procedure, the surgeon can address the ptotic gland by either attempting a sling suture, such as the Giampapa suture from the submental region to each mastoid fascia, or performing partial resection of the submandibular gland. The gland can be approached through the

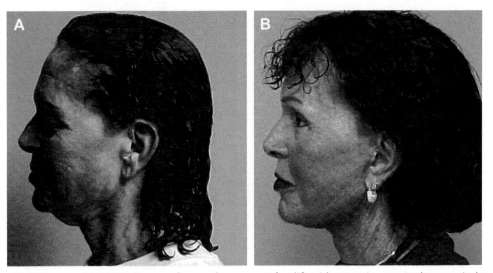

Fig. 8. (*A*) A 61-year-old woman 8 years after a subcutaneous facelift with extensive pre- and postauricular scarring. (*B*) Same patient after a revisional facelift with SMAS elevation and plication as well as endoscopic brow lift.

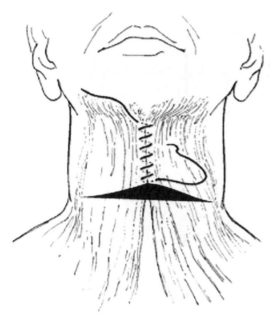

Fig. 9. Platysmal plication and lateral myotomy. (*From* Sykes JM. Rejuvenation of the aging neck. Facial Plast Surg 2001;17:103, Thieme-connect; with permission.)

subplatysmal dissection, whereby the cervical fascia is carefully penetrated over the bulge of the gland. The most inferior and anterior portion of the gland is then gently grasped, and the

excessive portion of the gland is removed. This procedure has to be done with extreme care and under excellent visualization because branches of the facial artery and vein and the mandibular branch of the facial nerve are close by and have to be preserved. This procedure should be reserved for the experienced surgeon who is very familiar with the anatomy.

PRESENCE OF UNUSUAL RHYTIDS

Facial rhytids are not removed by facelifts or neck lifts, whether it is primary or revisional surgery. The rhytids are improved and redraped. Regarding nasolabial folds, Dr Howard Tobin (author's mentor) often calls them "undefeated nasolabial folds" and says, "nothing will remove them, but we can improve them." (Howard Tobin, MD, Abilene, TX, personal communication, 2000).

Occasionally, patients present for reoperation with unnatural-looking rhytids, which occur as a result of an exaggerated rotation of the cervicofacial flap, causing the rhytids to run in an upward direction. This condition is compounded by the fact that with aging, the patients lose some of the skin elasticity and have more actinic damage because of continued sun exposure, leading to inelastic poor-quality skin with keratotic changes and hyperpigmentation. Therefore, at the secondary procedure the surgeon should be aware of the direction of flap rotation to not

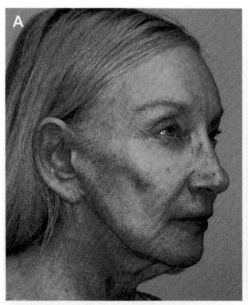
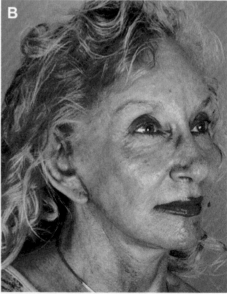

Fig. 10. (*A*) A 70-year-old woman 6 years after primary brow lift, facelift, upper and lower blepharoplasty, and cheek augmentation. (*B*) Same patient 6 months after revisional face and neck lifts and full-face trichloroacetic acid peel.

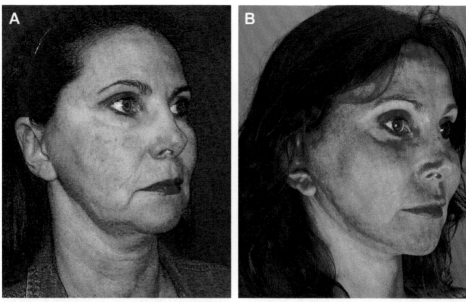

Fig. 11. (*A*) A 50-year-old woman 3 years after primary face and neck lifts. (*B*) Same patient 3 months after a facial tuck and full-face CO_2 laser resurfacing.

exaggerate the abnormal rhytids. Furthermore, laser skin resurfacing and/or chemical peels are useful adjuncts to the secondary procedure; these techniques can correct the actinic changes and improve some of the fine lines and rhytids (**Fig. 10**). When combining revisional surgery with laser resurfacing or chemical peeling, the skin dissection is kept to the minimum and the lift must rely mostly on the rotation of the deeper musculofascial structure. This method works well because most of the patients presenting for the secondary procedure have little skin laxity. On smokers, is advisable to do shorter skin flaps and rely mostly on the SMAS and platysma dissection. The skin flap in reoperations should be more resistant to vascular compromise, especially because it was delayed during the primary procedure.[7]

FACE TUCK

A common question presented by patients is "How long will my facelift last?" A recent article tried to answer this question for a single surgeon.[11] The author's standard answer is "The changes that one will make to your face are permanent but you will continue to age." Patients who want to maintain their lifted appearance are better served with a face tuck within the first 2 to 3 years after the primary procedure (**Fig. 11**).

In that period, the scar tissue is still fairly resilient and the pull in the periauricular area can be easily transmitted to the jowl and neck. When the wait for the secondary procedure is longer, a combination of skin elevation, SMAS dissection and plication, as well as platysmal manipulation followed by careful skin redraping often leads to considerable improvement and a satisfied patient.

SUMMARY

The complexity of the revisional facelift or neck lift is directly related to the way the primary procedure was performed. With so many techniques now available to the facial cosmetic surgeon, such as the subcutaneous facelift,[12] variations of SMAS or extended SMAS procedures,[13–15] lateral SMASectomy,[16] deep plane and composite ryhtidectomy,[17,18] subperiosteal facelift,[19,20] and short-scar facelifts,[21] the revisional procedure should be directed to the specific problems that the patient exhibits, such as laxity in the upper face, laxity in the neck, jowling, or deepening of the nasolabial folds. In general, it is more prudent to restore contour within the deep layer support by the elevation of the SMAS and platysma rather than by rotating skin flaps in an exaggerated manner in a cephalad direction producing a tight unnatural look. In addition, it is extremely important that the posterior hairline and the temporal hairline are correctly aligned at the time of closure.

REFERENCES

1. Guyuron B. Secondary rhytidectomy. Plast Reconstr Surg 2004;114(3):797–800.

2. Tobin HA, Cuzalina A, Tharanon W, et al. The biplane facelift: an opportunistic approach. J Oral Maxillofac Surg 2000;58:76–85.

3. Mitz V, Peyronie M. The superficial musculo-aponeurotic system (SMAS) in the parotid and cheek area. Plast Reconstr Surg 1976;58:80.

4. Jost G, Levet Y. Parotid fascia and face lifting: a critical evaluation of the SMAS concept. Plast Reconstr Surg 1984;74:42–51.

5. Little JW. Applications of the classic dermal fat graft in primary and secondary facial rejuvenation. Plast Reconstr Surg 2002;109:788–804.

6. Stuzin MJ. Reoperations and refinements after rhytidectomy. In: Nahai F, editor. The art of aesthetic surgery: principles and techniques. St Louis (MO): QMP; 2005. p. 1286–326.

7. Guyuron B, Bokhari F, Thomas T. Secondary rhytidectomy. Plast Reconstr Surg 1997;100(5):1281–4.

8. Sarver MD, Proffit RW, Ackerman LJ. Evaluation of facial soft tissues. In: Rudolph P, Alvis K, editors. Contemporary treatment of dentofacial deformities. St Louis (MO): Mosby; 2003. p. 98–126.

9. Ellenbogen R, Karlin J. Visual criteria in restoring a youthful neck. Plast Reconstr Surg 1980;66:826–37.

10. Cuzalino A, Koehler J. Submentoplasty and facial liposuction. Oral Maxillofac Surg Clin North Am 2005;17(1):85–98.

11. Sundine JM, Kretsis V, Connell B. Longevity of SMAS facial rejuvenation and support. Plast Reconstr Surg 2010;126(1):229–39.

12. Duffy MJ, Friedland JA. The superficial-plane rhytidectomy revisited. Plast Reconstr Surg 1994;93:1392–403.

13. Connell BF, Semlacher RA. Contemporary deep layer facial rejuvenation. Plast Reconstr Surg 1997;100:1513–23.

14. Baker TJ, Stuzin JM. Personal technique of face lifting. Plast Reconstr Surg 1997;100:502–8.

15. Stuzin JM, Baker TJ, Gordon HL, et al. Extended SMAS dissection as an approach to midface rejuvenation. Clin Plast Surg 1995;22:295–311.

16. Baker DC. Lateral SMASectomy. Plast Reconstr Surg 1997;100:509–13.

17. Hamra ST. The deep-plane rhytidectomy. Plast Reconstr Surg 1990;86:53–9.

18. Hamra ST. Composite rhytidectomy. Plast Reconstr Surg 1992;90:1–13.

19. Ramirez OM, Maillard GF, Musolas A. The extended subperiosteal face lift: a definitive soft-tissue remodeling for facial rejuvenation. Plast Reconstr Surg 1991;88:227–36.

20. Tobin HA. The extended subperiosteal coronal lift. Am J Cosmet Surg 1993;10:47–57.

21. Tonnard P, Verpaele A. The MACS-lift short scar rhytidectomy. Aesthetic Plast Surg 2007;27:188–98.

Reoperative Temporomandibular Joint Surgery

Luis G. Vega, DDS[a],*, Rajesh Gutta, BDS, MS[b],
Patrick Louis, DDS, MD[c]

KEYWORDS

- TMJ reoperation • TMJ failures • TMJ arthrocentesis
- TMJ arthroscopy • TMJ diskoplasty • TMJ diskectomy

Temporomandibular joint (TMJ) surgery is perhaps one of the most controversial and challenging topics in oral and maxillofacial surgery. Although clear indications for TMJ surgery exist (**Boxes 1** and **2**), in numerous circumstances, multiple surgical procedures are suggested for the same TMJ condition. Clinicians are faced not only with the critical task of recognizing when or when not to operate but they also have to establish what is the most effective surgery to treat a particular patient. Unfortunately, TMJ surgeries are not always successful, and the patient's preoperative symptoms persist or may even increase after surgery. There are many potential pitfalls that can occur during any phase of the treatment that can lead to complications, less than desirable results, and short- or long-term failures. Unsatisfactory results can occur for multiple reasons, including misdiagnosis of the original pathologic condition, incorrect selection of surgical technique, technical failures, complications, systemic disease, and unrealistic expectations. This article focuses on the reoperation of the TMJ primarily in cases of internal derangement and specifically discusses TMJ arthrocentesis, arthroscopy, modified condylotomy, and open joint procedures.

PATIENT EVALUATION
History and Physical Examination

History and physical examination of the patient undergoing reoperative TMJ surgery do not differ much from the patient who needs primary TMJ surgery. Readers are referred to a comprehensive review on this topic published by Moore[1] in the *Oral and Maxillofacial Surgery Clinics of North America*. Special considerations must be taken to review all data from previous failed surgical and nonsurgical therapies in an effort to elucidate possible contributing factors for the unsatisfactory result. The patient's level of cooperation, perceptions, and expectations are vital to the surgeon's evaluation of the degree to which the current result can be improved.

Imaging

When reoperation is needed in our patients, most times adequate imaging studies that have been already obtained need to be reevaluated. In certain cases, the need for reoperation occurs several years after the original surgery and further imaging studies may be required for better diagnosis. The same holds true for referred patients for whom no imaging is available. Magnetic resonance

[a] Division of Oral and Maxillofacial Surgery, Department of Surgery, University of Florida, Health Science Center at Jacksonville, 653-1 West 8th Street, Jacksonville, FL 32209, USA
[b] Division of Oral and Maxillofacial Surgery, Department of Surgery, University of Cincinnati, 222 Piedmont Avenue, Cincinnati, OH 45219, USA
[c] Oral and Maxillofacial Residency Program, Department of Oral and Maxillofacial Surgery, School of Dentistry, University of Alabama at Birmingham, 1919 7th Avenue South, Birmingham, AL 35294, USA
* Corresponding author.
E-mail address: luis.vega@jax.ufl.edu

Oral Maxillofacial Surg Clin N Am 23 (2011) 119–132
doi:10.1016/j.coms.2010.12.001
1042-3699/11/$ – see front matter © 2011 Elsevier Inc. All rights reserved.

imaging continues to be the study of choice to evaluate the possibility of internal derangement, whereas plain films and computed tomographic scans are used to examine morphologic bony changes or TMJ replacements. Mercuri and Anspach[2] suggested several critical points to consider when doing a radiographic reevaluation of an alloplastic TMJ replacement (**Box 3**, **Fig. 1**).

SURGICAL GOALS AND DEFINITION OF SUCCESS

The goals of reoperative TMJ surgery are the same as primary surgery: (1) relief or reduction of temporomandibular pain, (2) improved range of motion and/or function, (3) limited period of disability, (4) appropriate understanding by patients of treatment options and acceptance of treatment plan, (5) appropriate understanding and acceptance by patients of favorable outcomes and known risks and complications.[3]

Studies in TMJ surgery contain a wide range of definitions of success or improvement.[4] Efforts to standardize clinical outcomes and criteria for success have been reported in the literature.[5] A definition of favorable therapeutic outcomes for TMJ surgery was published in 2007 by the American Association of Oral and Maxillofacial Surgeons (AAOMS) and is provided in **Box 4**.

ESTABLISHING REASONS FOR REOPERATION

Establishing the possible cause of the unsatisfactory outcome allows the surgeon to plan better for reoperation. Several causative factors have been described in the literature[2,6] and are discussed in the following sections.

Misdiagnosis of the Original Pathologic Condition/Patient Selection

Even after significant advances in the classification and understanding of the pathophysiology of TMJ disorders, misdiagnosis still plays an important role as a source of surgical failure. A thorough history and physical examination should allow the clinician to identify patients with nonoperative conditions such as myofascial pain, central neurogenic pain, and so forth, and patients with a pathologic condition related to a different anatomic structure than the TMJ (eg, parotid gland tumor).

Patient selection is not easy; the patient must show severe symptoms to be considered for surgery. Patients with mild or moderate symptoms

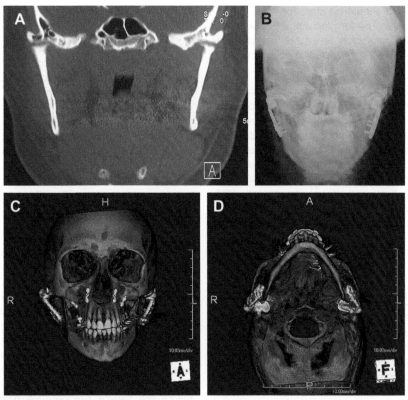

Fig. 1. Radiographic examination includes the reevaluation of imaging of previous stages of treatment. Failed alloplastic TMJ prosthesis. (*A*) Original computed tomographic (CT) scan showing signs of bilateral severe TMJ degeneration. (*B*) Postoperative plain film showing placement of bilateral stock prostheses. (*C, D*) New 3-dimensional CT scan reconstructions for reevaluation of the prostheses 5 years after placement.

may be more suitable for nonsurgical therapies. The literature also suggests that the likelihood of improvement in function and pain management decreases after multiple surgical procedures.[7]

Box 4
AAOMS favorable therapeutic outcomes for TMJ surgery

- A level of pain that is of little or no concern to the patient and preferably measured objectively (eg, visual analog scale)
- Improved mandibular function that is compatible with mastication, deglutition, speech, and oral hygiene
- A stable occlusion
- Acceptable clinical appearance
- Limited period of disability
- Patient acceptance of procedure and understanding of outcome

Data from American Association of Oral and Maxillofacial Surgeons. Parameters of care: clinical practice guidelines for oral and maxillofacial surgery (AAOMS ParCare07). 2007.

Additional considerations should be given to patients with psychiatric disorders, drug-dependent behavior, or unrealistic expectations.

Inappropriate Procedure

Another challenge in the surgical management of TMJ disorders is the lack of one universally accepted surgical protocol. Multiple procedures have been described in the literature to treat the same condition, with similar success rates.[8,9] The lack of high levels of evidence with randomized clinical trials comparing surgical treatments with placebo or no treatment makes it difficult to conclusively determine the efficacy of different TMJ surgical procedures. However, in a meta-analysis of surgical treatment of TMJ articular disorders, Reston and Turkelson[10] demonstrated that TMJ surgery seems to provide some benefit to patients in whom nonsurgical management failed. They also concluded that the most reliable evidence supports the effectiveness of minimally invasive surgical therapies, such as arthrocentesis or arthroscopic lysis and lavage, for the treatment of patients with disk displacement without reduction. Still, it should be clear for the clinician that, for example, performing an arthrocentesis for TMJ fibrous ankylosis is a poor selection of surgical technique for that specific condition.

Surgeon's Experience

The importance of proper training and constant involvement in TMJ surgery cannot be overemphasized. Occasional or inexperienced TMJ surgeons can take incorrect decisions in the operating room. Such decisions could lead to complications that later require further surgery. Furthermore, Kirk and Kirk[11] suggested that training of TMJ surgeons must include knowledge of the 3-dimensional functional and biomechanical principles that influence the TMJ system to allow better diagnosis and selection of the initial surgical modality.

Complications

Several reviews on TMJ surgery complications have been published in the literature.[12,13] Although the incidence of reoperation due to complications is unknown, not all complications require reoperation. Complications such as infection, heterotopic bone formation, and hardware failure are some of the indications for reoperation that have been described in the literature.[2,6]

Systemic Disease

Several systemic diseases are known to affect the TMJ, including rheumatoid arthritis, psoriatic arthritis, and ankylosing spondylitis. Although the primary surgical management of these disease processes may require minimally invasive techniques such as arthrocentesis or arthoscopic lysis and lavage, progression of the disease will eventually demand more invasive procedures such as diskectomies or total joint replacement. Furthermore, in a pilot study in which clinical and laboratory analyses were used for risk assessment criteria for TMJ surgical therapy, Halpern and colleagues[14] suggested that surgical failure may be secondary to autoimmune dysfunction with a predisposition to multisystem disease.

Improper Postoperative Care

The role of postoperative care in the success of the TMJ surgery is as essential as the surgery itself. Even when the best surgical procedure is performed, if no postoperative care is enforced, the likelihood of failure increases. Necessary physiotherapy to ensure adequate rehabilitation needs to be implemented, and patient compliance is vital.[15]

REOPERATIVE SURGICAL OPTIONS
Arthrocentesis

Arthrocentesis is a simple, minimally invasive, and low-risk surgical procedure that was described by Murakami and colleagues[16] and later modified by Nitzan and colleagues.[17] Tozoglu and colleagues[18] reviewed the different modifications of this procedure. Arthrocentesis has been described as highly diagnostic and therapeutic. It has been used with good success on patients with anterior disk displacement without reduction and anchored disk phenomenon and to a lesser extent in patients with osteoarthritis.[19] In a comprehensive literature review on TMJ arthrocentesis by Al-Belasy and Dolwick,[20] an overall success rate of 83.2% in cases of closed lock was reported. How arthrocentesis works is still unknown, but it is thought that the procedure reduces the friction between the articular surfaces, breaks up fine adhesions, and washes out chemical mediators of pain and inflammation.[19,20] Medications such as sodium hyaluronate,[21] steroids,[20] and morphine[22] have been used, but evidence for their effectiveness is still inconclusive. Nishimura and colleagues[23] suggested that possible prognostic factors for arthrocentesis failure are severe preoperative pain, relapse in the amount of mouth opening within 1 week after the procedure, and preoperative bony changes in the condyle. In addition, synovial fluid research has shown an increased level of inflammatory mediators in unsuccessful cases treated with arthrocentesis.[24,25]

The role of reoperative TMJ arthrocentesis is yet to be established. Following successful protocols in other joints, several investigators[26,27] have studied the effect of a cycle of 5 arthrocenteses with the implementation of hyaluronic acid (once weekly) on patients with osteoarthritis and reported good preliminary results. Furthermore, in a pilot study, Guarda-Nardini and colleagues[28] used the same protocol in patients with disk displacement with reduction, with relative good short-term results. Additional research is needed to determine the efficacy of reoperative arthrocentesis in other clinical situations such as previous failed arthrocentesis or patients who present with new symptoms several years after a successful TMJ surgery (eg, new onset of closed lock in a patient who previously had a successful TMJ arthroscopy or diskoplasty).

Surgical considerations
The surgical technique for reoperative TMJ arthrocentesis is basically the same as the primary surgery with the only difference that joint palpation

may be more difficult because of scarring from previous surgery.

Arthroscopy

TMJ arthroscopy is a minimally invasive technique with a high diagnostic and therapeutic value and was originally described for the lysis of adhesions and joint lavage under direct visualization. After technological advances, it has allowed surgeons to develop operative techniques with minimal morbidity for the management of several TMJ conditions such as TMJ disk displacements, osteoarthritis, chronic dislocations, and other pathologic entities including synovial chondromatosis. Several investigators have proved the value of TMJ arthroscopy especially for the treatment of TMJ internal derangements.[29–33] An analysis of 4561 patients in a systematic review of TMJ arthroscopy revealed that 80% of the patients reported improvement in pain and functional symptoms after the procedure.[34] There are many different approaches and philosophies regarding the arthroscopic management of TMJ conditions. Because repositioning of the disk within the joint has not been proved to be essential for a successful outcome, the surgeon must take a decision how best to approach the patient's problem. In a prospective study to determine the efficacy of TMJ arthroscopic lysis and lavage correlated with Wilkes classification, Smolka and colleagues[35] found no significant difference between the success rates for Wilkes stages II to V. They concluded that when surgery is indicated, TMJ arthroscopy should be performed as a standard operation for internal derangement in all Wilkes stages. In a retrospective case series that included 344 joints, González-García and colleagues[36] reported no statistical differences in the outcome between arthroscopic lysis and lavage and operative arthroscopy for patients with chronic closed lock. Similar conclusions were obtained by Miyamoto and colleagues[37] and White.[38]

Few reports in the literature have analyzed the incidence and the role of reoperative arthroscopy. Indresano[39] compared his experience of TMJ arthroscopy lysis and lavage (103 patients) with operative arthroscopy (121 patients) and found lower incidence of reoperation in operative arthroscopy (9%) than arthroscopic lysis and lavage (37%). Abd-Ul-Salam and colleagues[40] reviewed 450 TMJ arthroscopies and reported that the reoperation rate was 20%. Most of the failed joints were classified as Bronstein-Merrill stages IV to V during the first arthroscopic procedure. Further analysis showed that repeat arthroscopies were performed within 6 to 12 months after the primary surgery. In addition, 10% of the patients after the second surgical arthroscopy underwent further surgical intervention.

Mancha de la Plata and colleagues[41] studied the role of a second TMJ arthroscopy after an unsuccessful TMJ arthroscopy. They analyzed 550 patients who underwent TMJ arthroscopy, and the incidence of reoperation was found to be 10.9%. Ten of the 60 patients who required reoperation underwent open joint procedures based on the unfavorable clinical evolution and severe articular changes (Bronstein-Merrill stages IV–V). Forty-six of the 50 remaining patients underwent a second operative arthroscopy, whereas only 4 had an arthroscopic lysis and lavage. The second arthroscopy was performed within 12 to 72 months after the primary TMJ arthroscopic procedure. The most common finding was chondromalacia, followed by adhesions. Worsening of the Bronstein-Merrill staging after the first TMJ arthroscopy was also found. In addition, pain and function had a statistically significant improvement after the second procedure and it was maintained at a 2-year follow-up. Finally, 8 patients (16%) had an unsuccessful result after their second arthroscopy and required further open joint surgery.

These previous studies may suggest that although many surgeons would consider a different operation if TMJ arthroscopy has failed, there is some literature to suggest that a second TMJ arthroscopy may be of benefit because it takes advantage of the strengths of the original procedure. One must consider the time frame in which the failure occurred. If the patient did not receive any relief from the primary procedure, a different procedure should be contemplated. The Bronstein-Merill stage at the time of the original operation may play a role in helping the surgeon make a decision. Further studies should determine the effectiveness of reoperative TMJ arthroscopy in other clinical situations such as a previous failed condylotomy or patients who present with new symptoms several years after a successful TMJ surgery (eg, new onset of closed lock in a patient who previously had a successful TMJ diskoplasty).

Surgical considerations

If reoperative TMJ arthroscopy is planned after a failed TMJ arthroscopy, the basic surgical technique is essentially the same as that of primary surgery. A normal diagnostic sweep should be performed; findings and staging should be further documented. If deemed necessary, the surgeon should consider arthroscopic operative techniques that are beyond the scope of this article.

In the presence of a previous open joint procedure, scar tissue and possibly the lack of mandibular mobility make the identification of key anatomic landmarks, the palpation of the articular surfaces, and ultimately the joint puncture more challenging. Cases of fibrous ankylosis are particularly challenging, and care must be taken to avoid further damage of the articular surfaces and adjacent structures. Once within the joint, a diagnostic sweep must be done. Often visualization is difficult because of important anatomic alterations. Lysis of adhesions or other operative arthroscopic techniques can also be implemented.

Condylotomy

Modified condylotomy is an extra-articular operation that does not directly involve the articular surfaces. Essentially, the procedure consists of an intraoral vertical ramus osteotomy in which the medial pterygoid muscle is detached to allow for 3 to 4 mm of condylar sag. Ideally, the downward position of the condylar segment increases the joint space, reducing the load on the retrodiskal tissue and relieving the pain and dysfunction.[42] Modified condylotomy has been used for anterior disk displacement with reduction (94% successful)[43] and anterior displacement without reduction (87% successful).[44] Two interesting facts about this procedure are (1) it is claimed that it can result in a more normal disk-condyle relationship[45] and (2) it seems to positively affect the progression of the disease.[46]

The incidence of reoperation after modified condylotomy has been reported to be between 4.4% and 5.1%.[47–49] In a retrospective study, Hall and Werther[49] reviewed 361 joints, and the incidence of reoperation was 4.4%. Although the reoperation rate varied according to the disk status, the differences were not statistically significant (anterior disk displacement with reduction, 3.9%; anterior disk displacement without reduction, 6.5%). The period between modified condylotomy and reoperation ranged from 1 to 63 months. Diskectomy was performed in 10 joints, and 5 other joints had a modified condylotomy redone. One patient required a modified condylotomy as a third surgical procedure, 8 months after a diskectomy. Two possible risk factors for failure were identified: loss of superior joint space and persistent disk displacement. The role of modified condylotomy in the treatment of previous failed TMJ arthrocentesis, arthroscopy, or open joint procedures is yet to be determined.

There are 3 potential complications in modified condylotomy that may require reoperation: excessive condylar sag with condylar dislocation, malocclusion, and fracture of the condylar segment.

Excessive condylar sag with condylar dislocation

Avoidance of excessive condylar sag with or without condylar dislocation can be achieved with judicious detachment of the medial pterygoid muscle. As a general rule, it requires more muscle detachment in young individuals than in older patients. If excessive movement is found intraoperatively, stabilization with either wires or a miniplate can be obtained. If the dislocation is found during the healing process, prompt surgical repositioning of the condylar segment and stabilization with wires or a miniplate must be achieved (**Fig. 2**). If uncorrected, this complication can result in postoperative pain and malocclusion.

Malocclusion

Significant malocclusion is uncommon after modified condylotomy. However, 22% of patients with anterior disk displacement without reduction reported that their bite felt worse after a modified condylotomy. All but 1 of these patients required only minor occlusal equilibration. One patient elected to undergo Le Fort I and bilateral sagittal split osteotomies to correct a 3-mm overjet after a bilateral modified condylotomy.[44] Special attention must be paid to the postoperative use of elastics to avoid this problem. Postsurgical orthodontic evaluation may be useful to avoid further surgery.

Fracture of the condylar segment

This complication is seldom reported in the literature and is related mostly to bad surgical technique or the surgeon's inexperience. Inadequate visualization and lack of identification of the key landmarks may lead to an improper osteotomy that when manipulated can fracture. The fracture segments are then treated in a similar fashion as a regular mandibular fracture using closed or open reduction and internal fixation techniques (**Fig. 3**). Better visualization to avoid this problem can be achieved by using endoscopy or the LeVasseur-Merrill retractor (**Fig. 4**). This device is hooked around the posterior border of the mandible at the level of the occlusal plane, allowing the osteotomy to be consistently placed approximately 7 mm anterior to the posterior border. In an anatomic study of the position of the mandibular foramen in relation to the LeVasseur-Merrill retractor, da Fontoura and colleagues[50] showed that the mandibular foramen was located within 7 mm of the posterior edge of the mandible in only 3.3% of the rami. When properly placed, the LeVasseur-Merrill retractor was effective in avoiding the inferior alveolar nerve in 98.9% of the analyzed rami.

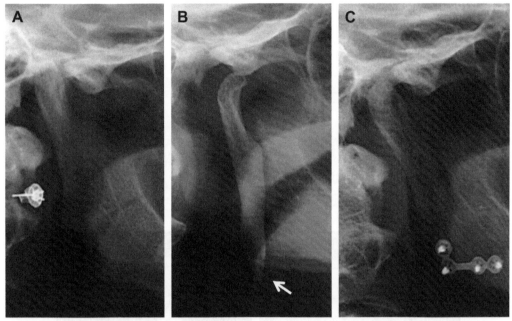

Fig. 2. Excessive condylar sag after modified condylotomy. (*A*) Preoperative radiograph. (*B*) Postoperative radiograph showing excessive condylar sag (*arrow*) after a modified condylotomy. (*C*) Radiograph taken after reoperation to stabilize the condylar segment with a miniplate.

Surgical considerations

If reoperative modified condylotomy is used as a second procedure after failed TMJ arthrocentesis, arthroscopy, or open joint surgery, the technique is basically the same as in primary surgery. The only significant difference is that condylar sag may be more difficult to achieve due to capsular scarring. In such cases, a predictable downward position of the condylar segment can be maintained by wires or miniplate fixation.

When the procedure is essentially redone, it should focus on the adequate repositioning of the condylar segment. Key landmarks must be properly identified and visualized, including posterior ramus, mandibular angle, and sigmoid notch. Special attention must be taken to the width of the osteotomy to avoid injury to the inferior alveolar nerve as a result of anatomic variations after the original surgery.

Open Joint Procedures

Open joint procedures were the first procedures performed for TMJ repair. Classically, they include diskoplasty, diskectomy, and TMJ replacements, but many other variations of these techniques have been described in the literature and are not covered in this article. Studies have suggested that success rates with this type of procedure are similar to more conservative procedures such as TMJ arthrocentesis, arthroscopy, and even modified condylotomy.[8,9,51,52] Still, some investigators[11,53,54] have advocated open joint procedures as first-line treatment. According to Dimitroulis,[55] 3 main controversies exist in open joint surgery: (1) the role of disk repositioning surgery in light of the results of TMJ arthrocentesis and arthroscopic lysis and lavage, (2) the necessity for disk replacement after diskectomy, and (3) the use of alloplastic TMJ replacements for end-stage TMJ disease.

Diskoplasty

The technique usually involves plication of the disk posteriorly by using sutures. Other techniques involve resection of the posterior disk attachment and repair by suturing the disk in a more posterior position. The literature reports a success rate of 80% to 95% with these procedures, but Dolwick[56] suspects that the reported successes may have been overstated.

In a retrospective study of 186 joints treated with diskoplasty, Kirk[57] demonstrated that surgical failure seemed to increase in patients with Wilkes stage III disease, especially when the degree of qualitative tissue changes, advancing arthrosis, or associated risk factors (decreased joint space, skeletal malocclusion, missing posterior support) were present in increasing frequency. Studying the clinical outcome of diskoplasty after a failed TMJ arthroscopy, Van Sickles and Dolezal[58] found

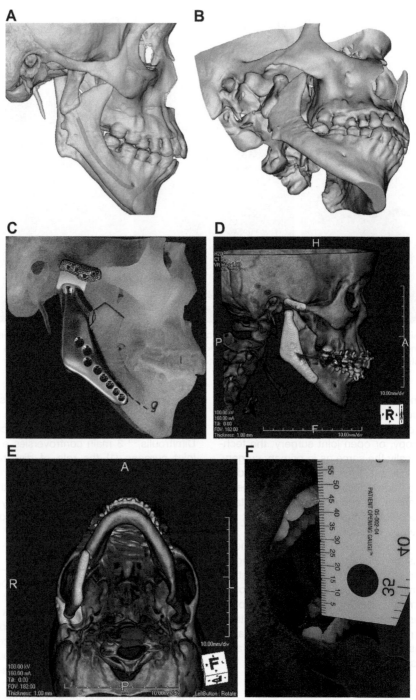

Fig. 3. Alloplastic TMJ replacement for complications caused by modified condylotomy. A 35-year-old woman had a condylar segment fracture during a right mandibular modified condylotomy. Surgeons unsuccessfully tried to stabilize the segments. One year later, the patient presented to the authors' institution complaining of pain and dysfunction. After clinical and radiographic evaluation, it was established that the patient required an allo-plastic TMJ replacement. (*A*, *B*) Three-dimensional (3D) computed tomographic (CT) scan reconstructions after failed modified condylotomy. Note the lack of bone stock in the mandibular ramus and the level of dislocation of the condylar segment. (*C*) Custom-made alloplastic TMJ prosthesis that included the creation of a new mandib-ular angle for mandibular symmetry. (*D*, *E*) Postoperative 3D CT scan reconstructions showing good prosthesis placement and achievement of mandibular symmetry. (*F*) Patient's postoperative maximum interincisal opening 9 months after the TMJ replacement surgery.

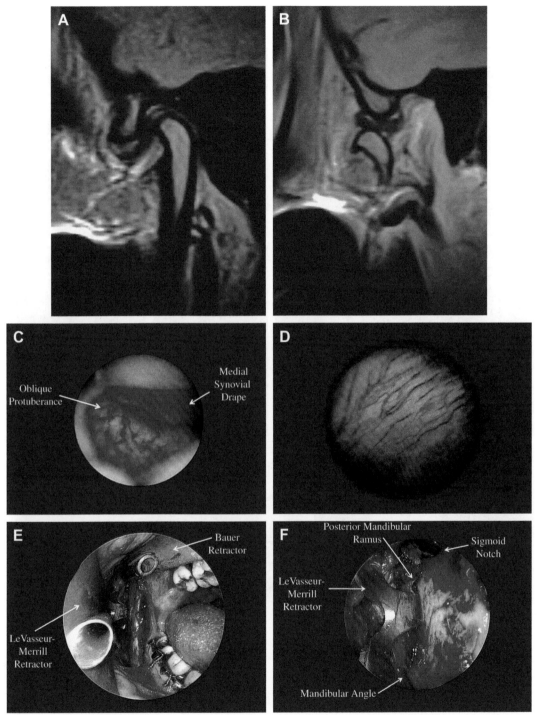

Fig. 4. Modified condylotomy after a failed TMJ arthroscopy. After nonsurgical management failed, a 32-year-old woman underwent a TMJ arthroscopy for TMJ internal derangement. Arthroscopic findings show significant synovitis but no adhesions. During the next 5 months of postoperative conservative treatment, patient continued to have moderate to severe pain and dysfunction. After further discussion of the risks, complications, and limitations of different TMJ surgical options, the patient decided to undergo an endoscopically assisted modified condylotomy, with success at 18 months' follow-up. (*A*) Closed and (*B*) open TMJ magnetic resonance images depicting an anterior disk displacement with reduction. (*C*) Arthroscopic view showing significant synovitis in the posterior recess. (*D*) Close-up of synovitis at the medial synovial drape. (*E*) Retractor placement for endoscopically assisted modified condylotomy. (*F*) LeVassuer-Merrill retractor in place showing the posterior ramus, sigmoid notch, and mandibular angle. (*G*) Angled oscillating saw blade in proper position against the LeVassuer-Merrill retractor. (*H*) Osteotomy completed. (*I*) Detachment of medial pterygoid muscle. (*J*) Checking for condylar sag with the amount of downward displacement of the condylar segment. (*K*) Wire fixation. (*L*) Postoperative radiograph.

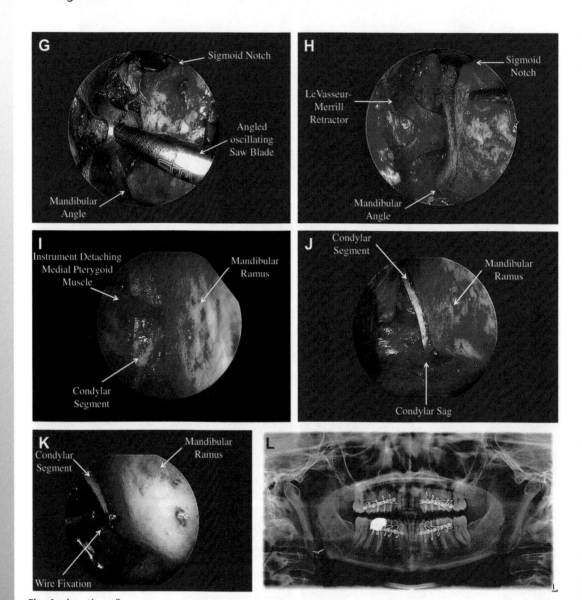

Fig. 4. (continued)

improvement in 5 of the 9 patients studied and they suggested caution when offering this option to patients. Further studies are needed to determine the value of reoperative TMJ diskoplasty.

Surgical considerations

In cases in which the primary surgery was TMJ arthrocentesis, arthroscopy, or modified condylotomy, the technique for reoperative diskoplasty is the same as that for primary diskoplasty.

In comparison, when the technique is used for revision diskoplasty, the surgeon will likely encounter variations in the anatomic landmarks that will make a safe surgical approach more challenging. The focus should be on proper positioning of the disk. It is important to mobilize the disk before suturing. Releasing the lateral attachment and stretching the anterior attachment of the disk before suturing usually provide mobilization. Any disk that cannot be mobilized before repair is likely to fail secondary to suture tearing with a subsequent disk perforation. Other techniques can also be considered, such as disk fixation with anchor implants.[59,60] Once the disk has undergone deformation from being dislocated for an extended period, it is difficult to maintain it in its posterior position. In addition, when diskoplasty fails, consideration should be given to arthroscopy or diskectomy. Further research is needed to establish the role of reoperative diskoplasty.

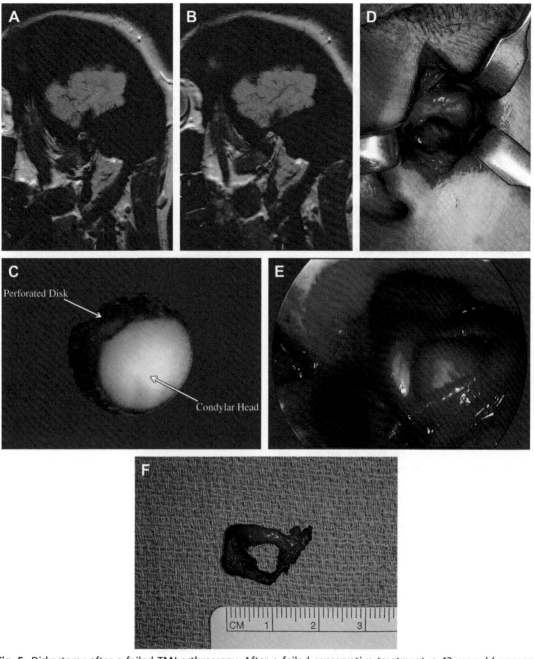

Fig. 5. Diskectomy after a failed TMJ arthroscopy. After a failed conservative treatment, a 43-year-old woman underwent a right TMJ arthroscopic lysis and lavage for pain and dysfunction caused by TMJ internal derangement. Arthroscopic findings showed a perforated disk. After 8 months of postoperative nonsurgical treatment, the patient's pain failed to improve. After discussion of the risks, complications, and limitations of different TMJ surgical options, the patient decided to undergo a diskectomy for the Wilkes stage V internal derangement, with success at 2 years' follow-up. (*A*) Closed and (*B*) open TMJ magnetic resonance images showing an anterior disk displacement with limited reduction. (*C*) Arthroscopic view of the condylar head through the perforated disk. (*D*, *E*) Intraoperative and close-up photographs depicting the perforated disk. (*F*) Surgical specimen of a large irreparable disk perforation.

Diskectomy

Diskectomy is probably the most common and most studied TMJ procedure.[61] Diskectomy is performed for articular disks that are deformed or with unsalvageable perforations. It has the advantage that eliminates unfavorable mechanical interferences. Many alloplastic implants and autogenous materials have been used for disk replacement, but no ideal material has been identified. Furthermore, the literature has failed to demonstrate the advantages of autogenous tissues for disk replacement when compared with diskectomy.[62]

It has been suggested that failures after diskectomies are caused by inadequate control of the joint load during the first 6 to 12 months after the procedure and poor physiotherapy.[61]

In a retrospective study of 117 joints treated with diskectomy, Kirk[57] showed that the presence of osteoporosis or other medical conditions that may influence the quality of articular bone surface seems to be a significant surgical risk factor. Eriksson and Westesson[63] reported in a 5-year clinical and radiographic follow-up study that the incidence of reoperation was 5%. In another study to subjectively and objectively assess the temporalis muscle flap in previously operated TMJs (mostly diskectomies with Proplast implant), Smith and colleagues[64] found an improvement of 65% in pain and functional levels.

In general, if diskectomy fails, prosthetic joint replacement is recommended. As with previous TMJ procedures, if diskectomy is used to reoperate on a patient after another failed TMJ procedure, the technique is basically the same as that of a primary diskectomy (**Fig. 5**).

Alloplastic Reconstruction

Alloplastic TMJ replacement has been used to treat patients with end-stage TMJ disease, with long-term successful outcomes.[65] In the patient operated multiple times, alloplastic TMJ replacement has been used as salvage surgery with the goals of (1) decreasing or eliminating the pain, (2) increasing mandibular mobility, and (3) restoring mandibular asymmetry and occlusion.

Several excellent reviews on revision surgery, surgical failures, and management of infections in alloplastic TMJ replacement have been reported in the literature, and the readers are referred to them for further review.[2,6,66]

SUMMARY

It is not realistic to expect 100% success rates in TMJ surgery. Correct diagnosis, careful patient selection, surgeon's experience, and proper postoperative care are some of the key features to achieve surgical success. The lack of high levels of evidence with randomized clinical trials comparing surgical treatments with placebo or no treatment makes it difficult to conclusively determine the efficacy of different TMJ surgical procedures. When contemplating surgical failure and the necessity for reoperation, the surgeon must take into account all the different variables of the disease process to select the best surgical solution with the highest probability of success.

REFERENCES

1. Moore LJ. Evaluation of the patient for temporomandibular joint surgery. Oral Maxillofac Surg Clin North Am 2006;18(3):291–303.
2. Mercuri LG, Anspach WE. Principles for the revision of total alloplastic TMJ prostheses. Int J Oral Maxillofac Surg 2003;32(4):353–9.
3. American Association of Oral and Maxillofacial Surgeons. Parameters of care: clinical practice guidelines for oral and maxillofacial surgery (AAOMS ParCare07). 2007.
4. Kropmans TJ, Dijkstra PU, Stegenga B, et al. Therapeutic outcome assessment in permanent temporomandibular joint disc displacement. J Oral Rehabil 1999;26(5):357–63.
5. Holmlund AB. Surgery for TMJ internal derangement. Evaluation of treatment outcome and criteria for success. Int J Oral Maxillofac Surg 1993;22(2):75–7.
6. Quinn P, Giannakopoulos H, Carrasco L. Management of surgical failures. Oral Maxillofac Surg Clin North Am 2006;18(3):411–7.
7. Bradrick J, Indresano A. Failure rates or repetitive temporomandibular joint surgical procedures. J Oral Maxillofac Surg 1992;50(Suppl 3):145.
8. Hall HD, Indresano AT, Kirk WS, et al. Prospective multicenter comparison of 4 temporomandibular joint operations. J Oral Maxillofac Surg 2005;63(8):1174–9.
9. Ng CH, Lai JB, Victor F, et al. Temporomandibular articular disorders can be alleviated with surgery. Evid Based Dent 2005;6(2):48–50.
10. Reston JT, Turkelson CM. Meta-analysis of surgical treatments for temporomandibular articular disorders. J Oral Maxillofac Surg 2003;61(1):3–10 [discussion: 10–2].
11. Kirk WS, Kirk BS. A biomechanical basis for primary arthroplasty of the temporomandibular joint. Oral Maxillofac Surg Clin North Am 2006;18(3):345–68.
12. Dolwick F. Complications of temporomandibular joint surgery. In: Kaban L, Pogrel A, Perrot D, editors. Complications in oral and maxillofacial surgery. 1st edition. Philadelphia: WB Saunders; 1997. p. 89–103.

13. Keith DA. Complications of temporomandibular joint surgery. Oral Maxillofac Surg Clin North Am 2003; 15(2):187–94.

14. Halpern LR, Chase DC, Gerard DA, et al. Temporomandibular disorders: clinical and laboratory analyses for risk assessment of criteria for surgical therapy, a pilot study. Cranio 1998;16(1): 35–43.

15. Israel HA, Syrop SB. The important role of motion in the rehabilitation of patients with mandibular hypomobility: a review of the literature. Cranio 1997; 15(1):74–83.

16. Murakami KI, Iizuka T, Matsuki M, et al. Recapturing the persistent anteriorly displaced disk by mandibular manipulation after pumping and hydraulic pressure to the upper joint cavity of the temporomandibular joint. Cranio 1987;5(1):17–24.

17. Nitzan DW, Dolwick MF, Martinez GA. Temporomandibular joint arthrocentesis: a simplified treatment for severe, limited mouth opening. J Oral Maxillofac Surg 1991;49(11):1163–7 [discussion: 1168–70].

18. Tozoglu S, Al-Belasy FA, Dolwick MF. A review of techniques of lysis and lavage of the TMJ. Br J Oral Maxillofac Surg 2010. DOI:10.1016/j.bjoms.2010.03.008.

19. Nitzan DW. Arthrocentesis-incentives for using this minimally invasive approach for temporomandibular disorders. Oral Maxillofac Surg Clin North Am 2006; 18(3):311–28.

20. Al-Belasy FA, Dolwick MF. Arthrocentesis for the treatment of temporomandibular joint closed lock: a review article. Int J Oral Maxillofac Surg 2007; 36(9):773–82.

21. Alpaslan GH, Alpaslan C. Efficacy of temporomandibular joint arthrocentesis with and without injection of sodium hyaluronate in treatment of internal derangements. J Oral Maxillofac Surg 2001;59(6): 613–8 [discussion: 618–9].

22. Kunjur J, Anand R, Brennan PA, et al. An audit of 405 temporomandibular joint arthrocentesis with intra-articular morphine infusion. Br J Oral Maxillofac Surg 2003;41(1):29–31.

23. Nishimura M, Segami N, Kaneyama K, et al. Prognostic factors in arthrocentesis of the temporomandibular joint: evaluation of 100 patients with internal derangement. J Oral Maxillofac Surg 2001;59(8): 874–7 [discussion: 878].

24. Nishimura M, Segami N, Kaneyama K, et al. Comparison of cytokine level in synovial fluid between successful and unsuccessful cases in arthrocentesis of the temporomandibular joint. J Oral Maxillofac Surg 2004;62(3):284–7 [discussion: 287–8].

25. Kaneyama K, Segami N, Sato J, et al. Factors in arthrocentesis of the temporomandibular joint: comparison of bradykinin, leukotriene B4, prostaglandin E2, and substance P level in synovial fluid between successful and unsuccessful cases. J Oral Maxillofac Surg 2007;65(2):242–7.

26. Guarda-Nardini L, Stifano M, Brombin C, et al. A one-year case series of arthrocentesis with hyaluronic acid injections for temporomandibular joint osteoarthritis. Oral Surg Oral Med Oral Pathol Oral Radiol Endod 2007;103(6):e14–22.

27. Manfredini D, Bonnini S, Arboretti R, et al. Temporomandibular joint osteoarthritis: an open label trial of 76 patients treated with arthrocentesis plus hyaluronic acid injections. Int J Oral Maxillofac Surg 2009;38(8):827–34.

28. Guarda-Nardini L, Manfredini D, Ferronato G. Short-term effects of arthrocentesis plus viscosupplementation in the management of signs and symptoms of painful TMJ disc displacement with reduction. A pilot study. Oral Maxillofac Surg 2010;14(1):29–34.

29. Moses JJ, Poker ID. TMJ arthroscopic surgery: an analysis of 237 patients. J Oral Maxillofac Surg 1989;47(8):790–4.

30. McCain JP, Sanders B, Koslin MG, et al. Temporomandibular joint arthroscopy: a 6-year multicenter retrospective study of 4,831 joints. J Oral Maxillofac Surg 1992;50(9):926–30.

31. Stegenga B, de Bont LG, Dijkstra PU, et al. Short-term outcome of arthroscopic surgery of temporomandibular joint osteoarthrosis and internal derangement: a randomized controlled clinical trial. Br J Oral Maxillofac Surg 1993;31(1):3–14.

32. Sorel B, Piecuch JF. Long-term evaluation following temporomandibular joint arthroscopy with lysis and lavage. Int J Oral Maxillofac Surg 2000;29(4):259–63.

33. Murakami K, Segami N, Okamoto M, et al. Outcome of arthroscopic surgery for internal derangement of the temporomandibular joint: long-term results covering 10 years. J Craniomaxillofac Surg 2000; 28(5):264–71.

34. Montini R, Hayes C, Antczak-Bouckoms A, et al. Systematic review of arthroscopic treatment of temporomandibular joint disorder [abstract #1340]. J Dent Res 2002;81:A-184.

35. Smolka W, Yanai C, Smolka K, et al. Efficiency of arthroscopic lysis and lavage for internal derangement of the temporomandibular joint correlated with Wilkes classification. Oral Surg Oral Med Oral Pathol Oral Radiol Endod 2008;106(3):317–23.

36. González-García R, Rodríguez-Campo FJ, Monje F, et al. Operative versus simple arthroscopic surgery for chronic closed lock of the temporomandibular joint: a clinical study of 344 arthroscopic procedures. Int J Oral Maxillofac Surg 2008;37(9):790–6.

37. Miyamoto H, Sakashita H, Miyata M, et al. Arthroscopic surgery of the temporomandibular joint: comparison of two successful techniques. Br J Oral Maxillofac Surg 1999;37(5):397–400.

38. White RD. Arthroscopic lysis and lavage as the preferred treatment for internal derangement of the temporomandibular joint. J Oral Maxillofac Surg 2001;59(3):313–6.

39. Indresano AT. Surgical arthroscopy as the preferred treatment for internal derangements of the temporomandibular joint. J Oral Maxillofac Surg 2001;59(3):308–12.

40. Abd-Ul-Salam H, Weinberg S, Kryshtalskyj B. The incidence of reoperation after temporomandibular joint arthroscopic surgery: a retrospective study of 450 consecutive joints. Oral Surg Oral Med Oral Pathol Oral Radiol Endod 2002;93(4):408–11.

41. Mancha de la Plata M, Muñoz-Guerra M, Escorial Hernandez V, et al. Unsuccessful temporomandibular joint arthroscopy: is a second arthroscopy an acceptable alternative? J Oral Maxillofac Surg 2008;66(10):2086–92.

42. McKenna SJ. Modified mandibular condylotomy. Oral Maxillofac Surg Clin North Am 2006;18(3):369–81.

43. Hall HD, Navarro EZ, Gibbs SJ. One- and three-year prospective outcome study of modified condylotomy for treatment of reducing disc displacement. J Oral Maxillofac Surg 2000;58(1):7–17 [discussion: 18].

44. Hall HD, Navarro EZ, Gibbs SJ. Prospective study of modified condylotomy for treatment of nonreducing disk displacement. Oral Surg Oral Med Oral Pathol Oral Radiol Endod 2000;89(2):147–58.

45. Werther JR, Hall HD, Gibbs SJ. Disk position before and after modified condylotomy in 80 symptomatic temporomandibular joints. Oral Surg Oral Med Oral Pathol Oral Radiol Endod 1995;79(6):668–79.

46. McKenna SJ, Cornella F, Gibbs SJ. Long-term follow-up of modified condylotomy for internal derangement of the temporomandibular joint. Oral Surg Oral Med Oral Pathol Oral Radiol Endod 1996;81(5):509–15.

47. Upton LG. The case for mandibular condylotomy in the treatment of the painful, deranged temporomandibular joint. J Oral Maxillofac Surg 1997;55(1):64–9.

48. Albury CD. Modified condylotomy for chronic nonreducing disk dislocations. Oral Surg Oral Med Oral Pathol Oral Radiol Endod 1997;84(3):234–40.

49. Hall HD, Werther JR. Results of reoperation after failed modified condylotomy. J Oral Maxillofac Surg 1997;55(11):1250–3.

50. da Fontoura RA, Vasconcellos HA, Campos AE. Morphologic basis for the intraoral vertical ramus osteotomy: anatomic and radiographic localization of the mandibular foramen. J Oral Maxillofac Surg 2002;60(6):660–5 [discussion: 665–6].

51. Holmlund AB, Axelsson S, Gynther GW. A comparison of discectomy and arthroscopic lysis and lavage for the treatment of chronic closed lock of the temporomandibular joint: a randomized outcome study. J Oral Maxillofac Surg 2001;59(9):972–7 [discussion: 977–8].

52. Undt G, Murakami KI, Rasse M, et al. Open versus arthroscopic surgery for internal derangement of the temporomandibular joint: a retrospective study comparing two centres' results using the Jaw Pain and Function Questionnaire. J Craniomaxillofac Surg 2006;34(4):234–41.

53. Holmlund A. Disc derangements of the temporomandibular joint. A tissue-based characterization and implications for surgical treatment. Int J Oral Maxillofac Surg 2007;36(7):571–6.

54. Miloro M, Henriksen B. Discectomy as the primary surgical option for internal derangement of the temporomandibular joint. J Oral Maxillofac Surg 2010;68(4):782–9.

55. Dimitroulis G. The role of surgery in the management of disorders of the temporomandibular joint: a critical review of the literature. Part 2. Int J Oral Maxillofac Surg 2005;34(3):231–7.

56. Dolwick MF. Disc preservation surgery for the treatment of internal derangements of the temporomandibular joint. J Oral Maxillofac Surg 2001;59(9):1047–50.

57. Kirk WS. Risk factors and initial surgical failures of TMJ arthrotomy and arthroplasty: a four to nine year evaluation of 303 surgical procedures. Cranio 1998;16(3):154–61.

58. Van Sickels JE, Dolezal J. Clinical outcome of arthrotomy after failed arthroscopy. Oral Surg Oral Med Oral Pathol 1994;78(2):142–5.

59. Mehra P, Wolford LM. The Mitek mini anchor for TMJ disc repositioning: surgical technique and results. Int J Oral Maxillofac Surg 2001;30(6):497–503.

60. Sembronio S, Robiony M, Politi M. Disc-repositioning surgery of the temporomandibular joint using bioresorbable screws. Int J Oral Maxillofac Surg 2006;35(12):1149–52.

61. McKenna S. Discectomy for the treatment of internal derangements of the temporomandibular joint. J Oral Maxillofac Surg 2001;59(9):1051–6.

62. Kramer A, Lee J, Beirne OR. Meta-analysis of TMJ discectomy with or without autogenous/alloplastic interpositional material: comparative analysis of function outcome. J Oral Maxillofac Surg 2004;62 (Suppl 1):49–50.

63. Eriksson L, Westesson PL. Discectomy as an effective treatment for painful temporomandibular joint internal derangement: a 5-year clinical and radiographic follow-up. J Oral Maxillofac Surg 2001;59(7):750–8 [discussion: 758–9].

64. Smith JA, Sandler NA, Ozaki WH, et al. Subjective and objective assessment of the temporalis myofascial flap in previously operated temporomandibular joints. J Oral Maxillofac Surg 1999;57(9):1058–65 [discussion: 1065–7].

65. Mercuri LG, Edibam NR, Giobbie-Hurder A. Fourteen-year follow-up of a patient-fitted total temporomandibular joint reconstruction system. J Oral Maxillofac Surg 2007;65(6):1140–8.

66. Wolford LM, Rodrigues DB, McPhillips A. Management of the infected temporomandibular joint total joint prosthesis. J Oral Maxillofac Surg 2010;68(11):2810–23.

Reoperative Midface Reconstruction

Julio Acero, MD, DMD, PhD, FDSRCS, FEBOMFS[a,b,]*,
Eloy García, MD, FEBOMFS[c,d]

KEYWORDS

- Reoperative secondary reconstruction • Midface
- Head neck reconstruction

The midface is a critical region of the human body, concerning aesthetic and function. Anatomic structures, including the maxilla, palate, orbit, cheek, upper lips, eyelid, and nose, are part of the central face. Because of the complex surgical anatomy, defects after resection of the midface are often challenging situations for the reconstructive surgeon.[1] Functional and aesthetic deformities after loss of midfacial structures as a result of complex trauma or tumor resection may include large oronasal and oroantral fistulae, loss of eye support, alterations of the masticatory function because of loss of tooth-bearing bone segments, and loss of midfacial soft tissues coverage, including cheek, upper lip, and nose. Functional impairment affecting vision, oral alimentation, deglutition, and speech can be related to these deformities. The objectives of the reconstructive maxillofacial surgeon should be to restore the midfacial projection, providing support for the orbit or filling the orbital cavity in case of exenteration to separate the oral cavity from the nasoantral tract, thus restoring palatal competence, and to provide a support for a functional dentition.[1] Reconstruction of the facial soft tissues and avoidance of sequela, such as ectropion, are also goals of the midfacial reconstruction. Lack of reconstruction or failure of a primary reconstructive surgery frequently leads to a severe aesthetic sequela that causes functional impairment, critically affecting the quality of life of the patient who has not undergone reconstruction (**Fig. 1**).

The algorithm for reconstruction of the midfacial defects is usually based on the extent of the resection. This concept can be considered as the key of the reconstruction either in cases of primary repair of a defect after oncologic excision or in situations of reoperative reconstruction. In most cases of midface ablation, the loss of structure mainly affects the maxilla. Different classifications of the maxillary defect have been described, although this issue remains controversial. Spiro and colleagues[2] proposed the terms limited, subtotal, and total maxillectomies to designate those resections affecting 1, 2, and more maxillary walls. Cordeiro and Santamaría,[3] based on this concept, described 4 types of maxillary defects:

Type I: Limited maxillectomy. Includes resection of 1 or 2 walls, excluding the palate

Type II: Subtotal maxillectomy. Includes resection of the maxillary arch, palate, and anterior and lateral walls, with preservation of the orbital floor

Type III: Total maxillectomy. Includes resection of the 6 maxillary walls, either with orbital content preservation (IIIa) or with orbital exenteration (IIIb)

Type IV: Orbitomaxillectomy. Includes resection of the orbital contents with preservation of the palate.

[a] Department of Oral and Maxillofacial Surgery, Gregorio Marañon Hospital, Complutense University, Doctor Esquerdo 46, 28007 Madrid, Spain
[b] Department of Oral and Maxillofacial Surgery, Quirón University Hospital, Diego de Velazquez 1, 28223 Pozuelo Madrid, Madrid, Spain
[c] Department of Oral and Maxillofacial Surgery, Clinic i Provincial Hospital, Villarroel, 170, 08036 Barcelona, Spain
[d] San Juan de Dios Hospital, Central University Barcelona, Passeig Sant Joan de Déu, 2 08950 Esplugues de Llobregat, Barcelona, Spain
* Corresponding author. Velazquez 27, 2 iz., Madrid 28001, Spain.
E-mail address: J-acero@terra.es

Oral Maxillofacial Surg Clin N Am 23 (2011) 133–151
doi:10.1016/j.coms.2010.10.004
1042-3699/11/$ — see front matter © 2011 Elsevier Inc. All rights reserved.

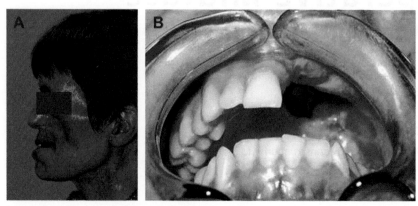

Fig. 1. (*A*) Left maxillectomy. Severe aesthetic sequela after failure of primary reconstruction. (*B*) Lack of reconstruction after maxillectomy. Oroantral communication.

Brown and colleagues[4] classified the defects after maxillectomy according to the vertical and horizontal components of the defect. Classes 1 to 4 define the vertical component. Class 1 involves maxillectomy without oroantral fistula. Class 2 is defined as a low maxillectomy not including the orbital floor. Class 3 includes high maxillectomy involving the floor of the orbit. Class 4 refers to radical maxillectomy, including orbital exenteration with or without extension to the surrounding structures (ethmoid bone, cranial basis). The horizontal or palatal component of the defect is classified as a, b, or c (a, unilateral alveolar maxillectomy; b, subtotal bilateral alveolar maxillectomy; c, total bilateral alveolar maxillary resection). This classification is widely used as a basis to define the reconstructive protocol after maxillectomy, although midfacial skin or orbito-maxillary resections not involving the palate are not included. Minor or extensive soft tissue defects occasionally affecting the surrounding bone structures can respect the lower maxillary area while affecting important structures, such as the nose and orbital region.

Although immediate single-stage reconstruction is mainly accepted as the preferred method of restoration in the head of the neck to prevent important sequela, reoperative reconstruction can be indicated if primary reconstruction is not performed or if primary reconstruction is performed but fails. Secondary or delayed reconstruction of the midface is a challenging issue because of the complexity of this region complicated with the presence of scarring, tissue atrophy, collapse of the midfacial projection, lack of soft tissue elasticity, and poor vascularity.[5] These effects are worsened by adjuvant oncologic treatment, such as radiotherapy, and frequently result in an unacceptable facial deformity and a diminished capacity for normal speech, chewing,

and deglutition, with a severe impact in the patient's social life. This article reviews the different clinical situations that can lead to the indication of a reoperative reconstruction after previous oncologic ablative procedures affecting the midface and discusses the problems related to these situations and the surgical techniques that are available to resolve them.

RELEVANT ANATOMY
Anatomic Changes After Midfacial Oncologic Resection

The central portion of the face includes important structures such as the maxilla, palate, orbit, cheek, upper lips, eyelid, and nose. The maxilla provides the structural support to the midface. This bone, located between the skull base and the occlusal plane, can be described as a hexahedron geometric structure with 6 walls.[3] The roof of the maxilla is part of the orbital floor. The medial wall is the lateral wall of the nasal cavity, including part of the lacrimal system. The lower part forms the anterior portion of the hard palate and the alveolar ridge, supporting the teeth. The maxillary antrum is contained within the central portion of this bone. The palate separates the oral cavity of the nasoantral cavities. The maxilla provides anchorage to the upper dentition and supports the masticatory forces. The maxilla is involved together with other bones located in the midface, such as the malar bone and ethmoid, in the anatomy of the orbit, thus providing support to the globe of the eye. Soft tissue midfacial structures and its musculature are also supported by the maxilla. Aesthetic appearance, including facial expression of the individual, is critically related to the anatomy of the midface.[3,6]

Knowledge of the normal anatomy is a basic principle concerning reconstruction of the head of the neck. The goal of primary or secondary repair after oncologic resection of the midface is to restore the normal anatomy and function. Reoperative reconstructive surgery is performed in a previously surgically altered area, which poses an additional challenge for the reconstructive surgeon.[5] Patients undergoing secondary reconstruction present a bone and/or soft tissue defect associated with fixed and contracted soft tissues of the midface and scars related to previous incisions intra- and/or extraorally. These changes make the evaluation of the defect difficult to plan the restoration of the anatomy, influence the quality of the reconstruction, and increase the risk of complications. Microvascular free flaps are valuable tools for reoperative reconstruction of major midfacial defects. An adequate vessel selection is critical for the flap viability, especially concerning reconstruction of the midface, because of the distance to the neck, the usual location for the recipient vessels. A previous neck dissection reduces the availability of suitable recipient vessels, which can increase the risk of flap failure. An alternative could be the use of the temporal artery and vein as the recipient vessels, but these vessels are frequently unavailable after previous surgery in this area. The impact of previous radiotherapy on the quality of the tissues and the vasculature can also have an impact on secondary reconstruction. Problems caused by the anatomic changes on reoperative reconstruction are reviewed later.

REOPERATIVE MIDFACE RECONSTRUCTION
When and How to Do It

Indications
Immediate single-stage reconstruction is accepted generally as the first-choice strategy of restoration after oncologic resection affecting the head and neck. Despite this concept, reoperative reconstruction of the midface may be necessary under different circumstances:

> Lack of primary reconstruction
> Poor result after primary reconstruction
> Failure after immediate repair of the defect (partial or complete flap loss)
> Other major complications (Orocutaneous fistula, bony nonunion)
> Inadequate result of the primary reconstruction because of poor planning.
> Planned multistage midfacial reconstruction or refinements (elective procedure to refine a previous surgery)
> Tumor recurrence.

Minor postoperative complications after a primary surgery can lead to the necessity of performing reoperative procedures, such as evacuation of a hematoma or scar revision. These situations should be treated according to the general principles in surgery and are not reviewed in this article.

Absence of indication of primary reconstruction or inability to perform immediate repair because of technical problems or because of the general status of the patient leads to important functional and aesthetic sequela in the midface depending on the type and extension of the resection. Frequently, prosthetic obturators were indicated in oral rehabilitation after maxillary resection involving the hard palate. Obturation of the defect is simple but is often associated with poor hygiene and lack of comfort and is a poor solution in case of extensive defects. One of the advantages often stated is the accessibility for inspection to detect recurrent disease. This advantage has not shown to influence survival in comparison with the current diagnostic methods, such as endoscopy, computed tomography (CT), magnetic resonance imaging, or positron emission tomography. Mobility of the prosthesis, inadequate oral-nasal sealing, rhinolalia, inability to effectively chew, and poor aesthetic result may indicate a secondary reconstruction after prosthetic obturation in nonreconstructed defects after maxillary resection.

Immediate repair with pedicled flaps, especially after the incorporation of microsurgical tissue transfer, has dramatically improved the reconstruction of complex defects of the head and neck. Microvascular free flaps placement shows a reduced complication rate, and success rate are in excess of 95%.[7,8] Still, even in most experienced centers, complications and flaps failures occur. Complication rates after head and neck microsurgical reconstruction may oscillate between 17% and 29% of the cases.[9,10] The rate of complications in the recipient site is lower after microvascular tissue transfer than that related to pedicled flap reconstruction. Cigarette smoking and preoperative comorbidity are factors correlated with flaps complication. Salvage of a flap in case of failure after immediate reconstruction can be possible in case of early recognition of flap compromise and rapid reoperative procedure; the chance of surgical salvage is low after the first 48 hours. Successful salvage rates after reexploration of free flaps in the head and neck range from 30% to 60% of the cases, but references in the literature do not specify salvage rates for midfacial microvascular reconstruction.[7,11] Partial or total failure of a flap after immediate reconstruction of a midfacial defect can lead to aesthetic or functional morbidity, thus making additional reoperative reconstructive procedures necessary.

Less frequently, reoperative midfacial reconstruction is related to a previously planned multistage reconstruction or technical elective refinements after primary reconstruction. Nose reconstruction with frontal pedicle flap is a classical example of this indication (**Fig. 2**). Tumor relapse in a previously reconstructed patient is frequently a challenging situation, especially after previous major ablation and reconstructive surgery. Morbidity of salvage surgery after recurrent oral cancer seems to be reduced in case of free flap reconstruction.[12]

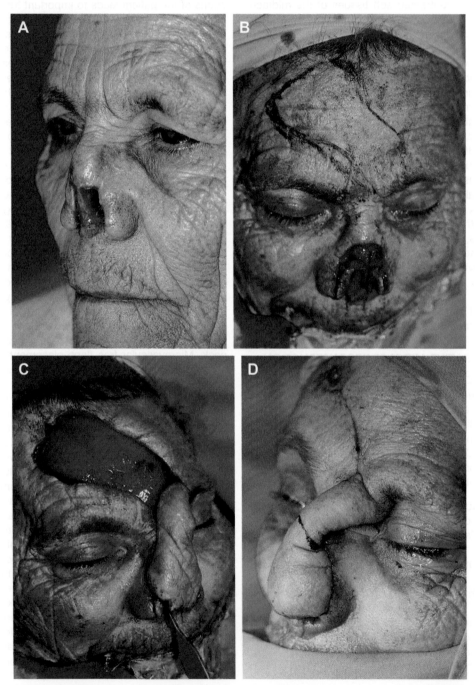

Fig. 2. (*A*) Planned multistage reconstruction of the nose after oncologic resection without primary repair. (*B, C*) Paramedian forehead flap transfer. (*D, E*) Secondary resection of the pedicle and debulking. (*F, G*) Final result.

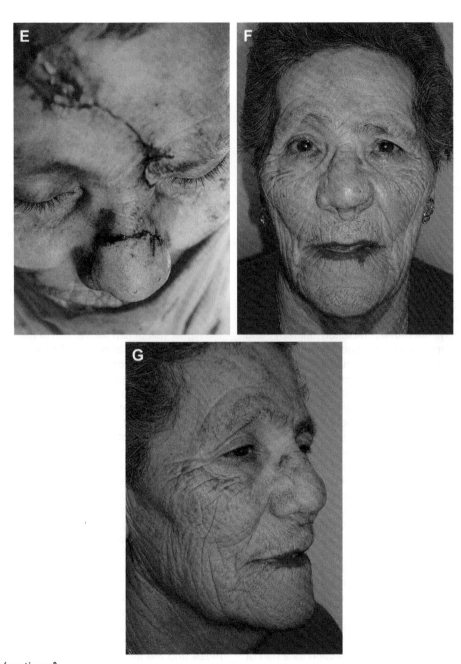

Fig. 2. (*continued*)

Problems and limitations

Secondary reconstruction of midfacial defects can be successfully performed; however, both the surgical team and the patient should be aware of its limitations. Although little evidence appears in the literature concerning this issue, it is clear that reoperative reconstruction of the midface is a surgical challenge facing different problems related to the locoregional anatomic situation after previous treatment. Anatomic changes after previous operative procedures have been reviewed earlier. Functional results of the secondary procedure can be limited because of loss of function after primary surgery related to progressive scarring, fibrosis, and the development of compensatory mechanisms that may make recovering normal swallowing or speech function as well as facial mobility difficult. Soft tissue retraction, neural lesions, and the influence of the gravitational force can lead to negative results regarding soft tissue position and dynamics, resulting in sequela, such as ectropion, after soft tissue reoperative repair of the midfacial skin or eyelids. Concerning free tissue transfer, it seems that the success rate for a second free flap may be similar to that of primary microvascular flap surgery but technical limitations due to the situation of the recipient site, including tissue scarring and vessels depletion after a previous surgery, make secondary reconstruction technically more difficult.[5] Scarring related to previous treatment may cause a collapse of the midfacial structures, making it difficult to define the planning objectives to restore the ideal anatomy and interfering during the dissection of anatomic structures in the midface. The identification of the facial nerve branches can become additionally difficult because of scarring involving the lateral aspect of the midface, thus increasing the possibility of postoperative facial palsy. Moreover, radiation therapy and chemotherapy could have been administered as an adjunctive therapy in association with previous surgical procedures. Success of reoperative reconstruction in an irradiated patient demands a high surgical skill. The negative effect of previous radiotherapy on the tissues, including vasculature of the head and neck, appears to be well established. Radiotherapy causes intimal fibrosis and early arteriosclerosis.[13] Local complication rate in the recipient site is higher in irradiated patients. Although the negative impact of radiation therapy in the outcome of microvascular tissue transfer has been pointed out,[11] there is still a controversy because some investigators did not find this association.[14] Thus, microvascular flaps, despite the higher technical demands, are a good option in irradiated patients in comparison with pedicled flaps in the reoperative reconstruction of major midfacial defects.

After primary oncologic surgery, the patient frequently has a neck dissection or a previous free or pedicled flap. Neck dissection as a part of the procedure has been performed during the surgical treatment of malignant tumors of the lower third of the face more frequently than in case of midfacial tumors, although an increasing tendency to perform neck dissection in this type of tumors has been registered because of the evidence of a higher rate of cervical subclinical positive nodes than previously described in maxillary carcinomas.[15] Despite the higher technical demands, reoperative free flap reconstruction after previous neck dissection does not seem to have a negative impact on the flap success rate in general, although there is a lack of studies on this factor focused in midfacial reconstruction.[16] Knowledge of the recipient vessels used in a previous reconstruction is important to plan a second microvascular flap. Planning of reoperative reconstruction is reviewed later in this article. Use of recipient vessels in the contralateral neck can be an alternative, mainly in case of lower facial defects, but it is not a favorable option in case of reoperative reconstruction of the midface because of the distance. Recipient vessel depletion can be a problem especially after radical neck dissection. The external carotid artery and its lingual branches are frequently preserved after radical neck dissection and can be used within the ipsilateral neck. However, the external and internal jugular veins are sacrificed in these cases and isolation of a recipient vein after radical neck dissection is usually more difficult than after a previous selective neck dissection. Cephalic vein transposition or vein grafts can be an alternative in case of lack of adequate recipient veins but because of the higher risk of flap failure, use of flaps containing long pedicles is advocated for reoperative midfacial reconstruction, especially after primary ipsilateral neck dissection. The use of the temporal vessels could be an alternative but these vessels are frequently not available because of the previous treatment. Jacobson and colleagues[17] reviewed a series of 14 patients undergoing head and neck microvascular reconstruction at a vessel-depleted neck because of previous radiation or chemotherapy and multiple surgeries. Recipient arteries used were the transverse cervical artery, internal mammary artery, and thoracoacromial artery. Venous anastomoses were performed using mainly the cephalic vein, whereas the internal mammary vein and the transverse cervical vein were alternative in fewer cases. Vein grafts were used in 3 arterial and 1 venous anastomosis. Only 3 cases of maxillary reconstruction are included in this group. In all 3 cases, reconstruction was achieved using the reverse flow scapular flap with the cephalic vein for the venous anastomosis and the thoracodorsal artery as the donor artery. Use of flow-through flaps, including those based in the radial or peroneal artery, may be an alternative to vascularize a tandem free flap in case of frozen neck.[18]

Preoperative planning

Workup Reoperative midfacial reconstruction demands careful clinical analysis and knowledge of the previous procedures. Careful planning aims to minimize the surgical steps necessary to achieve the best result. Accurate assessment of the degree of anatomic distortion; quality of the tissue in the involved area, including the situation of the scars; and availability of healthy surrounding tissues and recipient vessels should be performed in case of microvascular reconstruction planning.[19] Evaluation of the general status of the patient should include information on age, history of tobacco and alcohol abuse, nutritional situation, and presence of comorbidity. Workup is necessary to exclude unresectable situation in case of recurrence or distant metastasis.[12]

Assessment of the defect Complex defects in the midfacial area can include defects of the skin, musculature, innervations, and mucosa. Defect evaluation requires assessment of the surface and volume of missing tissue. CT scan, including 3-dimensional (3D) reconstruction, is a valuable tool in the evaluation of the craniomaxillofacial situation before reoperative reconstruction. Modeling enables measurement of the defect but may also facilitate 3D design of the flap. Models can be prepared preoperatively or intraoperatively by simply taking an impression of the defect using plastic material, such as alginate or polymethyl methacrylate. Introduction of computed 3D modeling has allowed to perform the virtual planning of the reconstruction aiming to define the ideal objectives. Virtual planning can minimize the negative results related to subjective factors

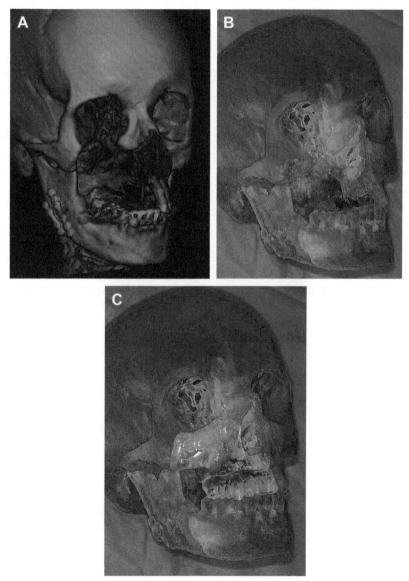

Fig. 3. (*A*) 3D CT reconstruction showing right midfacial defect after maxillectomy. (*B, C*) Stereolithographic model showing planning of the ideal reconstruction.

in reoperative surgery through mirror duplication of the image of the contralateral side in case of hemifacial defects. The 3D images can be converted into a 3D model using stereolithographic techniques (**Fig. 3**). 3D models can be transferred to the donor site to raise a tailored flap.[20]

Assessment of recipient vessels Assessment of recipient vessels is a critical issue in case of reoperative free flap reconstruction. Knowledge of surgical procedures is mandatory, including the type of neck dissection and anastomosis that were performed in case of previous free tissue transfer. Angiography of the external carotid artery system can be helpful in the preoperative evaluation in case of reoperative reconstruction, but its value to explore the venous situation is limited.[5] CT scan with contrast or magnetic resonance angiography can provide valuable information on the situation of the potential recipient vessels, including venous anatomy (**Fig. 4**).

Treatment Options

Treatment options for reoperative reconstruction of the midface are based on the same principles that are applied to the treatment of primary defects while taking into account the problems and limitations related to a prior treatment, which have been reviewed earlier in this article.

Midfacial reconstruction after oncologic resection has evolved from the prosthetic replacement to the complex microvascular reconstructions. Surgical options to repair a defect in this region can include local or regional soft tissue flaps, although these types of flaps are limited for the reconstruction of major defects. Development of microvascular free flaps was a tremendous revolution, allowing the transfer of an adequate amount of well-vascularized bone and/or soft tissue without the limitation of a fixed pedicle, thus allowing for a better 3D fitting of the flap.[1,6,21,22] All these advantages are critical in the reconstruction of previously operated and irradiated midfacial defects. New reconstructive methods are currently under development. In the future, tissue engineering may contribute to the ideal regeneration of head and neck defects. Facial transplantation has opened a new path in this field, having been applied to the reconstruction of very complex defects in various cases, some of them affecting the midface with good results.[23] This method is not currently a routine procedure, and its indications seem to be highly restricted. Facial transplantation should not be indicated in patients affected by malignant tumors because the effects of immunosuppression in these cases are not clear, although it can be an option in case of reoperative reconstruction of defects after treatment of complex benign tumors affecting the midface.

The different treatment options, including the most suitable microvascular flaps used for reoperative reconstruction of the midface, are reviewed in the following sections.

Maxillofacial prosthesis

In the past, the main method of rehabilitation after maxillectomy was based on the use of prosthesis with a palatal obturator. This method, designed for functional restoration of a maxillectomy defect using the remaining bone and soft tissues and dentition to support an obturator bulb, is simple but can be related to a poor result in terms of quality of life (**Fig. 5**). Okay and colleagues[24]

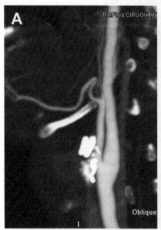
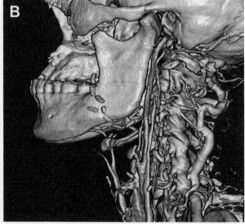

Fig. 4. (*A, B*) CT angiography showing the vascular situation of the neck after failure of a primary maxillary reconstruction with an iliac crest free flap. External carotid artery and its lingual branch are preserved, whereas the facial and thyroid arteries are not available. Imaging of the internal jugular vein shows a poor venous situation.

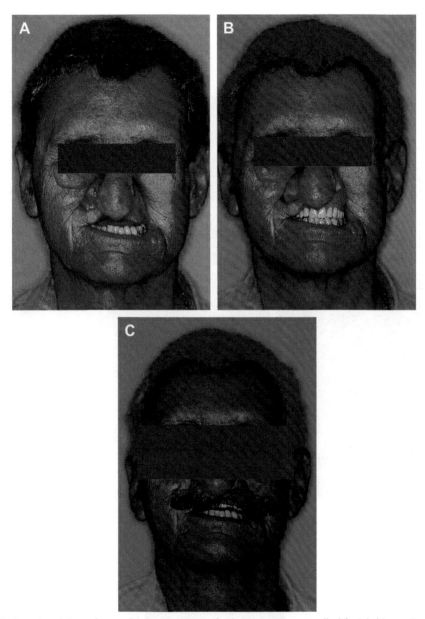

Fig. 5. (A–C) Complex defect after multiple resections of relapsing, not-controlled facial skin carcinoma that led to the patient's death. Poor result after rehabilitation of the defect with a palatal obturator and facial prostheses.

systematized prosthodontic guidelines for functional restoration of the maxillectomy defect. Poor retention, lack of adequate hygiene, and oronasal regurgitation are frequent problems, although some controversy on this issue still remains.[25] Moreover, obturation with dental prosthesis cannot resolve adequately large defects after maxillectomy.[1,4,24] At present, functional rehabilitation after maxillary excision can be achieved with dental prosthesis based on dental implants but frequently associated with reconstruction of the defect with microvascular flaps.

Complex defects not suitable for flap reconstruction, affecting structures such as the nose and orbit, can be resolved by using maxillofacial prostheses that currently are mainly anchored by dental implants fixed in the remaining skeleton.

Local and regional flaps
The goal of salvage reconstruction is to select the simplest reconstructive option that has the highest chance to restore form, function, and aesthetics.[8] Structures such as lips, eyelids, and nose should be reconstructed using local flaps whenever

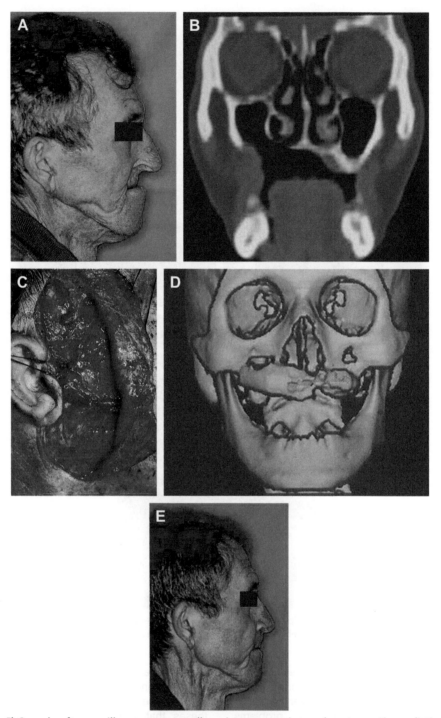

Fig. 6. (*A*, *B*) Sequela after maxillary squamous cell carcinoma resection and postoperative radiation therapy. Large oroantral fistula and loss of midfacial projection. (*C*, *D*) Reoperative reconstruction with an iliac free flap transfer with anastomosis to the temporal vessels. (*E*) Final result.

possible. These are unique anatomic structures extremely difficult to reconstruct in case of major resection. Although microvascular free flaps can provide large amounts of soft tissue, they usually fail to achieve adequate aesthetic and functional results for reoperative reconstruction of the eyelids, lips, and nose. Use of local flaps provides a better aesthetic because of a better skin color and texture match. Moreover, the main goal in these situations should be to restore the oral sphincter function and to protect the cornea. Local flaps can be used for this purpose, whereas free flap should be used to repair the remaining defects in the neighbor areas.[26] Secondary correction of a retracted lower eyelid can be a difficult trend. Split-thickness skin grafts, upper lid pedicle flaps, and suspension techniques are used for this purpose. Eyelid tissue−based flaps are more effective than other flaps in case of secondary procedures to correct eyelid defects. Musculocutaneous flaps transferred from the upper lid are effective for the correction of lower eyelid ectropion (Tripier flap). Secondary nasal reconstruction

is also a challenging situation. Multistage reconstruction based on the principle of nasal aesthetic subunits repair is often planned to achieve the best aesthetic outcome; the paramedian forehead flap is the most commonly used flap. Nose reconstruction needs to be supported in a stable maxillary platform around the base. Cartilage and bone grafts are used to create hard tissue architecture during the intermediate procedures. Further operations are required to resect the pedicle and for the debulking of the flap (see **Fig. 2**).[26–28]

Different local and regional pedicled flaps are available to restore other defects, such as oroantral fistula (buccal fat pad, buccinators flap, nasolabial flap, temporalis muscle flap) or midfacial skin moderate defects (frontal flap, cervicofacial rotation-advancement flap), whereas traditional methods, such as the forehead flap, have been abandoned because of its morbidity. Distant pedicled flaps, such as the pectoralis, latissimus dorsi, or trapezius myocutaneous flaps, are useful in the secondary repair of lower cervicofacial defects, especially in case of vessel-depleted neck but

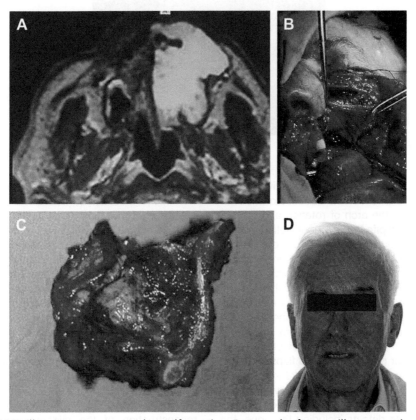

Fig. 7. (A−E) Maxillary intraosseous vascular malformation. Poor result after maxillectomy and primary repair with a temporalis muscle flap. (F−I) Reoperative reconstruction 7 years later with an iliac crest free flap and secondary dental implants placement. Temporal artery and vein were used as the recipient vessels.

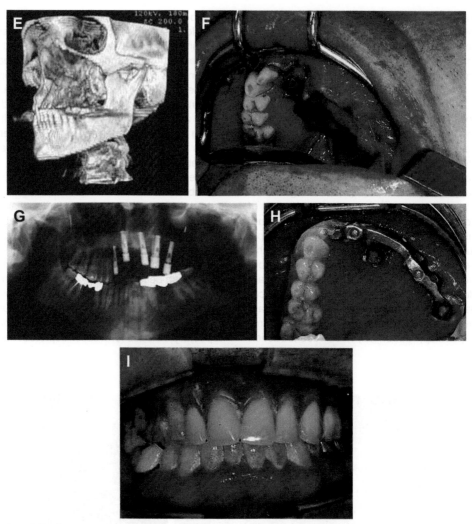

Fig. 7. *(continued)*

have a very limited value in reoperative reconstruction of midfacial defects because of the limitation related to the arch of rotation and lack of adaptability.[8] Despite being a poor option, sometimes, distant pedicled flaps can be considered as an emergency procedure to cover extensive defects in the midface after failure of other regional or free flaps.[29] Pedicled flaps, such as the temporoparietal fascia flap or the temporalis muscle flap, can also be used to cover free bone grafts or synthetic implants, such as titanium mesh, for the correction of upper midfacial defects.

Use of local or regional pedicled flaps is limited in case of severe soft tissue contracture and loss of soft tissue bulk, especially in heavily irradiated patients.[30,31] In these cases and in extensive or major composite defects including the bone, the reoperative reconstruction should be accomplished by means of microvascular free flaps.

Secondary free flap reconstruction

Donor site selection is based on the type and extension of the defect (soft tissue or composite soft tissue/bone defect) as well as on the patient's comorbidities. Long-pedicle free flaps are the best choice for reoperative reconstruction in the midfacial region because of the distance to the recipient vessels. Secondary free flap reconstruction seems to be a highly reliable procedure (failure rate 1.4%) but complications are not uncommon. Various free tissue microvascular transfers have been described for midfacial reconstruction, including radial forearm, rectus abdominis, fibula, latissimus dorsi, anterolateral thigh flap (ALT), scapular system, and iliac crest free flap.[22,32–36] There is a lack of information in the literature on reoperative reconstruction of the midface with free flaps because most series are related to secondary reconstruction in the head and neck as a whole, referring only a low number of cases with secondary midfacial reconstruction. Iseli and colleagues[37] reviewed 71 secondary free flap procedures in the head and neck. The radial forearm flap was most commonly used, followed by the fibula flap, rectus abdominis, ALT flap, and latissimus. Among the described flaps, the skin island of the flap can sometimes be too bulky for intraoral reconstruction. The iliac crest free flap is a good option to reconstruct major defects of the maxilla and palate, although big disadvantages

are the short pedicle and the poor quality of the skin island, which is too bulky. Raising the iliac crest bone flap combined with the internal oblique muscle allows for reconstruction of composite defects.[4,5,34,36] The iliac crest flap can provide support to the globe of the eye and restore the midfacial projection (**Figs. 6** and **7**). Moreover, the iliac bone is of excellent quality for implants placement. As in primary reconstruction, indication of bone repair is based on the horizontal extent of the defect and the necessity of bone for

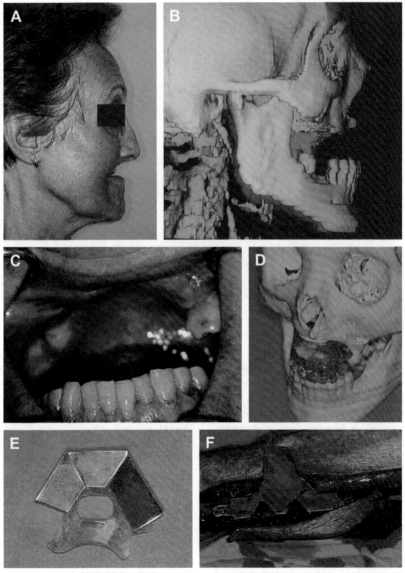

Fig. 8. (*A–C*) Sequela after bilateral alveolar maxillary resection caused by squamous cell carcinoma. Primary closure of the defect without bone reconstruction. Postoperative radiation therapy. (*D–I*) Secondary reconstruction with a prefabricated fibula flap according to the 3D model planning. Anastomoses were performed, with the facial artery and vein as the recipient vessels. (*J, K*) Delayed implant placement. Vestibuloplasty and debulking of the flap were performed before the prosthetic rehabilitation. (*L*) Final aspect of the patient.

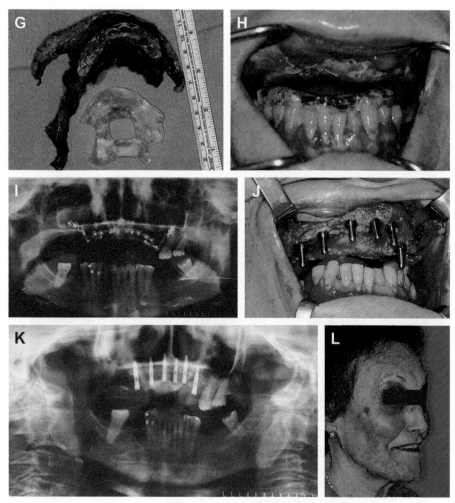

Fig. 8. (*continued*)

dental implant rehabilitation. According to Okay and colleagues[24] and Brown and colleagues,[4] lateral lower defects without significant volume defect do not need bone reconstruction. In these cases, if reconstruction with soft tissue pedicled flaps is not feasible, a forearm fasciocutaneous flap can be an option to seal the oroantral fistula, providing a thin and pliable soft tissue surface for the palate. Extended horizontal defects need bone reconstruction to recover the midfacial projection and to provide support for dental implant secondary rehabilitation. Vascularized osseocutaneous forearm flap can be an option in case of composite lower maxillary defects, but it shows a high donor site morbidity. The fibular free flap is an excellent option in this type of defects, providing a long fragment of bone and the possibility to include the soft tissue component, which is very useful in case of secondary defects reconstruction. The bone flap can be

preshaped according to the 3D model planning to achieve an optimal result (**Fig. 8**). Moreover, the fibula flap offers a long pedicle, especially useful in cases of reoperative midfacial reconstruction.[5,38] The fibula flap is also suitable for dental implant rehabilitation.[39] Secondary soft tissue procedures, such as vestibuloplasty, skin or mucosa grafts, or flaps debulking, are usually necessary to refine the results.

Free flaps based in the subscapular system can provide a large soft tissue component associated with a scapular bone flap that can be rotated with great 3D freedom, allowing for the reconstruction of complex composite defects. Another advantage of this type of flaps is the length of the pedicle, including the possibility of using the thoracodorsal artery. Moreover, the subscapular system of vessels offers the possibility to raise a chimeric flap, including the scapular, latissimus, and serratus flaps, for the reconstruction of highly complex defects, thus avoiding the necessity to use various simultaneous free flaps, which is advocated in complex cases by some authors.[40] Disadvantages of the scapular flaps are that the amount of bone is limited and that it cannot be harvested simultaneously with the ablative procedure as a 2-team approach.[1] Secondary reconstruction of large volume defects not needing osseous reconstruction can be performed very successfully using soft tissue free flaps, such as rectus abdominis, latissimus dorsi, or ALT flap, according to the same principles applied to the midfacial primary reconstruction. All these flaps allow to restore the volume deficiencies and to obliterate the dead space to seal the intracranial structures providing a barrier to separate them from the nasopharyngeal tract in case of extensive midfacial defects affecting the cranial basis (**Fig. 9**). Providing a large well-vascularized soft tissue flap is especially critical in reoperative reconstructions of craniofacial defects in irradiated patients. Intraoral lining can be provided by the skin island or after reepithelization of the muscle fascia, which is advocated to avoid malposition of the skin island intraorally because of the gravitational forces. The ALT flap is ideal under these circumstances because of the long pedicle (10–15 cm), its low morbidity, and the possibility to harvest the flap according to the volume and surface requirements and, thus, has been proposed to replace other flaps, such as the radial forearm or the latissimus dorsi flap.[41]

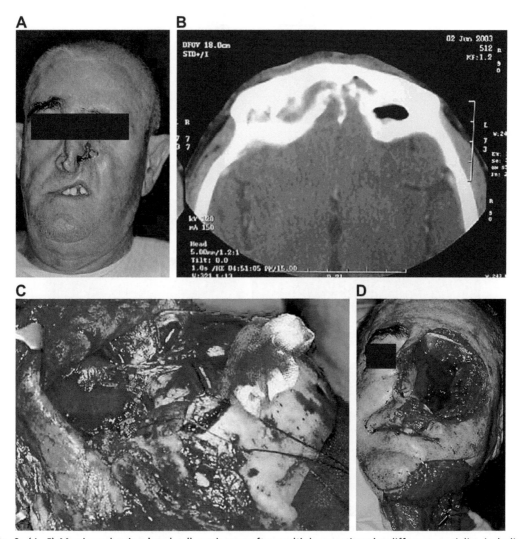

Fig. 9. (*A, B*) Massive relapsing basal cell carcinoma after multiple resections by different specialist, including orbit exenteration. Tumor invasion of the frontal and ethmoidal sinus. (*C–E*) Large craniofacial combined resection. (*F*) Reconstruction with a rectus abdominis musculocutaneous free flap. (*G*) Final result.

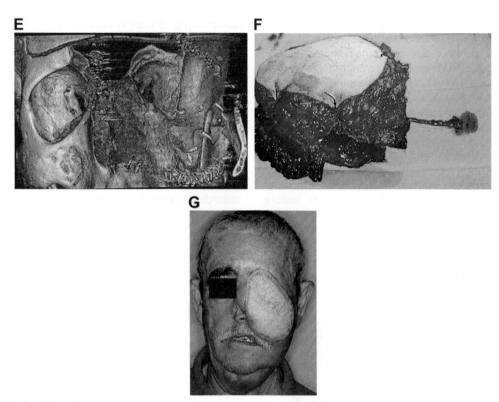

Fig. 9. (*continued*)

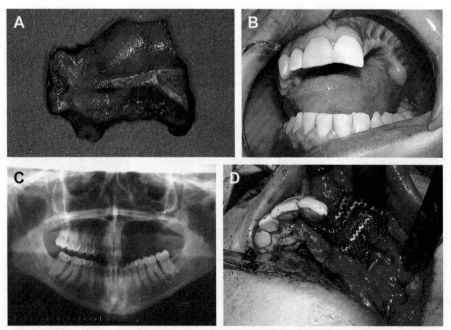

Fig. 10. (*A–C*) Maxillary alveolar defect after low maxillectomy caused by a myxoma. (*D, E*) Secondary repair 10 years after the primary resection using free, particulate, autologous iliac crest bone supported by a titanium mesh. (*F, G*) Excellent bone regeneration allowing for delayed dental implants placement. (*H, I*) Final intraoral and facial aspects of the patient.

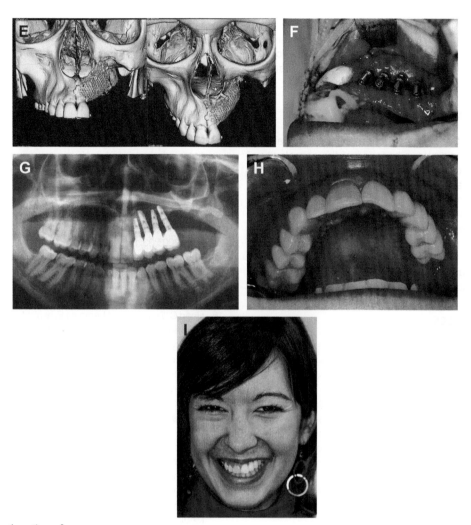

Fig. 10. (*continued*)

Adjunctive procedures

Ancillary techniques may contribute to a better result in case of midfacial reoperative reconstruction. Facial contouring with free bone grafts, mainly of calvarial origin, or synthetic implants (porous polyethylene, methyl methacrylate, titanium meshes) can be indicated in upper midfacial defects, especially in the orbital area, although previous radiation therapy may contraindicate this option, especially in case of communication with the oral cavity.[30,42] Disadvantage of the nonvascularized bone grafts is the frequent resorption. CT imaging and computed custom-designed prosthesis are valuable tools to obtain adequate contour in the fronto-orbital area.[43] Titanium meshes in combination with soft tissue coverage can also be used for this purpose and to provide support to the globe of the eye.[44] Lipostructure can be an alternative to fill selected residual defects after midfacial reconstruction. Results are quite predictable, and morbidity is less than in microvascular flaps in case of filling residual flattened areas.[45] Distraction osteogenesis used to repair bone defects in case of impossibility of bone flap reconstruction has been described mainly for mandibular repair but can also be an alternative in minor maxillary defects.[46] Oral rehabilitation with dental implants is a multistage procedure aiming to restore the masticatory function. Implants can be inserted during the primary reconstructive procedure but are often a delayed procedure (**Fig. 10**). Zygomatic implants can also support dental rehabilitation without any bone reconstruction, which can be a good alternative in selected cases in which bone reconstruction is not feasible.[31] Implant placement outcomes are good concerning osseointegration, but some degree of functional impairment remains in many cases because of soft tissue scarring and mobility restrictions. Radiation therapy seems not to interfere with implants placed primarily before the irradiation and secondarily restored but can affect the results in case of delayed implant placement.[47]

SUMMARY

Reoperative reconstruction of the midface is a challenging issue because of the complexity of this region and the severity of the aesthetic and functional sequela related to the absence or failure of a primary reconstruction. The different situations that can lead to the indication of a reoperative reconstructive procedure after previous oncologic ablative procedures in the midface are reviewed. Surgical techniques, anatomic problems, and limitations affecting the reoperative reconstruction in this region of the head and neck are discussed.

REFERENCES

1. Futran ND. Retrospective case series of primary and secondary microvascular free tissue transfer reconstruction of midfacial defects. J Prosthet Dent 2001; 86:369–76.
2. Spiro RH, Strong EW, Shah J. Maxillectomy and its classification. Head Neck 1997;19:309–14.
3. Cordeiro PG, Santamaría E. A classification system and algorithm for reconstruction of maxillectomy and midfacial defects. Plast Reconstr Surg 2000; 105(7):2331–46.
4. Brown JS, Rogers SN, McNally DN, et al. A modified classification for the maxillectomy defect. Head Neck 2000;22:17–26.
5. Teknos TN, Chepeha DB, Wang SJ. Secondary oral cavity reconstruction. In: Day T, Girod D, editors. Oral cavity reconstruction. New York: Taylor & Francis Group; 2006. p. 383–90.
6. Futran N, Mendez E. Developments in reconstruction of midface and maxilla. Lancet Oncol 2006;7: 249–58.
7. Novakovic D, Patel RS, Goldstein DP, et al. Salvage of failed free flaps used in head and neck reconstruction. Head Neck Oncol 2009. DOI:10.1186/1758-3284-1-33. [Online].
8. Wang SJ, Teknos TN, Chepeha DB. Complications of free-tissue transfer. In: Eisele DV, Smith RV, editors. Complications in head and neck surgery. Philadelphia: Mosby Elsevier; 2009. p. 795–802.
9. Classen DA, Ward H. Complications in a consecutive series of 250 free flap operations. Ann Plast Surg 2006;56:557–61.
10. Singh B, Cordeiro PG, Santamaria E, et al. Factors associated with complications in microvascular reconstruction of head and neck defects. Plast Reconstr Surg 1999;103:403–11.
11. Pohlenz P, Blessmann M, Heiland M, et al. Postoperative complications in 202 cases of microvascular head and neck reconstruction. J Craniomaxillofac Surg 2007;35:311–5.
12. Kostrzewa JP, Lancaster WP, Iseli TA, et al. Outcomes of salvage surgery with free flap reconstruction for recurrent oral and oropharyngeal cancer. Laryngoscope 2010;120:267–72.
13. Mulholland S, Boyd JB, Mc Cabe S, et al. Recipient vessels in head and neck microsurgery: radiation effect and vessel access. Plast Reconstr Surg 1993;92:628–32.
14. Smolka W, Iizuka T. Surgical reconstruction of maxilla and midface: clinical outcome and factors relating to postoperative complications. J Craniomaxillofac Surg 2005;33:1–7.
15. Kruse A, Gratz K. Cervical metastases of squamous cell carcinoma of the maxilla: a retrospective study of 9 years. Head Neck Oncol 2009;1:28–32. DOI: 10.1186/1758-3284-1-28.
16. Head C, Sercarz JA, Abemayor E, et al. Microvascular reconstruction after previous neck dissection. Arch Otolaryngol Head Neck Surg 2002;128:328–31.
17. Jacobson AS, Eloy JA, Park E, et al. Vessel depleted neck: techniques for achieving microvascular reconstruction. Head Neck 2008;30(2):201–7.
18. Pribaz JJ, Taylor HOB. Reoperative issues following flap reconstruction in the head. In: Grotting JC, editor. Reoperative aesthetic & reconstructive plastic surgery. St Louis (MO): Quality Medical Publishing Inc; 2007. p. 829–58.
19. Grotting JC. What is reoperative plastic surgery? In: Grotting JC, editor. Reoperative aesthetic & reconstructive plastic surgery. St Louis (MO): Quality Medical Publishing Inc; 2007. p. 3–33.
20. Rohner D, Jaquiéry C, Kunz C, et al. Maxillofacial reconstruction with prefabricated osseous free flaps: a 3-year experience with 24 patients. Plast Reconstr Surg 2003;112(3):748–57.
21. Schliephake H. Revascularized tissue transfer for the repair of complex midfacial defects in oncologic patients. J Oral Maxillofac Surg 2000;58:1212–8.
22. Eckardt A, Fokas K. Microsurgical reconstruction in the head and neck region: an 18-year experience with 500 consecutive cases. J Craniomaxillofac Surg 2003;31:197–201.
23. Devauchelle B, Badet L, Lengelé B, et al. First human face allograft: early report. Lancet 2006; 368:203–9.
24. Okay DJ, Genden E, Buchbinder D, et al. Prosthodontic guidelines for surgical reconstruction of the maxilla: a classification system of defects. J Prosthet Dent 2001;86(4):352–63.
25. Rogers SN, Lowe D, McNally D, et al. Health-related quality of life after maxillectomy: a comparison between prosthetic obturation and free flap. J Oral Maxillofac Surg 2003;61:174–81.

26. Cordeiro PG, Disa JJ. Challenges in midface reconstruction. Semin Surg Oncol 2000;19:218–25.

27. Menick FJ. Defects of the nose, lip and cheek: rebuilding the composite defect. Plast Reconstr Surg 2001;120:887–98.

28. Li QF, Xie F, Gu B, et al. Nasal reconstruction using a split forehead flap. Plast Reconstr Surg 2006;118: 1543–50.

29. El-Marakby HH. The reliability of pectoralis major myocutaneous flap in head and neck reconstruction. J Egypt Natl Cancer Inst 2006;18:41–50.

30. Pollice PA, Frodel JL. Secondary reconstruction of upper midface and orbit after total maxillectomy. Arch Otolaryngol Head Neck Surg 1998;124:802–8.

31. Mucke T, Loeffelbein DJ, Hohlweg-Majert B, et al. Reconstruction of the maxilla and midface-Surgical management, outcome and prognostic factors. Oral Oncol 2009;45(12):1073–8.

32. McLeod AM, Morrison WA, McCann JJ. The free radial forearm flap with and without bone for closure of large opalatal fistulae. Br J Plast Surg 1987;40:391–5.

33. Brown JD, Burke AJ. Benefits of routine or maxillectomy and orbital reconstruction with the rectus abdominis free flap. Otolaryngol Head Neck Surg 1999;121:203–9.

34. Brown JS, Jones DC, Summerwill A, et al. Vascularized iliac crest with internal oblique muscle for immediate reconstruction after maxillectomy. Br J Oral Maxillofac Surg 2002;40:183–90.

35. Baliarsing AS, Kumar VV, Malik NA, et al. Reconstruction of maxillectomy defects using deep circumflex iliac artery-based composite flaps. Oral Surg Oral Med Oral Pathol Oral Radiol Endod 2010;109:e8–13.

36. Urken ML. Iliac crest osteocutaneous and osteomusculocutaneous. In: Urken ML, Cheney ML, Sullivan MJ, et al, editors. Atlas of regional and free flaps for head and neck reconstruction. New York: Raven Press; 1995. p. 261–90.

37. Iseli TA, Yelverton JC, Iseli CE, et al. Functional outcomes following secondary free flap reconstruction of the head and neck. Laryngoscope 2009; 119:856–60.

38. He Y, Zhu H, Zhang Z, et al. Three/dimensional model simulationand reconstruction of composite total maxillectomy defects with fibula osteomyocutaneous flap flow-through from radial forearm flap. Oral Surg Oral Med Oral Pathol Oral Radiol Endod 2009;108:e6–12.

39. Chang YM, Coskunfirat OK, Wei FC, et al. Maxillary reconstruction with a fibula osteoseptocutaneous free flap and simultaneous insertion of osseointegrated dental implants. Plast Reconstr Surg 2004; 113:1140–5.

40. Bianchi B, Ferrari S, Poli T, et al. Oromandibular reconstruction with simultaneous free flaps: experience in 10 cases. Acta Otorhinolaryngol Ital 2003; 23:281–90.

41. Chana JS, Wei FC. A review of the advantages of the anterolateral thigh flap in head and neck reconstruction. Br J Plast Surg 2004;57:603–9.

42. Rodriguez ED, Martin M, Bluebond-Langner R, et al. Microsurgical reconstruction of posttraumatic high-energy maxillary defects: establishing the effectiveness of early reconstruction. Plast Reconstr Surg 2007;120(Suppl 2):103S–17S.

43. Kokemueller H, Tavassol F, Ruecker M, et al. Complex midfacial reconstruction: a combined technique of computer-assisted surgery and microvascular tissue transfer. J Oral Maxillofac Surg 2008; 66:2398–406.

44. Zizelmann C, Gellrich NC, Metzger MC, et al. Computer-assisted reconstruction of orbital floor based on cone beam tomography. Br J Oral Maxillofac Surg 2007;45(1):79–80.

45. Coleman SR. Facial recontouring with lipostructure. Clin Plast Surg 1997;24:347–67.

46. González-García R, Naval-Gías L. Transport osteogenesis in the maxillofacial skeleton. Outcomes of a versatile reconstruction method following tumor ablation. Arch Otolaryngol Head Neck Surg 2010; 136:243–50.

47. Ihde S, Kopp S, Gundlach K, et al. Effects of radiation therapy on craniofacial and dental implants: a review of the literature. Oral Surg Oral Med Oral Pathol Oral Radiol Endod 2009;107:56–65.

Reoperative Mandibular Reconstruction

Phil Pirgousis, MD, DMD, FRCS, FRACDS(OMS),
Nathan Eberle, MD, DMD, Rui Fernandes, DMD, MD*

KEYWORDS

- Mandibular reconstruction • Reconstruction • Surgery
- Pedicle flap

Ideal reconstruction of the mandible is important for a multitude of reasons and has been and continues to be among the most common surgical challenges for reconstructive surgeons of the head and neck. Decades ago, it was deemed acceptable for a patient to undergo a large composite oncological resection without any type of reconstruction. Historically, pedicle flaps, such as the pectoralis major and deltopectoral myocutaneous flaps, were workhorse flaps for lower facial third head and neck reconstruction. Subsequent multiple permutations of these flaps included soft tissue and osseous components in an attempt to optimally replace composite defects.[1] Such pedicle flaps were usually transferred as part of a multistage surgical plan for the patients, which would also later include nonvascularized bone grafting, usually from the ilium or rib and a reconstruction bar.[2–4] This approach is somewhat appropriate for a patient who does not require adjuvant treatment or whose medical comorbidities preclude the ideal use of free tissue transfer. Such patients frequently endure suboptimal results, with a high incidence of complications after adjuvant radiotherapy and/or chemotherapy. However, at present, providing reliable expeditious treatment with minimal hospitalization and rapid postoperative recovery aimed at reestablishing the premorbid state of the patient has made free tissue transfer the gold standard for head and neck reconstruction of the mandible.[5–7]

Although microvascular reconstructive surgery is technically challenging and prone to more operator error than pedicle flaps, the success rate for free tissue transfers remains consistently between 96% and 99%.[5,6,8,9] That said, the question arises on the treatment method for the 1% to 4% of flaps that fail. When considering the reconstructive ladder, if transferring free tissue to reconstruct a defect of the mandible was the surgeon's plan A and it failed, then is plan B really to take a step down the reconstructive ladder to a regional flap or should plan B ideally be the same as plan A? In recent years, this old philosophy of plan B being different from plan A has been challenged so as to avoid consecutive failures. For most modern head and neck reconstructive surgeons, plan B would involve a staged reconstruction using a pedicle flap and then nonvascularized osseous reconstruction, with plan A involving vascularized composite free tissue transfer. However, this step down the reconstructive ladder is accompanied by functional and aesthetic compromises that would have otherwise been achieved by free tissue transfer.

The goals of reoperative mandibular reconstruction should be similar to, if not the same as, the initial reconstructive goals. The surgeon's goals should be to not only reestablish continuity of the mandible but also restore the patients' interrelated mandibular functions of speech, mastication, deglutition, airway patency, and facial aesthetics

Division of Oral and Maxillofacial Surgery, Department of Surgery, University of Florida College of Medicine, Jacksonvilla, FL, USA
* Corresponding author. Division of Maxillofacial Surgery, University of Florida, 653-1 West 8th Street, Jacksonville, FL 32209.
E-mail address: rui.fernandes@jax.ufl.edu

Oral Maxillofacial Surg Clin N Am 23 (2011) 153–160
doi:10.1016/j.coms.2010.11.001

because some or all of these functions are severely compromised after segmental loss of the mandible, regardless of the cause. The 4 major sources of vascularized bone routinely used to reconstruct large oromandibular defects include the fibula, ilium, scapula, and radius in that order of relative frequency used. Each donor site has its own unique advantages and disadvantages as related to the quality and quantity of tissue transferred as well as pedicle length, all of which are significant factors mandating careful consideration in reoperative reconstructive surgery. The remainder of this article outlines the relevant anatomy of the perimandibular region, reconstructive options including second free flaps, relevant workup, and complications pertaining to reoperative mandibular surgery.

SURGICAL ANATOMY

Regardless of the reconstructive plan, a firm grasp on the mandibular and perimandibular anatomy is critical in performing any type of reconstructive mandibular surgery. With respect to reoperative mandibular surgery, surgical access and exposure is fundamental. A transcervical approach to the mandible is necessary almost always. Rarely is the patient's previous surgery limited to a transoral approach. Prior surgical reconstructive attempts have significant effects on the design of neck incisions and potential vessel availability for microvascular anastamosis. However, in most reoperative mandibular reconstruction cases, patients have undergone at least 1 previous surgical procedure via a transcervical approach, and those treated for malignancy invariably had a type of neck dissection. The addition of adjuvant treatments, such as radiotherapy and chemotherapy, to the head and neck region further complicates the situation.

The mandible is a unique bone that provides both a horizontal and vertical buttress of the lower face. The horizontal portion is a horseshoe-shaped long bone comprising the alveolar bone or tooth-bearing portion and the thick cortical component or basal bone making up the remainder. The vertical buttress consists of the ascending vertical ramus with coronoid process and condyle, which enable the mandible to perform its masticatory functions and via its articulation with the skull base. Over the years, several investigators have proposed classification systems for mandibular defects, some systems were restricted to the osseous portion only, whereas other systems included the associated perimandibular soft tissue defects. Urken and colleagues[10] developed a detailed classification system for both hard and soft tissue mandibular defects, with the aim of identifying the ideal flap for a particular defect. Regardless of the classification system used, the quest for optimal aesthetic and functional reconstructive outcomes mandates a detailed analysis of the surgical defect such that the missing tissue elements form the basis of the most ideal donor site for reconstruction.

The perimandibular region has 2 fascial components consisting of a superficial and a deep layer. The superficial cervical fascia is immediately deep to the dermal plexus of skin and overlies the platysma muscle. The deep cervical fascia has 3 constituent layers: superficial, middle, and deep. Deep to the platysma is the superficial or investing layer of the deep cervical fascia. This layer is of critical importance to oromandibular reconstruction because it traverses the entire neck, while at the same time enveloping the sternocleidomastoid and trapezius muscles along with forming the capsule of the submandibular gland. This layer also has the marginal mandibular and cervical branches of the facial nerve, including the facial artery and vein. The marginal mandibular branch courses a predictable pattern in the submandibular triangle, where, in most cases, it courses posterior to the facial vessels. After dividing from the cervicofacial trunk of the facial nerve, the marginal mandibular branch courses just deep to the superficial layer of the deep cervical fascia. In the classic dissection of 100 cadaveric facial halves by Dingman and Grabb,[11] the marginal branch traveled up to 1 cm below the inferior border of the mandible in only 19% of cases. Thus, the nerve remains above the lower border of the mandible in most cases. Ziarah and Atkinson[12] dissected 76 facial halves to find the marginal branch coursed below the inferior border in 53% of cases, whilst in 6%, the nerve continued a maximal distance of 1.5 cm below the inferior border before turning upward to cross the mandible. The middle layer of the deep cervical fascia is also known as the pretracheal fascia or visceral fascia. This layer encircles the thyroid and parathyroid glands, esophagus, and trachea. The final layer is the deep layer of the deep cervical fascia, which includes the prevertebral and alar fascia.

When performing oromandibular reconstruction, familiarity with the submandibular triangle and its contents is paramount, which has, as its superior boundary, the inferior border of the mandible, whereas the anterior and posterior borders are formed by the anterior and posterior bellies of digastric muscle, respectively. The inferior limit includes the tendinous ring of the digastrics, with the deep aspect of the triangle formed by the mylohyoid muscle. The submandibular gland is located between the anterior and posterior bellies of digastric muscle and lateral to the mylohyoid muscle. The submandibular duct measuring approximately 5 cm in length exits from the posterosuperior portion of the gland and travels along the superior surface of the mylohyoid muscle to enter the sublingual space. As the duct traverses anteriorly, it passes over the lingual nerve in the sublingual space. At the base of the submandibular triangle, the hypoglossal nerve can be identified as it travels superficial to the hyoglossus muscle. The facial artery commonly arises from the external carotid artery independently but may also arise from a common trunk with the lingual artery. From its origin at the external carotid artery, it courses deep to the posterior belly of the digastric muscle and through the deep portion of the submandibular gland before crossing the inferior border of the mandible. The facial vein can be found superficial to the submandibular gland and it meets the posterior facial vein to form the common facial vein. In a patient without previous neck incisions, the facial

artery and vein are the most frequently used vessels for vascular anastomosis.

For many patients undergoing primary mandibular reconstruction, familiarity with the surgical anatomy of the submandibular triangle and its contents is vital. However, in patients in whom reoperative surgery is contemplated, a more thorough understanding of neck anatomy is crucial, particularly in the previously dissected neck, where there is often a paucity of vessels (**Fig. 1**A–C). In such cases, an alternative option for microvascular anastomosis is the superior thyroid artery that is located posterior and inferior to the hyoid bone. It is commonly the first branch off the external carotid artery. The artery courses in an anterior and inferior direction to loop around the omohyoid muscle before piercing the middle layer of the deep cervical fascia and entering the superior pole of the thyroid gland. The other vessel option for arterial anastomosis, if neither the facial nor the superior thyroid arteries are available, is the transverse cervical artery or the dorsal scapular arteries arising from the thyrocervical trunk (**Fig. 2**A–C). The transverse cervical branch can usually be found coursing

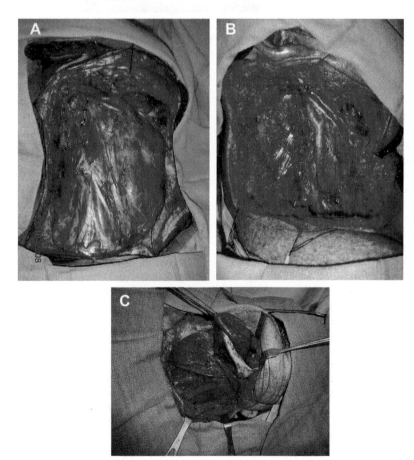

Fig. 1. (A–C) Example of radical neck dissections with resultant vessel depletion.

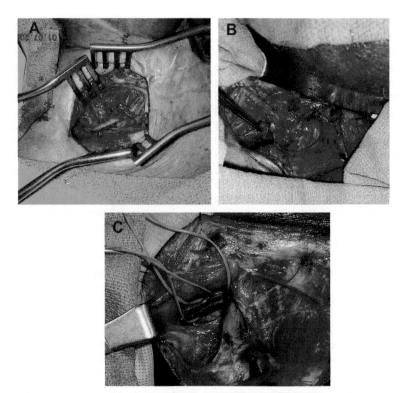

Fig. 2. (*A*) Dissected transverse cervical artery and vein in a patient with previous neck dissection. (*B*) Dissected dorsal scapular artery. (*C*) Dissected left transverse cervical artery and vein in a patient with vessel-depleted neck.

superficial to the brachial plexus and levator scapulae muscle, but in reoperative patients in whom prior neck dissection has been performed, the artery is often found in the supraclavicular fossa adjacent to the brachial plexus. The dorsal scapular artery lies deep to the levator scapulae muscle or occasionally arises directly from the subclavian artery. If none of these arteries are suitable for arterial anastomosis, the surgeon could use the lingual, inferior thyroid, superficial temporal, thoracoacromial, or internal mammary vessels, although, for geometric reasons, many of these vessels would not be ideal because flap pedicle length ultimately limits the appropriate recipient arteries (**Fig. 3**A, B). A final option for anastomosis in the ipsilateral neck would be an end-to-end anastomosis to the external carotid artery. In reoperative mandibular reconstruction, this artery often proves advantageous because of its large vessel caliber and superior blood flow. When no suitable ipsilateral vessels are available, the exploration and use of the contralateral neck vessels is preferred because the use of vein grafts in difficult reoperative cases has an increased risk of subsequent flap failure.

Finding a suitable vein for anastomosis in a previously operated patient can pose a challenge but rarely poses as much of a problem as finding a suitable artery. Venous options include the external jugular, facial, common facial, superficial temporal, transverse cervical, cephalic, and internal mammary veins. All of these veins are good options but they depend on the extent of previous neck surgery. The external jugular vein, when available, is a preferred option for end-to-end venous anastomosis in mandibular reconstruction because of its linear course and large caliber but is commonly sacrificed in head and neck oncological surgery. If no suitable recipient veins are available, end-to-side anastomosis to the internal jugular vein is possible, or in cases where this vein has been sacrificed, raising a cephalic vein with transfer into the neck may be necessary.

APPROACH TO THE MANAGEMENT OF FAILED FREE FLAPS

Salvage reconstruction after initial flap failure is extremely challenging for various reasons. Frequently, the most suitable flap has already been used in the first reconstruction, and recipient vessel availability for second free tissue transfer is limited. In addition, increased risk of wound infection and delayed healing are important sequelae of

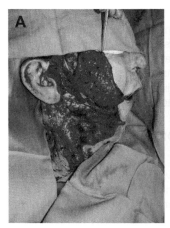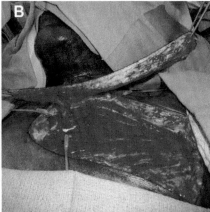

Fig. 3. (*A*) Use of the superficial temporal vessels for mandibular reconstruction in a multiple-operated patient. (*B*) Example of the internal mammary artery perforator vessels that may be used as recipient vessels in free flap reconstruction in vessel-depleted necks.

flap failure in the head and neck region, with possible disastrous consequences. The urgency for further surgical intervention and the nature of the contemplated method of surgical salvage must also be balanced by the general physical status of the patient.

Oliva and colleagues[13] summarized 3 critical issues that must be clarified once initial free flap nonviability is confirmed: (1) the reason or reasons for transplant failure, (2) the initial indication for free tissue transplantation, and (3) the status of the resultant wound. Only on careful evaluation of the above-mentioned issues can the surgeon and patient decide on an appropriate next course of action.

The important decisions that must be made are:

- The need for further reconstruction. Is the initial flap failure partial or total? Can the residual defect be treated conservatively? Or is a secondary skin graft, locoregional or is a distant flap warranted?
- Timing of reconstruction. Do critical structures require coverage? When major vessels and neurologic structures are exposed in the head and neck, immediate surgical intervention is mandatory to prevent further morbidity and mortality.
- When reconstruction is necessary, is a second free flap indicated? Or can successful salvage be accomplished with local or regional flaps? The nature of the defect and the tissue composition needing replacement frequently dictate the most appropriate reconstruction to achieve optimal functional outcomes.
- When a second free flap is necessary, what available donor sites remain? Do similar recipient tissues need replacement or can

the reconstructive goal be downgraded by the use of a simple free flap?
- If a second free flap is indicated, what recipient vessels are available? Is a vein graft required?

Answers to the final 2 questions ultimately determine the available options for reconstruction.

NEED FOR FURTHER RECONSTRUCTION

Unlike failed free tissue transfer in the extremities and trunk, reoperative surgery in cases of failed mandibular reconstruction is often inevitable. It is imperative that the reconstructive surgeon reappraises the initial indication for microvascular reconstruction. After careful evaluation of the residual defect, if the indications and reconstructive goals remain unchanged, then second free tissue transfer can be pursued. If only partial flap loss is evident after adequate debridement of the failed flap, then the defect may be successfully reconstructed with a combination of local, regional, and/or nonvascularized bone grafts. However, a second free flap should be attempted in cases of complete flap loss when free tissue transfer is appropriate and if the patient can withstand a second such procedure. Timely wound healing and residual defect repair is uniquely important to the patient undergoing head and neck oncological surgery such that delays in commencement of adjuvant treatments are avoided.

TIMING OF RECONSTRUCTION

Immediate or delayed second free tissue transfer remains a heavily debated topic.[14,15] The nature of the defect at hand inevitably determines the urgency of reconstruction. In the head and neck, an exposed skull base defect may lead to patient death as a result of meningitis and sepsis. Similarly, the exposure of major neck vessels to air and saliva in failed oromandibular reconstruction predisposes to vessel rupture and life-threatening hemorrhage. Oliva and colleagues,[13] in their series, reported an initial mean delay of a second free flap of 248 days from initial surgery. In later cases, this time period decreased dramatically to 7.2 days and finally to immediate second free flaps at exploration when salvage was unsuccessful. In the series by Fearon and colleagues,[14] 3 of 7 patients endured 2-week delays between initial and second free flaps, with the remaining patients ranging from 5 weeks to 21 months. Also, Wei and colleagues[15] reported a mean delay of 12 days (range 2–60 days) between the initial failure and the subsequent second free flaps in 17 of 42 head and neck reconstructive failures. Specifically, in cases of initial flap failure for oromandibular defects, early second free flap attempts are preferable to delayed reconstruction pending individual patient considerations.

SECOND FREE FLAP OUTCOMES

Numerous investigators have reported impressive results with second free flaps after initial flap failures.[13–19] In 2001, Wei and colleagues[15] reported the largest series to date for second free flap management of the initial free flap defect in 3361 head and neck and extremity reconstructions. Complete and partial flap failures occurred in 101 cases (3% failure rate). Of 1235 head and neck free flaps, 42 flap failures (3.4%) were identified. Of these 42 patients with flap failures, 17 received second free flaps, with only 1 flap loss in this group (94.1% success rate). These outcomes clearly showed both the feasibility and safety of second free flap management of the failed initial free flap in the head and neck reconstruction. The investigators noted greater complication rates with salvage regional flaps compared to second free flaps, with one-third of the flaps requiring replacement with another free flap. Based on their findings, they advocate repeat free flap mandibular reconstruction from the contralateral donor site or alterative donor site that is most familiar to the reconstructive microsurgeon. In their opinion, the only definitive contraindication to the above-mentioned treatment is a patient with a physically deteriorating state. Furthermore, they do not recommend the use of the original recipient vessels because these vessels expectedly have inherent vasculitis. Contralateral recipient neck vessels were used in 35% of second free flap cases. In 1999, Heinz

and colleagues[20] reported a significantly increased treatment cost associated with second free flaps (2.5 times). Despite this increased financial burden associated with second free flaps, the advantages in terms of functional superiority when compared with salvage locoregional flaps clearly outweighs the disadvantages (**Fig. 4**A–E).

ADJUNCTIVE WORKUP INVESTIGATIONS/ TOOLS

The preoperative workup of patients undergoing reoperative mandibular reconstruction varies somewhat based on the surgical plan. If free tissue transfer is the chosen method of reconstruction, the patient often has had appropriate preoperative imaging for that specific donor site (ie, computer tomographic [CT] angiogram of the lower extremities for fibula flap) based on the comorbidities of the patient. Contrast angiographic studies of the neck vasculature may also prove invaluable particularly when prior neck dissection has been performed or the initial surgery was performed at another institution (**Fig. 5**). Most reconstructive surgeons would also reimage the residual mandibular defect with a combination of a panoramic radiograph, a CT scan and, in some cases, a stereolithographic model. Computer software advances and computer-aided planning have added another dimension to the surgeon's accuracy and precision of reconstruction. Clinical photographs are valuable for both surgical planning and medicolegal purposes. Depending on the preoperative dental state, dental models mounted on an articulator can also prove useful, especially if it is the desire of the patient to be prosthetically rehabilitated after surgery. Stereolithographic models allow preoperative contouring of titanium reconstruction bars that can be sterilized for use in the operating room, saving significant time. Also, the contralateral possibly unaffected side of the mandible can be visualized in 3-dimensional rendition to optimize facial symmetry. In cases when a CT with model has been obtained, virtual surgery can be performed, with the CT scan of the patients allowing preoperative surgical guide fabrication based on computer-generated desired virtual outcomes.

COMPLICATIONS

Complications resulting from reoperative mandibular reconstruction can arise from multiple sources. It is imperative that all surgeons embarking on reoperative mandibular reconstruction analyze why the initial operation failed, especially when a second vascularized bone flap is intended. If

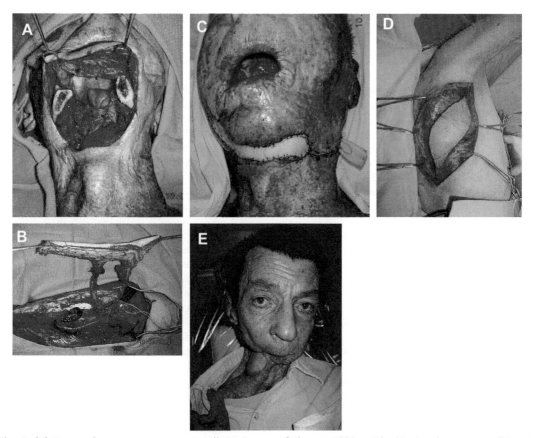

Fig. 4. (*A*) Resected recurrent squamous cell carcinoma of the mandible with skin involvement resulting in a through and through defect. (*B*) An anterolateral (ALT) thigh flap is harvested to reconstruct the defect. (*C*) Inset of the ALT flap that eventually failed. (*D*) Harvesting of a latissimus flap as a second flap to salvage the reconstruction. (*E*) Patient after latissimus flap salvage surgery.

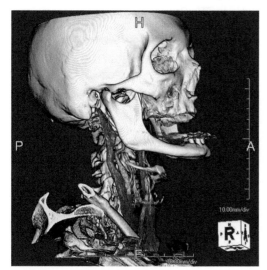

Fig. 5. Example of a CT angiogram of the neck to assess the vasculature during a workup of a patient for free tissue transfer.

initial flap failure was related to the medical comorbidities of the patient, then a thorough patient workup is critical to avoiding a repeat failure. However, if the failure was a result of poor surgical technique, then clear identification of such errors is critical before undertaking additional microsurgical reconstruction.

SUMMARY

Reoperative mandibular reconstruction poses many unique challenges to the head and neck reconstructive surgeon. Restoring proper form and function of the oromandibular complex via further surgical intervention is vital to not only facial aesthetics but also basic functions of daily life. A well-planned and executed surgery is essential to restore patients to their premorbid state with good long-term success. The use of free tissue transfer has revolutionized the reconstruction of previously operated patients, providing superior vascularity to locoregional flap alternatives together with enabling the replacement of both soft and hard tissues to restore the functional and aesthetic components of the oromandibular complex. Achieving excellent results in these patients is paramount to their quality of life, which ultimately form the basis for successful rehabilitation and reintegration into society.

REFERENCES

1. Ariyan S. The pectoralis major myocutaneous flap. Plast Reconstr Surg 1979;63:73–81.
2. Lawson V. Oral cavity reconstruction using pectoralis major muscle and amnion. Arch Otolaryngol Head Neck Surg 1985;111:230–3.
3. Robertson M, Allison R. The pectoralis major muscle in head and neck reconstruction. Head Neck Reconstr 1986;56:753–7.
4. Ariyan S. The viability of rib grafts transplanted with the periosteal blood supply. Plast Reconstr Surg 1980;65:140–51.
5. Urken ML, Weinberg H, Buchbinder D, et al. Microvascular free flaps in head and neck reconstruction. Arch Otolaryngol Head Neck Surg 1994;120:633.
6. Nakatsuka T, Harii K, Asato H, et al. Analytic review of 2372 free flap transfers for head and neck reconstruction following cancer resection. J Reconstr Microsurg 2003;19:363.
7. Shestak KC, Jones NF. Microsurgical free-tissue transfer in the elderly patient. Plast Reconstr Surg 1991;88:259.
8. Kroll SS, Schusterman MA, Reece GP, et al. Choice of flap and incidence of free flap success. Plast Reconstr Surg 1996;98:459.
9. Nahabedian MY, Singh N, Deune EG, et al. Recipient vessel analysis for microvascular reconstruction of the head and neck. Ann Plast Surg 2004;52:148.
10. Urken ML, Weinberg H, Vickery C, et al. Oromandibular reconstruction using microvascular composite free flaps. Arch Otolaryngol Head Neck Surg 1991; 117:733–44.
11. Dingman RO, Grabb WC. Surgical anatomy of the mandibular ramus of the facial nerve based on the dissection of 100 facial halves. Plast Reconstr Surg 1962;29:266.
12. Ziarah HA, Atkinson ME. The surgical anatomy of the cervical distribution of the facial nerve. Br J Oral Maxillofac Surg 1981;19:159.
13. Oliva A, Lineaweaver WC, Buncke HJ, et al. Salvage of wounds following failed tissue transplantation. J Reconstr Microsurg 1993;9:257–63.
14. Fearon JA, Cuadros L, May JW. Flap failure after microvascular free-tissue transfer: the fate of a second attempt. Plast Reconstr Surg 1990;86: 746–51.
15. Wei FC, Demirkan F, Chen HC, et al. The outcome of failed free flaps in head and neck and extremity reconstruction: what is next in the reconstructive ladder? Plast Reconstr Surg 2001;108:1154–60.
16. Okazaki M, Asato H, Takushima A, et al. Analysis of salvage treatments following the failure of free flap transfer caused by vascular thrombosis in reconstruction for head and neck cancer. Plast Reconstr Surg 2007;119:1223–32.
17. Abdel-Wahab Amin A, Baldwin BJ, Gurlek A, et al. Second free flaps in head and neck reconstruction. J Reconstr Microsurg 1998;14(6):365–8.
18. Bertino G, Benazzo M, Occhini A, et al. Reconstruction of the hypopharynx after free jejunum flap failure: is a second free jejunum transfer feasible? Oral Oncol 2008;44:61–4.
19. Lydiatt DD, Lydiatt WM, Hollins RR, et al. Use of free fibula flap in patients with prior failed mandibular reconstruction. J Oral Maxillofac Surg 1998;56: 444–6.
20. Heinz TR, Cowper PA, Levin LS. Microsurgery costs and outcomes. Plast Reconstr Surg 1999; 104(1):89–96.

Reoperative Maxillofacial Oncology

Daniel Petrisor, DMD, MD, Rui Fernandes, DMD, MD*

KEYWORDS

• Oropharyngeal • Recurrence • Radiotherapy • Locoregional

According to the Oral Cancer Foundation, approximately 36,000 people in the United States will be diagnosed with oral or oropharyngeal cancer in 2010.[1] In more than 90% of the cases of oral cavity and oropharyngeal cancers, histopathologic examination reveals squamous cell carcinoma (SCCA).[2] Management of oral SCCA is determined by many factors, but the primary modality of treatment remains surgery. Higher T and N status, and thus the higher stage of disease (stage III or IV), is generally treated with multimodal therapy using surgery and postoperative radiation therapy.

RECURRENCE

Treatment failure in oral SCCA can be divided into 5 categories: persistent disease, local recurrence, regional recurrence, distant metastasis, and the development of a second primary tumor. Locally persistent disease is defined as disease that had an incomplete response to definitive therapy or tumor that develops within 6 weeks of definitive therapy after a brief disease-free period.[3] Recurrent disease is defined as tumor that presents after a 6-week disease-free period. Recurrence can be further subdivided into recurrence at the tumor resection margins, local recurrence, or recurrence in the neck, regional recurrence. A second primary is a tumor that presents in an area different from the original or initial tumor.

The reality of oral cancer is that despite appropriate initial treatment, even if the resection margins are reported as histologically negative and even in the face of postoperative radiation therapy, oral SCCA recurs in 25% to 48% of cases.[4,5] Most patients whose cancer cannot be controlled experience local or regional recurrence, and its incidence is related mainly to the site of the tumor, clinical stage, and histopathologic characteristics.[4]

Numerous risk factors for recurrence have been investigated for oral SCCA, including advanced pathologic stage, histologic grade, tumor differentiation, pathologic lymph nodes, extracapsular spread, and margin status. Among them, the effect of margin status is well defined. Multiple studies suggest that 66% to 80% of patients with a positive resection margin will either develop a local recurrence or demonstrate persistent disease on reoperation.[6–8] A close, but clear, margin does not carry as high a recurrence rate as observed for patients with disease at the inked resection margin.[9,10] The most widely accepted definition of a close, but clear, margin is that the tumor is within 5 mm of the inked resection margin.[11] Nason and colleagues[11] analyzed a historical cohort of 277 surgically treated patients with oral SCCA and found that patients with margins of 5 mm or more had a 5-year survival rate of 73% when compared with those with margins of 3 to 4 mm (69%), 2 mm or less (62%), and involved margins (39%) (Table 1). After controlling for confounding variables (age, gender, stage), they found that each 1-mm increase in the clear surgical margin decreased the risk of death at 5 years by 8%. It was also noted that patients with positive surgical margins had a 2.5-fold increase in the risk of death at 5 years and those with close (≤3 mm) margins had a 1.5-fold increase in the risk of death when compared with patients with margins greater

Division of Oral and Maxillofacial Surgery, Department of Surgery, University of Florida, 653-1 West 8th Street, Jacksonville, FL 32209, USA
* Corresponding author.
E-mail address: rui.fernandes@jax.ufl.edu

Oral Maxillofacial Surg Clin N Am 23 (2011) 161–168
doi:10.1016/j.coms.2010.11.002
1042-3699/11/$ – see front matter © 2011 Elsevier Inc. All rights reserved.

Table 1
Relationship of the status of the surgical margin to the incidence of recurrence, sites of initial recurrence, and 5-year survival

	Margin Status					
	Involved (n = 61)	≤2 mm (n = 80)	3–4 mm (n = 95)	≥5 mm (n = 95)	All (n = 277)	P Value
Recurrence	27 (44.3)	33 (41.3)	10 (24.4)	24 (25.3)	94 (33.9)	.01
Site of Recurrence						
Primary Site	16 (26.2)	18 (22.5)	6 (14.6)	8 (8.4)	48 (17.3)	.04
Neck	14 (23.0)	13 (16.3)	5 (12.2)	13 (13.7)	45 (16.2)	.40
Metastases	3 (4.91)	6 (7.50)	1 (2.50)	4 (4.21)	14 (5.05)	.74
Survival at 5 years (%)						
Recurrence Free	48.3	48.5	69.5	70.5	59.4	.005
Overall	38.6	62.6	69.6	72.9	60.6	<.001

Numbers in parentheses are percentages.
Adapted from Nason RW, et al. What is the adequate margin of surgical resection in oral cancer? Oral Surg Oral Med Oral Pathol Oral Radiol Endod 2009;107(5):625–9; with permission.

than 3 mm. Hence, the investigators suggest that an adequate resection in oral cancer should provide a margin greater than 3 mm in width on permanent pathology section. Others suggest that histologically negative margins should be defined as no dysplasia, carcinoma in situ, or invasive carcinoma within 5 mm of the resection margin.[12] Regarding the relationship between the rate of locoregional recurrence and local regional factors, Koo and colleagues[4] noted that the resection margin status was a particularly important, and a potentially preventable, independent predictor for locoregional control (**Fig. 1**).

PATIENT SURVEILLANCE

The high rate of cancer recurrence among patients with oral SCCA points to the need for close posttreatment surveillance. Several studies have shown that most cancers recur within about 2 years after the initial treatment.[4,13] Hence, close follow-up of patients is important for the timely detection of recurrences. A common surveillance schedule is once every month during the first year, every second month during the second year, every third month during the third year, every sixth month during the fourth year, and once a year thereafter. After 5 years of follow-up, healthy patients are considered cured and, hence, they continue to be followed up yearly or are discharged.

Follow-up examinations clearly require close attention to both the primary site and the draining lymph nodes. Schwartz and colleagues[14] reported most recurrences at the primary site (58%), while the second most common pattern was

locoregional recurrence (26%). Similarly, Pathak and colleagues[15] in a review of 159 locoregional recurrences of SCCA of the lower gingivobuccal complex found that 56% were in the oral cavity, 20% were in the neck, and 24% involved both the neck and the primary site, with 79% of all recurrences being experienced within 18 months of surgery. Alternatively, Whitehurst and Droulias[16] found that most patients experienced recurrence regionally, with the remainder divided evenly between local and locoregional recurrences.

The clinical presentation of a patient with recurrent oral cavity SCCA can be variable, but most patients with persistent or recurrent disease complain of pain. Smit and colleagues[17] evaluated the role of pain as a sign of recurrent disease in patients with head and neck SCCA. They found that in 70% of all cases, tumor recurrence was preceded by pain complaints, whereas in their control group, only 2% had pain complaints. Thus, this symptom should be considered a warning sign, and patients with this symptom need to be followed up with a thorough head and neck examination.

As important as it is, the head and neck examination may offer limited information in the previously surgically treated or radiation-treated patient. This limitation may be even more pronounced in cases that were initially treated with combined modality therapy and significant posttreatment fibrosis has developed.[18] The use of a bulky flap to reconstruct the ablative defect can further obstruct the evaluation.[18] In this situation, imaging studies such as computed tomography or magnetic resonance imaging may be helpful to localize occult recurrences and can

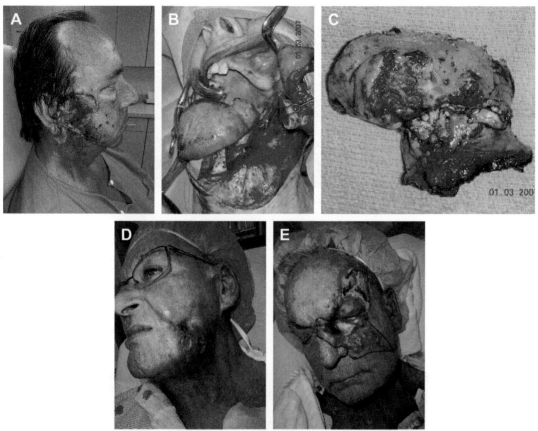

Fig. 1. (*A*) Recurrent carcinoma in the preauricular region with facial nerve involvement. (*B*) Recurrence at the base of tongue after initial treatment with primary radiation therapy. (*C*) Resected specimen showing the extent of disease to the base of tongue and lateral pharynx. (*D*) Large recurrent disease after failed primary radiotherapy for an SCCA of the floor of mouth. (*E*) Recurrent poorly differentiated carcinoma in an immunosuppressed patient who underwent a kidney transplant.

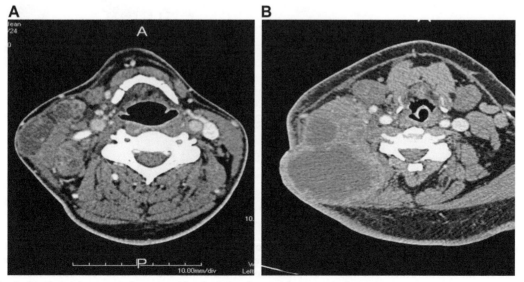

Fig. 2. (*A, B*) Axial computed tomography depicting large-volume neck disease.

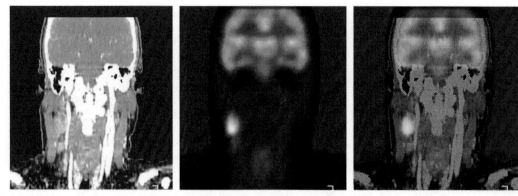

Fig. 3. PET/computed tomographic scan showing recurrent deep-neck disease.

serve to facilitate fine-needle aspiration cytology or biopsies during an evaluation under anesthesia (**Fig. 2**).

Because malignant cells are known to have an increased glycolytic metabolism, positron emission tomography (PET) with fluorodeoxyglucose (FDG) allows for evaluation of tumor recurrence in the face of distorted anatomy. In a prospective study, Krabbe and colleagues[19] found that ^{18}F FDG PET showed a sensitivity, specificity, positive predictive value, and negative predictive value of 100%, 43%, 51%, and 100%, respectively. In addition, for regular follow-up (ie, history and physical examination), these values were 0%,

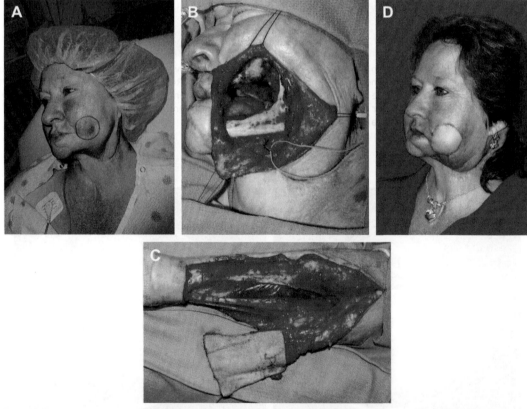

Fig. 4. (*A*) Recurrent disease in a patient with a history of buccal SCCA. Note the extent of recurrence with skin involvement. (*B*) Defect after a complete resection of the recurrent carcinoma. (*C*) Radial forearm free flap harvested for the reconstruction. The flap in deepitheliazed in the center and folded to reconstruct the buccal mucosal defect and the external skin defect. (*D*) The 2-week postoperative view of the patient.

60%, 0%, and 50%, respectively. PET scanning accounted for a change in diagnostics or treatment in 63% of the patients and regular follow-up in 25% of patients. They concluded that the best timing for a systemic ^{18}F FDG PET scan is between 3 and 6 months after treatment (**Fig. 3**).

TREATMENT OF RECURRENT DISEASE
Local Recurrence

Management of recurrent disease after previous surgical resection or combined modality treatment is a challenging clinical situation. Salvage of recurrence can be limited by many factors, including the extent of tumor involvement, previous adjuvant radiation therapy or chemotherapy, previous surgery and reconstruction, and the often poor general health of the patients at the time of recurrence. Most cases of recurrent oral SCCA that are treated for cure involve surgery as a major component of the salvage therapy.[18] Koo and colleagues[4] studied 127 patients surgically treated for SCCA of the oral cavity. Of these, 36 patients experienced recurrence and salvage treatment was attempted in 23 (64%). Of these 23 patients, 13 underwent salvage surgery with or without additional radiation therapy and 10 received chemotherapy and/or radiation therapy. It was

found that patients who underwent salvage surgery with or without postoperative radiotherapy had significantly improved salvage and total survival times compared with the patients who received chemotherapy and/or radiation therapy for their recurrence. Furthermore, the average salvage time in patients in whom the tumor recurred more than 6 months after their initial treatment was not significantly improved, even though the total survival time was improved by a statistically significant level. Thus, the early surgical salvage of locoregional recurrent SCCA of the oral cavity is the most reasonable option for patients.

Surgical resection of recurrent oral cancer with the intent to obtain clear margins can be confounded by factors such as radiation fibrosis, distorted tissue from previous surgery, and changes related to previous reconstruction. In this setting, initial margins of 2 cm are appropriate and should be followed by frozen sections to confirm the clear margins.[18] With the advent of microvascular reconstruction, functional reconstruction can be achieved even after wide margins of resection. As far as the management of the mandible is concerned, in cases in which previous treatment did not include the mandible, the same surgical protocols can be used for previously

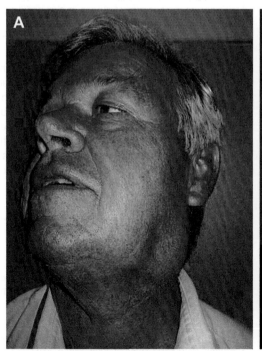
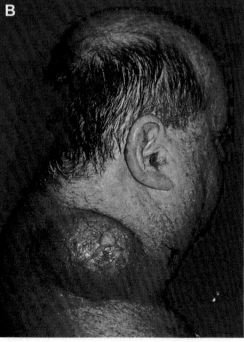

Fig. 5. (*A*) Patient with left upper jugular chain nodal recurrence. (*B*) Large neck recurrence with overlying skin involvement.

untreated and recurrent disease. For early tumors with minimal invasion, a rim or marginal resection is used with the saw cut angled to take into account the point of tumor entry, especially in tumors recurring adjacent to or abutting the mandible.[20] For advanced or deep tumors in the soft tissues abutting the mandible, a segmental resection is a safer option than a sagittal rim resection.[20] In cases in which a recurrent tumor is adherent to a previous rim resection site, a segmental resection should be completed (**Fig. 4**).

RECURRENT TUMOR IN THE NECK

Reoperative surgery for recurrent cancer in the neck can be a challenging undertaking. Treatment choices for managing neck recurrences depend to a large extent on the initial treatment of the primary tumor. Ferlito and colleagues[3] describe several clinical situations that are possible for recurrent disease in the neck as summarized in **Table 1**. If the initial treatment was surgery alone, surgery with adjuvant radiotherapy is often still possible and patients have an acceptable chance of regional control.[3,21] However, repeat neck dissection after previous surgery such as selective neck dissection or modified radical neck is challenging because recurrent disease is often within the soft tissues of the neck rather than within the nodes that are surrounded by fibrofatty tissue. Hence, if recurrent disease occurs within previously dissected neck levels, it will most likely be adherent to the great vessels of the neck, making complete resection difficult. If the recurrence presents at previously undissected levels, complete respectability may be possible. Lim and colleagues[21] reported on 236 patients who developed a recurrence after primary curative surgery with or without radiation therapy for head and neck SCCA. They found that the rate of isolated neck recurrence was 26% after primary surgical therapy and the overall salvage rate was 33% after salvage treatment. In addition, they concluded that previous treatment with surgery alone and a recurrent N1 tumor were independent predictive factors for a favorable outcome of salvage treatment (**Fig. 5**).

Patients initially treated with radiation therapy alone can also be treated with salvage surgery. The extent of surgical resection is often dictated by the location of the recurrence. Imaging studies should be reviewed to assess the location, extent, relationship to the carotid artery, and involvement of other soft tissues of the neck, such as the deep neck musculature. Edelstein describes certain

---

Box 1
Different possible clinical situations of neck tumor recurrence

- Neck recurrence after neck radiotherapy
- Neck recurrence after neck surgery

  Radical neck dissection

  Modified neck dissection

  Selective neck dissection

  Wide nodal resection

- Neck recurrence after combined therapy

  Surgery and radiotherapy

  Radiotherapy and surgery

  Chemoradiation

  Chemotherapy and surgery

- Neck recurrence in untreated neck
- Neck recurrence associated with local recurrence (locoregional recurrence)
- Neck recurrence associated with distant recurrence (regional and distant recurrence)
- Neck recurrence associated with local and distant recurrences (distant and locoregional recurrences)
- Neck recurrence associated with tracheostomal recurrence
- Ipsilateral neck recurrence
- Contralateral neck recurrence
- Bilateral neck recurrence

Data from Ferlito A, Shaha AR, Rinaldo A. Surgical management of recurrent tumor in the neck. Acta Otolaryngol 2002;122(1):121–6.

---

features of recurrent neck disease that may make reoperation contraindicated.[18] These features are summarized in **Box 1**. Even if a recurrent tumor is deemed resectable, the incidence of wound complications is high in patients who have been treated previously with a full course of radiation therapy, and the incidence of complications is even higher if the surgical procedure also includes treatment of the primary tumor (**Box 2**, **Fig. 6**).[3]

Box 2
Features that suggest tumor unresectability

- Carotid encasement/invasion/occlusion
- Dermal lymphatic invasion/dermal metastases
- Invasion of deep neck musculature/fixation to deep neck/brachial plexus invasion
- Base of skull invasion/extension/erosion

Data from Edelstein DR. Revision surgery in otolaryngology. New York: Thieme; 2009. xxii, p. 480.

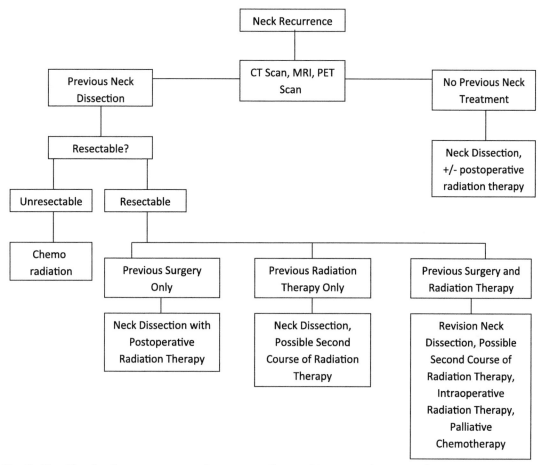

Fig. 6. Algorithm for the management of recurrence disease. CT, computed tomography; MRI, magnetic resonance imaging.

SUMMARY

Surgeons involved in the management of patients with malignancies must be facile with the diagnosis, surveillance, and work-up of possible recurrent disease. The reoperative intervention in these patients is often more challenging than the initial intervention because of several factors, including surgery in an irradiated field, surgery in a previously operated field, malnourishment of the patients because of their disease, and the availability of limited reconstructive options in these patients not only because of some of the already stated factors but also because of a paucity of recipient vessels and decreased donor site options. Irrespective of the challenges, surgeons are often the last resort for these patients, and as such they should be well versed on these issues and possessing of the necessary skill set to tackle these difficult patients.

REFERENCES

1. Available at: http://oralcancerfoundation.org. Accessed November 15, 2010.
2. Available at: www.cancer.org. Accessed November 15, 2010.
3. Ferlito A, Shaha AR, Rinaldo A. Surgical management of recurrent tumor in the neck. Acta Otolaryngol 2002;122(1):121–6.
4. Koo BS, Lim YC, Lee JS, et al. Recurrence and salvage treatment of squamous cell carcinoma of the oral cavity. Oral Oncol 2006;42(8):789–94.
5. Shah JP, Cendon RA, Farr HW, et al. Carcinoma of the oral cavity. Factors affecting treatment failure at the primary site and neck. Am J Surg 1976;132(4): 504–7.
6. Chen TY, Emrich LJ, Driscoll DL. The clinical significance of pathological findings in surgically resected margins of the primary tumor in head and neck

carcinoma. Int J Radiat Oncol Biol Phys 1987;13(6): 833–7.

7. Jones AS, Bin Hanafi Z, Nadapalan V, et al. Do positive resection margins after ablative surgery for head and neck cancer adversely affect prognosis? A study of 352 patients with recurrent carcinoma following radiotherapy treated by salvage surgery. Br J Cancer 1996;74:128–32.

8. Byers RM, Bland KI, Borlase B, et al. The prognostic and therapeutic value of frozen section determinations in the surgical treatment of squamous cell carcinoma of the head and neck. Am J Surg 1978; 136:525–8.

9. Loree TR, Strong EW. Significance of positive margins in oral cavity squamous carcinoma. Am J Surg 1990;160(4):410–4.

10. Sutton DN, Brown JS, Rogers SN, et al. The prognostic implications of the surgical margin in oral squamous cell carcinoma. Int J Oral Maxillofac Surg 2003;32(1):30–4.

11. Nason RW, Binahmed A, Pathak KA, et al. What is the adequate margin of surgical resection in oral cancer? Oral Surg Oral Med Oral Pathol Oral Radiol Endod 2009;107(5):625–9.

12. Kim DD, Ord RA. Complications in the treatment of head and neck cancer. Oral Maxillofac Surg Clin North Am 2003;15(2):213–27.

13. Wong LY, Wei WI, Lam LK, et al. Salvage of recurrent head and neck squamous cell carcinoma after primary curative surgery. Head Neck 2003;25(11): 953–9.

14. Schwartz GJ, Mehta RH, Wenig BL, et al. Salvage treatment for recurrent squamous cell carcinoma of the oral cavity. Head Neck 2000;22(1):34–41.

15. Pathak KA, Gupta S, Talole S, et al. Advanced squamous cell carcinoma of lower gingivobuccal complex: patterns of spread and failure. Head Neck 2005;27(7):597–602.

16. Whitehurst JO, Droulias CA. Surgical treatment of squamous cell carcinoma of the oral tongue: factors influencing survival. Arch Otolaryngol 1977;103(4):212–5.

17. Smit M, Balm AJ, Hilgers FJ, et al. Pain as sign of recurrent disease in head and neck squamous cell carcinoma. Head Neck 2001;23(5):372–5.

18. Edelstein DR. Revision surgery in otolaryngology. New York: Thieme; 2009. xxii, p. 480.

19. Krabbe CA, Pruim J, Dijkstra PU, et al. 18F-FDG PET for routine posttreatment surveillance in oral and oropharyngeal squamous cell carcinoma. J Nucl Med 2010;51:1164–5.

20. Brown JS, Kalavrezos N, D'Souza J, et al. Factors that influence the method of mandibular resection in the management of oral squamous cell carcinoma. Br J Oral Maxillofac Surg 2002;40(4):275–84.

21. Lim JY, Lim YC, Kim SH, et al. Factors predictive of successful outcome following salvage treatment of isolated neck recurrences. Otolaryngol Head Neck Surg 2010;142(6):832–7.

Reoperations in Cleft Lip and Cleft Palate Treatment

Rafael Ruiz-Rodríguez, DDS*,
Juan Carlos López-Noriega, DDS

KEYWORDS

- Revision cleft lip • Revision cleft palate
- Complications cleft lip/palate surgery

The surgical management of cleft lip and palate is a difficult and complex endeavor. Several surgical techniques for the treatment of this deformity have been described around the world; each one, when properly done by expert surgeons, renders good and predictable results most of the times. However, the fact that there are so many techniques means that there is no universal procedure that will always deliver great esthetic and functional results.

The integral management of the cleft lip and cleft palate deformities requires many different procedures such as cheiloplasty, palatoplasty, nasoalveolar fistula closure and bone grafting, pharyngoplasties, distraction osteogenesis, and orthognathic surgery. All these procedures are not related to improper management or complications but are inherent sequelae of the deformity.

One must remember that surgery is no magic, a defect so noticeable like a cleft lip is changed to a scar that will continue to be noticeable and stigmatize the patient. Scar revisions, dermabrasion, and use of fillers are some of the available procedures to make these scars less conspicuous; however, in certain occasions the primary repair renders untoward results that requires a more comprehensive surgical care.

Poor surgical results in the management of patients with cleft lip and palate are related to factors such as wide deformities, and severely displaced premaxilla as well as election of bad surgical technique, procedures not well performed, bad postoperative care, poor healing, and infection. In addition, it is very important to mention the steep learning curve in the surgical management of these deformities.

Bad results after a primary lip repair may present as poor lip esthetics, animation, and inappropriate function. Persistent rhinolalia and oronasal communication account for the more common unsatisfactory outcomes after primary palate repair.

The inadequate results in cleft lip and palate surgery can be:

1. Related to an adequately and precisely performed primary procedure. Unsatisfactory results related to well-performed techniques are associated with a severe deformity, bad postoperative care, infection, excessive scar retraction, and hypertrophic or keloid scars. The advantage in these cases is that all the anatomic structures for esthetics and function, such as the nasal ala, columella, Cupid bow, philtrum, and white roll, are still present and were not removed by mistake or lack of experience during the primary procedure. Usually simpler surgical solutions are used to repair these types of deformities.
2. Related to an inadequately performed primary procedure. This category of poor results is related to a badly selected, badly designed, or badly performed surgical procedure. As a consequence, irreplaceable anatomic structures are missing because of their removal or injury during surgery. It is important to note that these structures cannot be replaced and

Department of Oral and Maxillofacial Surgery, Faculty of Dentistry, Universidad Nacional Autónoma de México, Ciudad Universitaria, Mexico D.F. C.P. 06700, Mexico
* Corresponding author.
E-mail address: raruro@yahoo.com

Oral Maxillofacial Surg Clin N Am 23 (2011) 169–176
doi:10.1016/j.coms.2010.12.002

oralmaxsurgery.theclinics.com

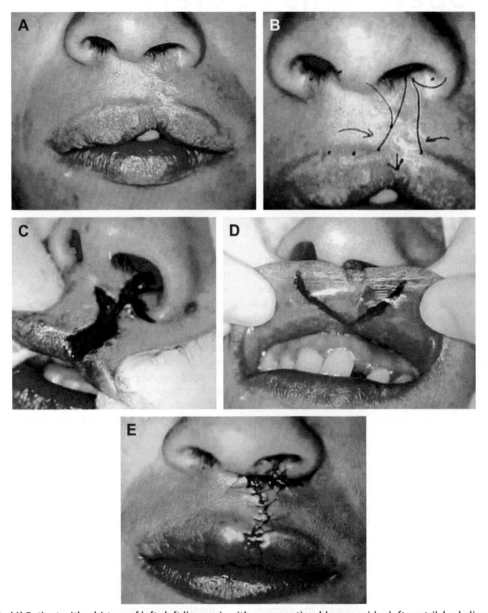

Fig. 1. (*A*) Patient with a history of left cleft lip repair with a very noticeable scar, wider left nostril, bad alignment of the white roll and whistle deformity. (*B*) Markings illustrating the Millard rotation and advancement flap technique for secondary correction of the cleft lip. (*C*) Flap rotation and advancement. (*D*) V-Y advancement of the upper lip oral mucosa to repair the whistle deformity. (*E*) Immediate postoperative picture showing correction of the above-mentioned problems.

should always be identified and preserved at the time of the primary repair. An example may be demonstrated by injury to the palatine artery during dissection, causing avascular necrosis of a portion of palatal flap and the subsequent development of large palatal fistulas.

The clinician must be aware that the best moment to obtain the best result is always during

the primary repair of the deformity. Secondary surgery is always more difficult; tissues are highly fibrous with poor vascularity, making dissection and re-creation of missing structures more challenging. The basic surgical principles to follow are (1) identification and preservation of all the vital anatomic structures for esthetics and function, such as the orbicularis oris muscle, the vermilion border, the white roll, and the descending palatine artery and (2) awareness of the extremely small

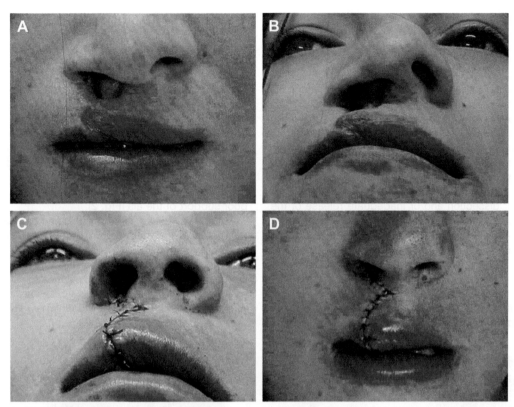

Fig. 2. (*A, B*) Patient with a history of right cleft lip repair with a residual nasal floor deformity, very noticeable scar, wider right nostril, and bad alignment of the vermilion border and white roll. (*C, D*) Postoperative pictures after a rotation and advancement flap technique improvement of the above-described problems.

working area where a slightly misplaced incision could remove an important piece of tissue that with time would develop as a very perceptible scar. It has been said that it is easier to fix a defect when excess of tissue is present rather that when the defect requires extra tissue. A good example of this statement is when during primary surgery an aggressive excision of tissue at the alar base results in an excessive narrowing of the nostril. The correction of this acquired defect is more difficult than correcting a wider nostril caused by a conservative approach that left more tissue, which allows for an easier secondary surgical correction.

REOPERATIONS IN CLEFT LIP SURGERY

It is always important to point out that the main objectives of reoperation in cleft lip surgery are the same as those in a primary surgery: reestablishment of normal esthetics and function by closure of the floor of the nose, reconstruction of the orbicularis muscle, placement of the Cupid bow in a horizontal position, mobilization of the philtrum to the midline, and maintenance of a thick vermilion border and the nasal symmetry.

As previously discussed, simple reoperations with relatively predictable results can be performed to correct minor deformities such as misalignments in the position of the white roll or vermilion border, nostril asymmetry, hypertrophic scar, whistle lip deformity, and short upper lip. A wider nostril may be corrected by performing a semilunar incision around the nasal alae with excision of a small amount of tissue to allow medial rotation of the nasal alae (Weir technique). Widening of the asymmetric nasal base is a more complex procedure. A small cheek transposition flap pedicled inferiorly is designed from the external portion of the alar base, just close to where the nasogenial groove stars. Medial rotation of the cheek tissue into the nasal vestibule allows for lateral advancement of the nasal ala, allowing widening of the nostril. Imperceptible misalignments when suturing the white roll may generate defects that become noticeable with patient growth; however, these defects can be corrected with a small Z-plasty. Vermilion border deficiencies and whistle lip deformities may be corrected by a submucosal graft or a V-Y advancement flap. Hypertrophic scars with shortening of the lip require an excision of the scar, usually with a rhomboid incision that would also allow lengthening of the lip. An advantage of all these procedures is that they carry little invasiveness and can be performed under local anesthesia or sedation.

When larger deformities are present, such as partial or complete dehiscence of the lip or nasal floor, severely hypertrophic or excessively contracted scar, and excessive resection of anatomic structures including the nasal alae, and philtrum, more intricate secondary surgical procedures may be necessary. Lip dehiscence is related to excessive suture tension normally caused by poor dissection and/or inadequate release of the subcutaneous tissue and muscle. Similarly, nasal floor dehiscence is linked to inadequate dissection of the mucosa flap from the nasal ala laterally and the nasal mucosa flap from the septum.

In general, the authors' approach is tailored to the patient's needs and existing anatomy. Most of these cases may be corrected using the same approach as doing a primary repair on an incomplete cleft lip. The authors' preference is to use Millard's rotation and advancement flap technique (**Fig. 1**). The 2 problems related to this technique are: (1) potential excessive nostril narrowing, which can be avoided by rotating and insetting the medial flap at the nasal base and not where the incision ends and (2) potential vertical scar contraction, which may be fixed by leaving the affected upper lip 1 to 2 mm longer than the unaffected side. There should be further consideration during reoperation for the correction of additional problems, such as repairing of the nasal floor, narrowing of the wider nostril, and correction of the poor support of the ala (**Fig. 2**).

Cases of bilateral cleft lip are commonly very challenging, especially when the premaxilla is extremely prominent or located in a more anterior and inferior position than normal. Good results are more difficult to achieve, and reoperations are common. Most of the times these cases necessitate the combination of several techniques in order to achieve acceptable results (**Fig. 3**).

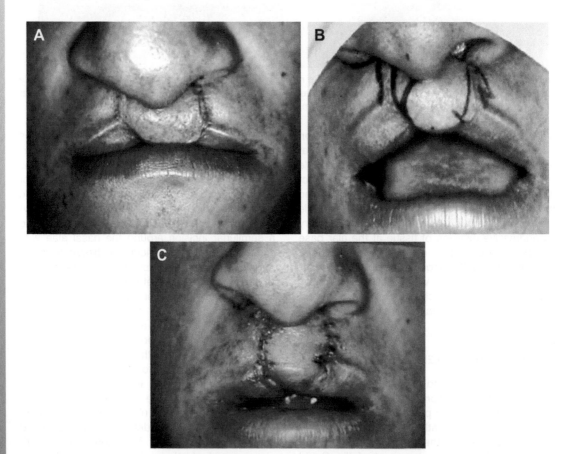

Fig. 3. (*A–C*) Patient with a history of bilateral cleft lip repair in which 2 techniques were used to correct the secondary deformities: a rotation with advancement flap on the right and the Tennison triangular flap on the left. These flaps were further combined with a large V-Y advancement of the vermilion border to create a normal and prominent tubercle and regular vermilion border.

In severe cases in which the philtrum is lost or is not useful because of multiple scars, an Abbe-Estlander flap represents a great alternative for reconstruction of the upper lip with low morbidity. This flap provides enough tissue for vertical lengthening and horizontal projection of the upper lip, simulating the philtrum and the Cupid bow. This technique allows rotation from the lower lip

of a full-thickness pedicle flap that includes skin, muscle, and oral mucosa. The pedicle flap can be V shaped or W shaped however, the authors prefer the W shape because it adapts perfectly well to the base of the columella. The flap must be dissected carefully to identify the lower labial artery that is located very close to the vermilion border. Also, the artery has to be maintained on

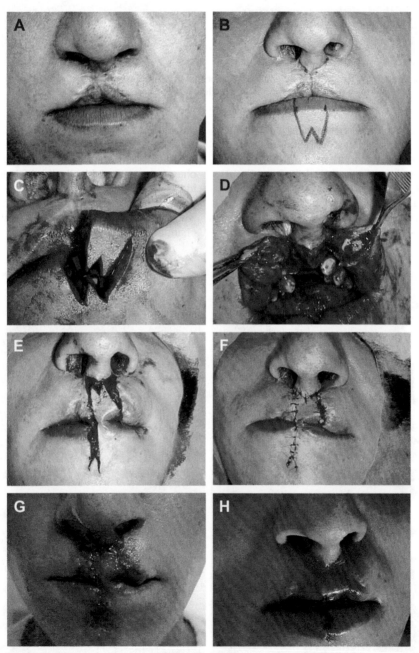

Fig. 4. Abbe flap (*A*) Patient with a history of bilateral cleft lip repair in which the philtrum was lost resulting in an absence of the Cupid bow, very noticeable scar, short upper lip, and whistle deformity. (*B*) Abbe flap markings. (*C*) Flap elevation preserving the vascular supply. (*D*) Preparation of the recipient bed. (*E*, *F*) Flap rotation, inset, and closure. (*G*, *H*) Flap takedown, and the immediate final result.

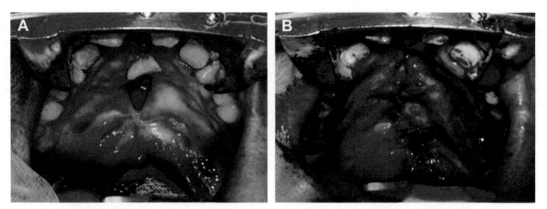

Fig. 5. (*A, B*) Midpalatal fistula repaired similar to a primary palatoplasty with the development of nasal and palatal flaps. The palatal flaps are fully mobilized to allow tension-free closure.

the pedicle side to preserve blood supply. The flap is rotated to the area of upper lip that has already been prepared by a good dissection of the orbicularis oris muscle and removal of the scar tissue. The muscle layer is sutured first followed by the oral mucosa and skin. The donor site on the lower lip is closed in the regular manner. After at least 2 weeks, a 2-0 silk suture is placed around the pedicle to test the flap revascularization. If no changes are noted, the flap pedicle can be cut. Additional time might be necessary if ischemic changes are noted. Mostly, this technique requires further scar revisions (**Fig. 4**). Counseling may be necessary for this procedure in male patients who grow a mustache because of hair orientation changes in the flap area.

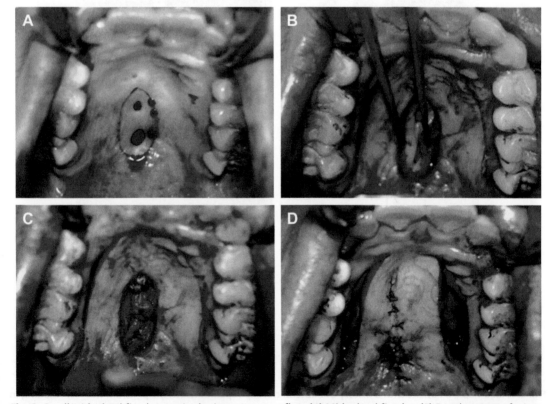

Fig. 6. Small midpalatal fistulas repaired using a turnover flap. (*A*) Midpalatal fistulas. (*B*) Development of a turnover flap with perifistular tissue. (*C*) Closure of the nasal floor. (*D*) Closure of the palatal mucosa. Note the releasing incision to allow mobilization and tension-free closure of the flaps.

REOPERATIONS IN CLEFT PALATE SURGERY

The main goal of cleft palate surgery is to isolate the oral cavity from the nasal cavity and provide good function of the soft palate. Proper closure and reconstruction of the palate and its musculature allows for normal deglutition and phonetics.

Similar to the cleft lip surgery, several surgical techniques have been described for the management of cleft palate. All these techniques are based on the development of 2 nasal flaps for nasal floor reconstruction and 2 palatal flaps for closure of the oral mucosa. In addition, on the soft palate, besides these 4 flaps, a good dissection and repair of the palatal muscles creates an extra layer of closure and promote good function of the oropharynx.

Suture failure, flap tension, bad postoperative care, or lesion of the descending palatine artery produce a partial or complete dehiscence on the repaired palate.

When the dehiscence is not due to tissue loss, repair may be achieved by using local tissues. Procedures for correction normally consist of careful dissection of the oral and nasal flaps, as in a primary repair, but with the inconvenience that the dissection is more difficult because of the hard fibrous scar tissue from the first surgery. Occasionally, to ensure proper tension-free closure, the foramen of descending palatine artery can be osteotomized, or a limited dissection of the artery out of the flap will allow better flap mobilization. Correct suturing is vital to avoid the recurrence of fistulas; nasal flaps are sutured together with knots facing the nasal cavity, and the palatal mucosa is closed with mattress sutures for wound margin eversion (**Fig. 5**). Small defects located in the middle of the palate are suitable for repair of the nasal floor using perifistular tissue (turnover flap) and palatal flaps (**Fig. 6**). When the fistula is located anteriorly and the rest of the palate is properly closed, a palatal rotational flap can be

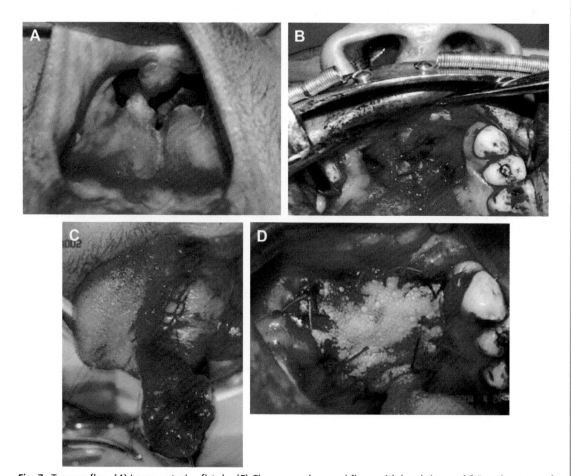

Fig. 7. Tongue flap. (*A*) Large anterior fistula. (*B*) Closure on the nasal floor with local tissues. (*C*) Development of a posterior base tongue flap. (*D*) Tongue flap in place.

used after a good closure of the nasal mucosa is done using perifistular tissue. Defects located on the soft palate require a dissection of the muscle layer to allow a proper function and an extra layer of closure.

A different approach is necessary when the dehiscence is because of the lack of tissue. Large anterior fistulas are commonly related to necrosis of the terminal segment of the palatal mucosa flaps, secondary to injury during dissection of the descending palatine artery. In these cases, repair is impossible to perform using surrounding tissues and tissues from other areas have to be transferred to the fistula. Pedicle flaps from the tongue are the most convenient sources of tissue and are preferred by the authors. The tongue has rich submucus vascular plexus that allows flaps to be raised safely based in any direction, anterior, posterior, or lateral, depending on the location of the fistula and the comfort of the patient. The flap has to be big enough to cover the fistula and as thick as 2 to 3 mm to ensure a good blood supply. After proper reconstruction of the nasal floor with a perifistular tissue dissection, the lingual flap is rotated, inset, and sutured, covering completely the defect. It is the authors' preference not to use maxillomandibular fixation (MMF) to preserve the integrity of the flap because of their experience that the lack of MMF allows the patient to have better feeding and oral hygiene and also allows for better postoperative flap monitoring. After 2 weeks, flap revascularization is tested by placing a tight suture around the pedicle for 5 to 10 minutes. If no changes are noted the flap can be released, but if the flap becomes pale one must wait for at least another 5 days before testing again. Further procedures such as thinning of the flap can be performed once the flap has healed (**Fig. 7**).

SUMMARY

If bad results in the patient with cleft lip and palate were either due to a bad surgical technique or due to complications in the postoperative care, the secondary management is very challenging. Poor tissue quality, lack of vital structures, and the surgeon's inexperience to identify and surgically correct the problem in a three-dimensional point of view accounts for some of the challenges when dealing with these deformities. Although many surgical resources exist for the management of these bad results, the surgeon must be aware that the best chance for optimal results is when the appropriate surgical technique is designed and performed during primary surgery. The value of knowledge and experience of primary surgery techniques cannot be overemphasized.

FURTHER READINGS

Buchbinder D, St Hilaire H. Tongue flaps in maxillofacial surgery. Oral Maxillofac Surg Clin North Am 2003; 15(4):475–86.

Cohen M. Residual deformities after repair of cleft of the lip and palate. Clin Plast Surg 2004;31(2):331–45.

Costello BJ, Ruiz RL, Fantuzzo JJ. Revision surgery for cleft malformations. In: Turvey T, editor. Oral and Maxillofacial Surgery, 2nd edition. vol. 3. St Louis (MO): Saunders; 2009. p. 828–47.

Doonquah L, Ogle OE. Scar revision of the cleft lip. Oral Maxillofac Surg Clin North Am 2002;14(4):425–37.

Lehman J. Closure of palatal fistulas. Oper Tech Plast Surg 1995;2(4):255–62.

Ogle OE. Keloids and hypertrophic scars. Oral Maxillofac Surg Clin North Am 1998;10(1):1–12.

Ogle OE. Management of oronasal fistulas in the cleft palate patient. Oral Maxillofac Surg Clin North Am 2002;14(4):553–62.

Reoperative Treatment of Obstructive Sleep Apnea

Mansoor Madani, DMD, MD[a,b,c,*], Farideh M. Madani, DMD[d], Dmitry Peysakhov, DMD[b]

KEYWORDS
- Obstructive sleep apnea • UPPP
- Maxillomandibular advancement • Radioablation

Choosing an appropriate method for the treatment of obstructive sleep apnea (OSA) requires a thorough understanding of the anatomic variations and abnormalities in various head and neck regions.[1–9] There are at least 10 different anatomic causes for OSA, including nasal cavity (deviated septum, enlarged nasal turbinates, polyps, or any other obstructive masses and nasal adhesions), soft palate and uvula (elongation or excessive vibrating flexibility), adenoids and tonsils (obstructive or chronically inflamed and enlarged), base of the tongue (macroglossia and retropositioning), narrowed and/or transversely deficient maxilla and mandible (retrognathism, micrognathism, and transverse maxillary deficiency), receded chin, lateral pharyngeal walls (pharyngeal muscle hypertrophy, constricted airway passage), and hyoid and epiglottis positions. Turbulent airflow and subsequent progressive vibratory trauma to the soft tissues of the upper airway are important factors contributing to snoring.[10] There is a complex interplay of the soft and hard tissue structures that contributes to upper airway obstruction. Besides this complex relationship, decreased dilating forces of the pharyngeal dilators and negative inspiratory pressure generated by the diaphragm are the 2 other factors involved in the development of OSA. These issues present a formidable challenge to the sleep apnea surgeon. Therefore, a surgeon should not promise any guarantees of curing OSA or even eliminating the sound of snoring with a single surgical procedure. Successful surgical outcomes depend on proper patient selection as well as choice of surgical procedures. The treatment failures of OSA are direct results of a combination of poor surgical planning, inadequate understanding of the contributing anatomic factors, and unrealistic patient expectation. To achieve success in OSA treatment, it is imperative to complete a thorough clinical evaluation, design a comprehensive treatment plan, and perform precise execution of a planned surgery.

PATIENT EVALUATION AND SELECTION

One of the most important aspects of surgical treatment is patient selection. Treatment of OSA is highly patient specific and depends on the combination of hereditary and acquired anatomic and lifestyle factors (**Box 1**). Each patient has a specific problem, and some may need a combination of procedures, whereas others may not be

[a] Department of Oral and Maxillofacial Surgery, Capital Health Regional Medical Center, 750 Brunswick Avenue, Trenton, NJ 08638, USA
[b] Temple University Hospital, 3401 North Broad Street, Philadelphia, PA 19140, USA
[c] Center for Corrective Jaw Surgery, Bala Institute of Oral and Facial surgery, 15 North Presidential Boulevard, Suite 301, Bala Cynwyd, PA 19004, USA
[d] Department of Oral Medicine, Robert Schattner Center, School of Dental Medicine, University of Pennsylvania, 240 South 40th Street, Philadelphia, PA 19104, USA
* Corresponding author. Center for Corrective Jaw Surgery, Bala Institute of Oral and Facial surgery, 15 North Presidential Boulevard, Suite 301, Bala Cynwyd, PA 19004.
E-mail address: drmadani@snorenet.com

Oral Maxillofacial Surg Clin N Am 23 (2011) 177–187
doi:10.1016/j.coms.2010.10.003
1042-3699/11/$ — see front matter © 2011 Elsevier Inc. All rights reserved.

Box 1
Surgical goals and outcome criteria

1. Choosing the most appropriate and individualized surgical procedures for each patient to eliminate mechanical ventilation during sleep
2. To increase the width of the airway at the oropharyngeal opening by squaring of the soft palate to improve its movement and closure
3. To reduce upper airway resistance to air movements by eliminating obstructions in the nasopharynx or oropharynx
4. To relieve symptoms such as snoring and daytime sleepiness and improve quality of life and restore uninterrupted breathing during sleeps
5. To achieve respiratory disturbance index (RDI) of less than 15
6. To achieve minimum oxygen saturation to above 90%

---

candidates for surgery at all. Evaluation usually begins by taking a detailed history from a patient and/or sleep partner and reviewing all pertinent clinical data, which include sleep studies and history of any previous treatments. Patients are usually asked to comment on the extent of loud snoring, daytime sleepiness, gasping for air, and periods of witnessed apnea as reported by the patient and the patient's bed partner, all of which are important indications for treatment.[11] Using an Epworth scale to determine the likelihood of sleep apnea is subjective but helpful in establishing a base to continue the evaluation.[12] This detailed examination determines which types of procedures suit the patient best. Another simple test to determine the possible origin of the sound of snoring is to ask the patient to imitate the snoring sound with the mouth slightly open. Usually a loud sound is detected from the vibration of the soft palate and the uvula. This sound could originate from the hypopharynx as well and is easily recognizable. The patient is then asked to make the snoring sound from the nose, with the lips completely sealed. Generally, in this case, patients with a nasal problem can make the sound. This sound is most commonly related to an obstruction in the nasal passage. In the authors' experience, up to 70% of snoring sounds in men results from the vibration of the uvula and the soft palate. Women, in more than 60% of occasions, have a nasal component of snoring.

Along with an initial clinical assessment, patient evaluation should include a comprehensive head and neck examination, which includes extraoral, intraoral, and airway examinations, and radiographic assessment. A thorough extraoral examination is extremely important and must also include the overall body mass index (calculated as weight in kilograms divided by height in meters squared) and neck circumference.[13] In contrast, a detailed intraoral examination allows identification of the potential sites of upper airway obstruction, including the nose, soft palate, lateral pharyngeal walls, and tongue base. Airway examination with a fiberoptic scope is an essential part of an overall assessment of the patient's anatomy. This evaluation enables the examiner to directly visualize the upper airway from the nose to the larynx and allows the assessment of the dimensions of the nasal, velopharyngeal, and hypopharyngeal regions. The use of fiberoptic nasopharyngoscopy and/or direct and indirect visualization of these areas has been highly recommended[14,15] throughout the literature but is rarely done by practitioners who perform nonsurgical treatment of sleep-related disorders.

After a thorough clinical examination, it is important to compare all the contributing clinical findings with radiographic imaging. Computed tomography (CT) or magnetic resonance imaging can precisely assess the dimension of the upper airway.[16] In practice, however, the most often used radiographic imaging is lateral cephalometric radiography, which has the advantages of ease of use, clarity, and low cost. Although a lateral cephalometric radiography is only a 2-dimensional method of evaluating a dynamic 3-dimensional area, it is a valuable study in identifying abnormal facial skeletal anatomy that may contribute to airway obstruction as well as the relation of the hard and soft tissues of the airway. In addition, it provides useful information on the size of the airway to include the posterior airway space behind the soft palate and the tongue base. The posterior airway space measurement on lateral cephalometric radiography has been shown to correlate with the volume of the hypopharyngeal airway on 3-dimensional CT scans.[17,18]

All of these diagnostic tools provide an examiner with the opportunity to come up with a list of specific abnormalities and problems that pertain to that particular patient, which in turn helps formulate a proper treatment plan. Clinicians must fit the appropriate treatment to the specific needs of the patient, which requires a detailed patient history and physical examination as well as an exhaustive explanation of the problem, treatment options, and possible complications. Teamwork with other specialists who use various methods of treatments for OSA yields successful outcomes. This team must include not only sleep specialists and dentists knowledgeable in fabricating oral appliances but also oral and maxillofacial surgeons, otolaryngologists, and even bariatric surgeons. Understanding the pathophysiology and the statistical probabilities associated with each procedure is essential for a successful outcome when treating patients with OSA. The resolution of symptoms with a surgical procedure does not necessarily equate to a resolution of OSA. Apnea could be improved with surgery, but significant apnea may persist. Because of this potential problem and the progressive nature of the disease, patients must always be monitored for a significant length of time, whether treated surgically or nonsurgically, with continuous positive airway pressure (CPAP) or oral appliances. This lack of follow-up, particularly when a patient is provided with CPAP or other positive airway pressure devices, is of major concern and the reason for failure of treatment of many patients with OSA.

SURGICAL PLANNING

Surgical planning for OSA must start with an appropriate diagnosis of the illness. This diagnosis includes obtaining a polysomnography in a laboratory or via portable units that can now accurately assess the degree of severity of apnea. The selection of the appropriate surgical procedures is based on numerous factors, including, but not limited to, patient's age, body mass index, neck size, and other relevant clinical findings as well as patient's health and their expectations. There are multiple factors that influence surgical outcomes, and a few are listed in **Table 1**. The goal of surgery may be different for patients. Many patients may only seek treatment of snoring issues, whereas others may elect surgical treatment because of intolerance of nonsurgical treatments, such as CPAP or oral appliances. In patients with severe blockage of the upper airway that is caused by nasal factors or enlarged uvula or tonsils, surgical correction may improve the ability to tolerate nonsurgical treatments, such as the reduction of therapeutic CPAP pressure or

improvement of nasal symptoms caused by CPAP use. Informing patients of the limitations of surgical procedures may prevent future reoperations or an unsatisfied patient. Informed consent must be obtained, and patients should be educated regarding the rationale of surgery as well as the associated risks and benefits.[19]

OSA and snoring originate from a variety of sources. When surgical intervention is required, and unless a specific anatomic obstruction has been clearly demonstrated, it must be assumed that all portions of the airway cause the problem. The surgical treatments may then range from treating the elongated and enlarged tissues in the nose and throat to orthognathic surgery to advance the jaws in order to increase the airway volume. The ultimate goal of any surgical treatment to correct the OSA is to open up the upper airway, such as the areas at the base of the tongue, by either osteotomy of the maxilla, mandible, and chin or partial glossectomy and genioglossal advancements with hyoid myotomy.[20] However, these procedures are certainly more invasive and complicated than the palatal and nasal procedures. In formulating a surgical plan, the most difficult task for the surgeon is to decide the procedure to be used. Indeed, information gathered from the preoperative assessment, including clinical examination, fiberoptic nasopharyngoscopy, and lateral cephalometric radiography, can provide useful information regarding the upper airway anatomy and the site of obstruction.

Surgical Options

Over the last several decades, many procedures have been introduced and performed to treat snoring and OSA. It started with the most drastic method of bypassing the airway with tracheotomy. Because this procedure is radical, at present, it is reserved only for the most severe forms of OSA.[21–23] Other procedures include uvuloplasty, uvulectomy,[24] uvulotomy, snare uvulopalatoplasty, and cautery-assisted palatal stiffening operation,

Table 1 Factors influencing sleep apnea surgery outcomes		
Factor	**Favorable**	**Unfavorable**
Age	Younger patients (<50 y)	Older patients (>50 y)
Body Mass Index	<27	>30
OSA Severity	Mild to moderate (RDI<25)	Severe (RDI>30)
Site of Obstruction	Oropharyngeal obstruction (with tonsils)	Hypopharyngeal
Tongue Size	Normal size	Hypertrophic
Neck Size	<17″	>17″

Common factors affecting long-term outcome: (1) other anatomic findings and variations, (2) aging, and (3) gaining weight after operation.

punctate diathermy of the soft palate,[25–27] and laser-assisted uvuloplasty, in which the focus was only on the removal or reduction of the uvula to open up the upper airway. The reoperations for these procedures were to remove more tissues, but in some cases, the excess removal has lead to velopharyngeal insufficiencies, vocal alterations, and even worsening of the OSA. One of the most effective soft tissue surgical corrective procedures was a traditional uvulopalatopharyngoplasty (UPPP), which was later modified by the authors to be performed by laser, hence named laser-assisted UPPP (LA-UPPP). The use of the HARMONIC scalpel (Ethicon, Endo-surgery, Cincinnati, OH, USA) has also been studied to perform harmonic-assisted UPPP or ultrasound-assisted UPPP.[10,28,29] The focus of these procedures was to remove a portion of the soft palate and uvula and at the same time perform tonsillectomy. These procedures were effective to treat mild to moderate OSA but were most effective in reducing the snoring sound. Reoperations were not necessary with these procedures. The uvulopalatal flap (UPF) is another available procedure, which involves suspension of the uvula superiorly toward the hard-soft palate junction after a limited resection of the uvula, lateral pharyngeal wall, and the mucosa. The procedure is reversible but rarely performed because it can increase the thickness of the soft palate.[24,30–38] Other recent soft tissue treatments include radiofrequency volumetric tissue reduction[39] or radiofrequency uvuloplasty procedures, including somnoplasty, coblation, and radioablation of the base of the tongue, soft palate, and nasal turbinate.[40–46]

Almost all of the procedures described use heat to create vacuolar degeneration and scar formation in the soft tissues to reduce vibration or motion of the structures treated, thereby reducing snoring and possibly opening up the upper airway. Although nasal radioablations are effective in opening up the nasal passages, in the authors' experience, the radioablation procedures on the soft palate and base of the tongue have more than 65% relapse potential after 5 years.

Nasal surgeries, such as septoplasty and inferior turbinate resection, rarely provide relief from snoring when used alone. In the authors' experience, they reduce the sound of snoring only up to 25% and do not cure sleep apnea to any greater degree. However, nasal procedures often improve patient tolerance and response to nasal CPAP. They are best used as an adjunct to more definitive surgical procedures. For these reasons, the authors initially offer a palatal procedure in combination with turbinate radioablation procedures to most patients who desire surgical treatment. Although

maxillomandibular advancement (MMA) is more invasive than soft tissue procedures, it has been hailed as the most effective surgical technique to significantly address the upper airway obstruction in patients with OSA. Patients with severe OSA, morbid obesity, or significant hypopharyngeal obstruction, such as severe mandibular deficiency, or those who wish to have the best chance for a cure with a single operation can certainly be considered as candidates for MMA as a primary surgical treatment option. It must be noted that this procedure can fail in obese patients with normal occlusion. Thus, as the severity of the OSA increases, so does the invasiveness of the procedures needed to achieve improvement. Clearly, surgery for treatment of snoring and OSA must be considered carefully on a case-by-case basis. Variations in the site of airway blockage as well as clinical measurement of abnormal anatomy determines the most appropriate course of surgical treatment.

Indications for Reoperation of Various Surgical Treatments

Nasal surgery

It is clear that the nasal obstruction, congestion, and blockage play an important role in patients with OSA. Inability to breathe through the nasal passages can even interfere with more conservative treatments, such as making the nasal CPAP delivery of the air more difficult. It is vital for surgeons as well as sleep specialists to assess this important structure and seek treatment before initiation of CPAP titration. The anatomic areas of the nose that may contribute to obstruction are the alar cartilages in the nasal valve region, the nasal septum, and the turbinates. The pathologic condition of this region, including the presence of nasal polyp, tumors, and other benign tissue enlargement, can play a crucial role. In some cases, nasal polyp surgery may need to be repeated because growth has been shown to recur after the initial surgery. Septoplasty to align the nasal septum may also need to be repeated because the cartilaginous portion of the septum can bend and blockage can recur. The nasal turbinate reduction, if performed by invasive open surgical reduction, has less chance of relapse but is more invasive than radioablation procedures, which have a higher chance of relapse. The major effects of nasal surgery are the subjective improvement of nasal patency and reduction of the nasal CPAP requirement. From experience, the nasal procedures alone have minimal long-term effect in treatment of OSA. It must be used in conjunction with other surgical procedures to achieve a successful outcome.[47–50]

UPPP

Ikematsu described UPPP in 1964 for the treatment of snoring. In 1981, Fujita introduced this procedure, with slight modifications, to the United States, for the treatment of snoring and OSA syndrome, which was further modified later.[51–60] The new procedure quickly became the gold standard for the treatment of oropharyngeal obstruction in OSA. During the procedure, as described by Fujita, the patient initially undergoes a tonsillectomy, which is followed by a partial removal of the soft palate, uvula, and pharyngeal arches in order to widen the oropharyngeal inlet.[61–65] The most serious perioperative complication reported with traditional UPPP is a 2% to 11% incidence of postoperative airway obstruction that has resulted in an approximately 1% perioperative mortality. Postoperative bleeding critical enough to require a return to the operating room occurs in 2% to 5% of cases. The most commonly reported short-term postoperative effect of the UPPP is severe pain that can last for several weeks. The most common long-term complications are velopharyngeal incompetence (VPI) and palatal dryness. Temporary postoperative VPI occurs in most patients, and studies have reported that 10% to 24% of patients continued to complain of intermittent nasopharyngeal regurgitation after traditional UPPP, even a year after surgery. In the same studies, up to 31% of patients complained of persistent palatal dryness. Less-frequent long-term complications include nasopharyngeal stenosis, long-term voice changes, and a partial loss of taste. In the authors' opinion, these complications could be reduced by a more careful and less-invasive soft tissue control. The limitations, complications, long recuperation time, and cost of UPPP have created a demand for a more effective, safer, economical, and comfortable alternative. LA-UPPP is an alternative to the traditional surgery in the operating room, which could also be performed in an in-office setting. This procedure is thought to be the most effective to eliminate the upper airway obstruction at the level of the nasopharynx and oropharynx, thereby reducing snoring significantly. However, it does not correct the hypopharyngeal obstruction. This modification of the traditional UPPP has significantly reduced and eliminated some of the potential complications, which included velopharyngeal insufficiency, stenosis, and dysphagia associated with an original procedure.[66,67] Reoperations in patients who have a persisting OSA but have already undergone UPPP must be avoided and can lead to more serious complications, such as worsened VPI and stenosis. The authors have performed radioablation and palatal implant placement in failed UPPP cases, with some success.

UPF

VPI is a recognized complication of traditional UPPP. In 1996, UPF was described as an alternative procedure to be performed in the operating room with the patient under general anesthesia, and it offered several theoretical advantages over traditional UPPP.[68] It involves stripping the superficial mucosal layer from the palatal midline lowered by uvula rotation and suturing it to the soft palate. The advantage of this procedure is that it is potentially reversible and in case of any complications, the uvula can be replaced to its original position. This procedure might offer less chance of nasopharyngeal stenosis and does not interfere with palatal dynamics as much as traditional UPPP. The ultimate goal of any surgical procedure designed to treat OSA is soft tissue reduction to open up the airway. In LA-UPPP, the amount of soft tissue ablated can be titrated such that the treatment can be discontinued once snoring is eliminated.

Pharyngoplasty/tonsillectomy

The pharyngoplasty procedure usually involves the removal of tonsillar tissues, but the uvula and the soft palate are preserved. The pharyngeal inlet is widened, and the airway collapsibility is reduced purely via suturing of the tonsillar wounds.[69–85] This procedure represents the most conservative pharyngeal surgery and has minimal side effects compared with other procedures. The advantage of pharyngoplasty is that in case of need for further operations such as UPPP, these procedures can be safely performed in an in-office setting because there is no more risk of tonsillar tissue bleeding.

Palatal radioablation, injection snoreplasty, and palatal implants

Recently, some procedures such as radioablation, palatal implants, and injection snoreplasty have received approval from the US Food and Drug Administration to treat OSA. The goal of these procedures is to stiffen up the soft palate, thereby reducing the vibrating effect of the soft palate and uvula. The potential disadvantage is that anatomic variations can limit their effectiveness. Radiofrequency treatments are designed to accomplish tissue volume reduction and at the same time reduce patients' discomfort, tissue damage, mucosal ulceration, and external scar formation.[41] Generally, radioablation procedures are less invasive and do not involve cutting tissues. Submucosal lesions (also known as ablations) are created without any need to remove tissues, thereby reducing the risk of complications and discomfort. The lesions created by these procedures are naturally resorbed in approximately

8 to 10 weeks, reducing excess tissue volume. These procedures are generally performed in an outpatient setting, and no general anesthesia is usually required. The key of the effectiveness of each procedure depends on the selection of patients, site of the lesions, number of repeated procedures, and the experience of the surgeons. At present, the most commonly used radiofrequency devices are the Coblation device (Arthrocare Corporation, Sunnyvale, CA, USA), and (Ellman International Inc, Oceanside, NY, USA) and (Elmed Inc, Addison, IL, USA). The long-term effect of injection snoreplasty is not yet known.[86] However, from extensive work with various radioablation systems, the authors' finding was conclusive that in many cases, radiofrequency treatment benefits were temporary and effective only in a selected number of patients with chronic snoring. These procedures were also found to be ineffective in patients who are obese or with OSA in addition to snoring. The advantage of these procedures is that if they prove to be ineffective, further more invasive procedures can be safely performed. With proper patient selection, these procedures may be very effective, but follow-up is always necessary.

MMA

Retrognathism, micrognathism, and transverse deficiencies of the maxillae and mandible are among the most frequent abnormalities found in patients with OSA.[87–91] These deformities result in diminished airway dimension, which leads to nocturnal obstruction. MMA is performed in an attempt to widen the airway while maintaining the existing occlusion or, optimally, to obtain class I occlusion. MMA is an extrapharyngeal operation that enlarges and stabilizes the velo-orohypopharyngeal airway, which can be safely combined with adjunctive nonpharyngeal procedures. It achieves the enlargement of the upper airway, including the nasal, pharyngeal, and hypopharyngeal airway expansions of the skeletal framework that encircle the airway. It also enhances the neuromuscular tone of the pharyngeal dilator musculature, such as soft palate and tongue base, via an extrapharyngeal operation, with minimal risks of postoperative edema-induced upper airway embarrassment or pharyngeal dysfunction.[92] Comparison of pre- and postoperative airway appearance based on fiberoptic nasopharyngoscopy and lateral cephalometric radiography have demonstrated that in addition to airway expansion by the forward movement of the maxillomandibular complex, the tension and collapsibility of the suprahyoid and velopharyngeal musculature may also be reduced, thus leading to the reduction of lateral pharyngeal wall collapse.[93]

To maximize the airway expansion, an advancement of 10 to 12 mm is usually recommended. However, it is important to achieve maximal advancement while maintaining a stable dental occlusion as well as balanced aesthetic appearance. MMA is more invasive than most soft tissue surgeries, and the associated surgical risks include bleeding, infection, malocclusion, trigeminal and facial nerve injuries, unfavorable splits, and relapse potential that can exist with any facial skeletal surgery. Particular attention is given in achieving rigid fixation and stabilizing the segments by placing adequate bone grafting where indicated (**Fig. 1**). MMA is a highly successful single-stage definitive treatment that can be easily combined with other soft tissue treatments previously described.

Advancement genioplasty/genioglossus advancement

One of the major areas of obstruction in patients with sleep apnea is the collapse of the tongue in the retropharyngeal space. The position of the mandible and tongue location during sleep determine the airway dimension. The collapsibility of the tongue can be improved with genioglossus advancement. The genioglossus is the primary muscle of the tongue and is attached to a small bony projection on the interior of the lower jaw. Anterior positioning of these structures has been shown to improve OSA. The genioglossus advancement procedure is limited to moving forward the geniotubercle with the genioglossus insertion without moving the mandible. This advancement places tension on the tongue musculature, thereby limiting the posterior displacement during sleep.[88,91,94–96] The genioglossus advancement procedure consists of a rectangular osteotomy on the symphysis of the mandible via an intraoral approach. The rectangle is advanced forward by the thickness of the mandible and partially rotated to prevent retraction back into the floor of the mouth. Incorporation of the geniotubercle during the procedure has been shown to be successful with this technique.[97] In general, genioglossus advancement is performed in conjunction with other surgical procedures, such as UPPP and hyoid advancement, to maximize improvement.[30,98–101] However, the results are unpredictable, and cases of relapse have been observed. Patients must be advised regarding the potential for relapse. Clearly, anatomic factors, body mass index, and OSA severity are all factors that influence surgical success. In general, the potential risks associated with genioglossus advancement are quite limited and include infection, hematoma, injury to the genioglossus muscle, and paresthesia of the lower teeth.

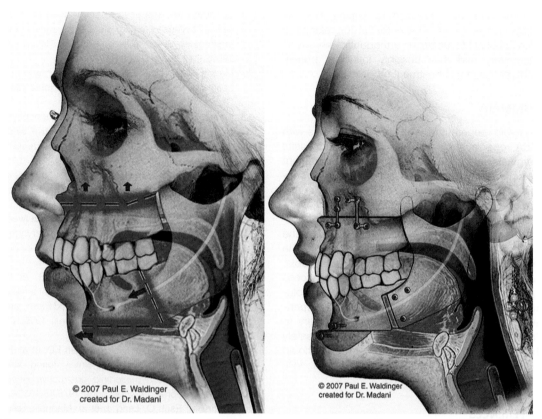

Fig. 1. Comparison of pre- and postoperative airway appearance based on fiberoptic nasopharyngoscopy and lateral cephalometric radiography has demonstrated that in addition to airway expansion by the forward movement of the maxillomandibular complex (*black arrows*), the tension and collapsibility of the suprahyoid and velopharyngeal musculature may also be reduced, thus leading to the reduction of lateral pharyngeal wall collapse. Particular attention is given in achieving rigid fixation and stabilizing the segments by placing adequate bone grafting where indicated. (*Courtesy of* Mansoor Madani, DMD, MD, Bala Cynwyd, PA, USA all rights reserved.)

Hyoid advancement

The tongue is a frequent cause of airway obstruction in OSA and can collapse toward the back of the throat during sleep, thereby contributing to OSA. The hyoid bone has a close relationship with the tongue base and pharyngeal musculature, thus portraying an integral aspect of the upper airway anatomy. The hyoid bone may be surgically repositioned anteriorly by attaching it to the thyroid cartilage to expand the airway. The procedure is usually performed in conjunction with genioglossus advancement so as to contribute to the improvement of OSA. However, some surgeons have elected to combine it with UPPP. An inherent problem with hyoid advancement is the requirement of an external incision on the neck, one aspect that may not be readily accepted by all patients. As with other surgical procedures for sleep apnea, the results of hyoid advancement are variable, ranging from 23% to 65%. In general, the associated surgical risks are low and may include

infection, seroma formation, and dysphagia, which are usually temporary, lasting for 7 to 10 days.

Maxillomandibular expansion

Patients with transverse deficiency of the maxilla generally present with a narrower hard palate and a deep palatal vault, impinging on the nasal cavity, thereby reducing nasal airflow. Studies have demonstrated that the expansion of the maxilla can improve OSA in children, adolescents, and adults.[102–108] The procedure consists of modified osteotomies to allow the widening of the maxilla and mandible with distractors or expansion devices. The advantages of surgical rapid palatal expansion are that it is simple, is much less invasive than MMA procedures, and could be safely performed in an in-office setting. Future reoperations, including hard and soft tissue surgery, could also readily be accomplished. However, with this procedure, the treatment time is lengthened, and patients need to keep the distractors in place for several months after the operation to ensure that the expansion is stable. The potential for relapse is also present. In addition, orthodontic therapy is mandatory and may possibly influence patient acceptance of this treatment modality.

SUMMARY

To avoid reoperations when treating patients with OSA, one must bear in mind that a successful surgical outcome depends on proper patient selection as well as the choice of surgical procedures. The adaptation of a sound and systematic approach to clinical evaluation, treatment planning, and surgical execution is necessary to maximize safety and improve surgical results and at the same time prevent the need for reoperations. The expectations of patients should be reasonable, and there should be no guarantee of success given for a surgical approach for complete resolution of OSA. From the authors' extensive experience using both soft and hard tissue surgery to treat snoring and OSA, reoperations can safely be performed if necessary, but patients should be cautioned of possible worsening of VPI, stenosis, and relapse potential.

REFERENCES

1. Schwab RJ, Gupta KB, Gefter WB, et al. Upper airway and soft tissue anatomy in normal subjects and patients with sleep-disordered breathing. Am J Respir Crit Care Med 1995;152:1673–89.
2. Hudgel DW, Hendricks C. Palate and hypopharynx—sites of inspiratory narrowing of the upper airway during sleep. Am Rev Respir Dis 1988;138:1542–7.
3. Isono S, Remmers JE, Tanaka A, et al. Anatomy of pharynx in patients with obstructive sleep apnea and in normal subjects. J Appl Phys 1997;82(4): 1319–26.
4. Kuna ST, Sant'Ambrogio G. Pathophysiology of upper airway closure during sleep. JAMA 1991; 266:1384–9.
5. Hamans EP, Van Marck EA, De Backer WA, et al. Morphometric analysis of the uvula in patients with sleep-related breathing disorders. Eur Arch Otorhinolaryngol 2000;257(4):232–6.
6. Metes A, Hoffstein V, Anderson D. Site of airway obstruction in patients with obstructive sleep apnea before and after uvulopalatoplasty. Laryngoscope 1991;101:1102–8.
7. Chaban R, Cole P, Hoffstein V. Site of the upper airway obstruction in patients with obstructive sleep apnea. Laryngoscope 1998;98:641–7.
8. Hudgel D. Variable site of airway narrowing among obstructive sleep apnea patients. J Appl Phys 1986;61:1403–9.
9. Sheppard JW, Thawley SE. Localization of upper airway collapse during sleep in patients with obstructive sleep apnea. Am Rev Respir Dis 1990;141:1350–5.
10. Madani M. Surgical treatment of snoring and mild obstructive sleep apnea. Oral Maxillofac Surg Clin North Am 2002;14:333–50.
11. Madani M, Madani F. Epidemiology, pathophysiology, and clinical features of obstructive sleep apnea. Oral Maxillofac Surg Clin North Am 2009; 21:369–75.
12. Johns MW. A new method for measuring daytime sleepiness: the Epworth sleepiness scale. Sleep 1991;14(6):540–5.
13. Davies RJ, Stradling JR. The relationship between neck circumference, radiographic pharyngeal anatomy, and the obstructive sleep apnoea syndrome. Eur Respir J 1990;3(5):509–14.
14. Aboussouan LS, Golish JA, Wood BG, et al. Dynamic pharyngoscopy in predicting outcome of uvulopalatopharyngoplasty for moderate and severe obstructive sleep apnea. Chest 1995;107: 946–51.
15. Borowiecki B, Pollack CP, Weitzman ED, et al. Fibro-optic study of pharyngeal airway during sleep in patients with hypersomnia obstructive sleep-apnea syndrome. Laryngoscope 1978;88:1310–3.
16. Mathru M, Esch O, Lang J, et al. Magnetic resonance imaging of the upper airway. Anesthesiology 1996;84:273–9.
17. Naganuma H, Okamoto M, Woodson BT, et al. Cephalometric and fiberoptic evaluation as a case-selection technique for obstructive sleep apnea syndrome (OSAS). Acta Otolaryngol Suppl 2002;547:57–63.
18. Strelzow VV, Blanks RHI, Basile A, et al. Cephalometric airway analysis in obstructive sleep apnea syndrome. Laryngoscope 1988;98:1149–58.
19. Ephros HD, Madani M, Geller BM, et al. Developing a protocol for the surgical management of snoring and obstructive sleep apnea. Atlas Oral Maxillofac Surg Clin North Am 2007;15(2):89–100.
20. Lowe AA. The tongue and airway. Otolaryngol Clin North Am 1990;23(4):677–98.
21. Campanini A, De Vito A, Frassineti S, et al. Role of skin-lined tracheotomy in obstructive sleep apnoea syndrome: personal experience. Acta Otorhinolaryngol Ital 2004;24:68–74.
22. Haapaniemi JJ, Laurikainen EA, Halme P, et al. Long-term results of tracheostomy for severe obstructive sleep apnea syndrome. ORL J Otorhinolaryngol Relat Spec 2001;63:131–6.
23. Kim SH, Eisele DW, Smith PL, et al. Evaluation of patients with sleep apnea after tracheotomy. Arch Otolaryngol Head Neck Surg 1998;124:996–1000.
24. Li HY, Li KK, Chen NH, et al. Three-dimensional computed tomography and polysomnography

findings after extended uvulopalatal flap surgery for obstructive sleep apnea. Am J Otol 2005;26:7–11.

25. Mair EA, Day RH. Cautery-assisted palatal stiffening operation. Otolaryngol Head Neck Surg 2000;122(4):547–56.

26. Wassmuth Z. Cautery-assisted palatal stiffening operation for the treatment of obstructive sleep apnea syndrome. Otolaryngol Head Neck Surg 2000;123(1Pt1):55–60.

27. Whinney JD, Williamson PA, Bicknell PG. Punctate diathermy of the soft palate: a new approach in the surgical management of snoring. J Laryngol Otol 1995;109:849–52.

28. Ephros HD, Madani M, Yalamanchili SC. Surgical treatment of snoring and obstructive sleep apnea. Indian J Med Res 2010;131:267–76.

29. Madani M. Laser assisted uvulopalatopharyngoplasty (LA-UPPP) for the treatment of snoring and mild to moderate obstructive sleep apnea. Atlas Oral Maxillofac Surg Clin North Am 2007;15(2):129–37.

30. Li KK, Powell NB, Riley RW, et al. Overview of phase I surgery for obstructive sleep apnea syndrome. Ear Nose Throat J 1999;78(11):836–45.

31. Guilleminault C, Kim Y, Palombini L, et al. Upper airway resistance syndrome and its treatment. Sleep 2000;23:S197–200.

32. Li KK, Troell RJ, Powell NB, et al. Uvulopalatopharyngoplasty, maxillomandibular advancement and the velopharynx. Laryngoscope 2001;111:1075–8.

33. Li HY, Li KK, Chen NH, et al. Modified uvulopalatopharyngoplasty: the extended uvulopalatal flap. Am J Otol 2003;24:311–6.

34. Li KK, Powell NB, Riley RW. Surgical management of obstructive sleep apnea. In: Lee-Chiong T Jr, Carskadon MA, Sateia MH, editors. Sleep medicine. Philadelphia: Hanley & Belfus Inc; 2001.

35. Li KK. Surgical management of obstructive sleep apnea. Clin Chest Med 2003;24:365–70.

36. Li KK. Obstructive sleep apnea—surgical treatment. In: Carney PR, Berry RB, Geyer JD, editors. Clinical sleep disorders. Philadelphia: Lippincott, Williams & Wilkins; 2004.

37. Li KK. Surgical therapy for obstructive sleep apnea syndrome. Semin Respir Crit Care Med 2005;26:80–8.

38. Li KK. Surgical therapy for adult obstructive sleep apnea. Sleep Med Rev 2005;9(3):201–9.

39. Powell NB, Riley RW, Troell RJ, et al. Radiofrequency volumetric tissue reduction of the palate in subjects with sleep disorder breathing. Chest 1998;113:1163–74.

40. Madani M. Radiofrequency treatment of the soft palate, nasal turbinates and tonsils for the treatment of snoring and mild to moderate obstructive sleep apnea. Atlas Oral Maxillofac Surg Clin North Am 2007;15(2):139–53.

41. Powell NB, Riley RW, Troell RJ, et al. Radio frequency volumetric reduction of the tongue. A porcine pilot study for the treatment of obstructive sleep apnea syndrome. Chest 1997;111:1348–55.

42. Powell NB, Riley RW, Guilleminault C. Radiofrequency tongue base reduction in sleep-disordered breathing: a pilot study. Otolaryngol Head Neck Surg 1999;120:656–64.

43. Li KK, Powell NB, Riley RW, et al. Temperature-controlled radiofrequency tongue base reduction for sleep-disordered breathing: long-term follow-up. Otolaryngol Head Neck Surg 2002;127:230–4.

44. Stuck BA, Maurer JT, Verse T, et al. Tongue base reduction with temperature-controlled radiofrequency volumetric tissue reduction for treatment of obstructive sleep apnea syndrome. Acta Otolaryngol 2002;122:531–6.

45. Tucker BT, Nelson L, Mickelson S, et al. A multi-institutional study of radiofrequency volumetric tissue reduction for OSAS. Otolaryngol Head Neck Surg 2001;125:303–11.

46. Fischer Y, Khan M, Mann WJ. Multilevel temperature-controlled radiofrequency therapy of soft palate, base of tongue, and tonsils in adults with obstructive sleep apnea. Laryngoscope 2003;113:1786–91.

47. Friedman M, Tanyeri H, Lim JW, et al. Effect of improved nasal breathing on obstructive sleep apnea. Otolaryngol Head Neck Surg 2000;122:71–4.

48. Verse T, Maurer JT, Pirsig W. Effect of nasal surgery on sleep-disordered breathing disorders. Laryngoscope 2002;112:64–8.

49. Lofaso F, Coste AD, Ortho MP, et al. Nasal obstruction as a risk factor sleep apnea syndrome. Eur Respir J 2002;16:639–43.

50. Young T, Finn L, Palta M. Chronic nasal congestion at night is a risk factor for snoring in a population-based cohort study. Arch Intern Med 2001;161:1514–9.

51. Fijita S, Conway W, Zorick F, et al. Surgical correction of anatomic abnormalities of obstructive sleep apnea syndrome: uvulopalatopharyngoplasty. Otolaryngol Head Neck Surg 1981;89:923–34.

52. Sher AE, Schechtman KB, Piccirillo JF. The efficacy of surgical modifications of the upper airway in adults with obstructive sleep apnea syndrome. Sleep 1996;19:156–77.

53. Fujita S. UPPP for sleep apnea and snoring. Ear Nose Throat J 1984;63:227–35.

54. Conway W, Fujita S, Zorick F, et al. Uvulopalatopharyngoplasty: one-year followup. Chest 1985;88:385–7.

55. Fujita S, Conway WA, Zorick FJ, et al. Evaluation of the effectiveness of uvulopalatopharyngoplasty. Laryngoscope 1985;95:70–4.

56. Koay CB, Freeland AP, Stradling JR. Short- and long-term outcomes of uvulopalatopharyngoplasty for snoring. Clin Otolaryngol 1995;20:45–8.

57. Wright S, Haight J. Changes in pharyngeal properties after uvulopalatopharyngoplasty. Laryngoscope 1989;99:62–5.

58. Croft CB, Golding Wood DG. Uses and complications of uvulopalatopharyngoplasty. J Laryngol Otol 1990;104:871–5.

59. Fairbanks DN. Uvulopalatopharyngoplasty complications and avoidance strategies. Otolaryngol Head Neck Surg 1990;102:239–45.

60. Haavisto L, Suopaa J. Complications of uvulopalatopharyngoplasty. Clin Otolaryngol Allied Sci 1994; 19:243–7.

61. Wareing MJ, Callan VP. Laser assisted uvulopalatoplasty: six and eighteen month results. J Laryngol Otol 1998;112:639–41.

62. Esclamando R, Glenn M. Perioperative complications and risk factors in the surgical treatment of obstructive sleep apnea syndrome. Laryngoscope 1989;99:1125–9.

63. Coleman JA Jr. Laser-assisted uvulopalatoplasty: long-term results with a treatment for snoring. Ear Nose Throat J 1998;77:22–4, 26–9, 32–4.

64. Krespi YP, Pearlman SJ, Keidar A. Laser assisted uvulopalatoplasty for the treatment of snoring. J Otolaryngol 1994;23:328–34.

65. Walker RP. Laser uvulopalatoplasty: techniques and results. Operative Techniques in Otolaryngology - Head Neck Surg 2000;11(1):2–6.

66. Madani M. Soft tissue surgeries to treat snoring and sleep apnea. American Association of Oral Maxillofacial Surgery Knowledge Update. 2006;4:402–19 (SLP 70–87).

67. Madani M. Complications of laser-assisted uvulopalatopharyngoplasty (LA-UPPP) and radiofrequency treatment of snoring and chronic nasal congestion: a 10-year review of 5,600 patients. J Oral Maxillofac Surg 2004;62:1351–62.

68. Powell NB, Riley RW, Guilleminault C, et al. A reversible uvulopalatal flap for snoring and obstructive sleep. Sleep 1996;19:593–9.

69. Cahali MB. Lateral pharyngoplasty: a new treatment for obstructive sleep apnea hypopnea syndrome. Laryngoscope 2003;113(11):1961–8.

70. Hultcrantz E, Linder A, Markstrom A. Tonsillectomy or tonsillotomy? A randomized study comparing postoperative pain and long-term effects. Int J Pediatr Otorhinolaryngol 1999;51(3):171–6.

71. Colreavy MP, Nanan D, Benamer M, et al. Antibiotic prophylaxis post-tonsillotomy: is it of benefit? Int J Pediatr Otorhinolaryngol 1999;50(1):15–22.

72. Boelen-van der Loo WJ, Scheffer E, de Haan RJ, et al. Clinimetric evaluation of the pain observation scale for young children in children aged between 1 and 4 years after ear, nose, and throat surgery. J Dev Behav Pediatr 1999;20(4):222–7.

73. Anand VT, Phillips JJ, Allen D, et al. A study of postoperative fever following pediatric tonsillectomy. Clin Otolaryngol 1999;24(4):360–4.

74. England RJ, Lau M, Ell SR. Angular cheilitis after tonsillectomy. Clin Otolaryngol 1999;24(4):277–9.

75. Drake-Lee A, Harris S. Day case tonsillectomy: what is the risk and where is the economic benefit? Clin Otolaryngol 1999;24(4):247–51.

76. Homer JJ, Williams BT, Semple P, et al. Tonsillectomy by guillotine is less painful than dissection. Int J Pediatr Otorhinolaryngol 2000;52(1):25–9.

77. Linder A, Markstrom A, Hultcrantz E. Using the carbon dioxide laser for tonsillotomy in children. Int J Pediatr Otorhinolaryngol 1999;50(1):31–6.

78. Saito T, Honda N, Saito H. Advantage and disadvantage of KTP-532 laser tonsillectomy compared with conventional method. Auris Nasus Larynx 1999;26(4):447–52.

79. Faulconbridge RV, Fowler S, Horrocks J, et al. Comparative audit of tonsillectomy. Clin Otolaryngol 2000;25(2):110–7.

80. Limb R, Walkley I. Adult day case tonsillectomy. Anaesth Intensive Care 2000;28(2):229–30.

81. Goldstein NA, Post JC, Rosenfeld RM, et al. Impact of tonsillectomy and adenoidectomy on child behavior. Arch Otolaryngol Head Neck Surg 2000;126(4):494–8.

82. Marshall T. How many tonsillectomies are based on evidence from randomized controlled trials? Br J Gen Pract 1999;49(443):487–8.

83. Panarese A, Clarke RW, Yardley MP. Early postoperative morbidity following tonsillectomy in children: implications for day surgery. J Laryngol Otol 1999;113(12):1089–91.

84. Raut VV, Yung MW. Peritonsillar abscess: the rationale for interval tonsillectomy. Ear Nose Throat J 2000;79(3):206–9.

85. Motamed M, Djazaeri B, Marks R. Acute pulmonary edema complicating adenotonsillectomy for obstructive sleep apnea. Int J Clin Pract 1999; 53(3):230–1.

86. Brietzke S, Mair E. Injection snoreplasty: how to treat snoring without all the pain and expense. Otolaryngol Head Neck Surg 2001;124:503–10.

87. Li KK, Riley RW, Powell NB, et al. Patient's perception of the facial appearance after maxillomandibular advancement for obstructive sleep apnea syndrome. J Oral Maxillofac Surg 2001;59:377–80.

88. Riley RW, Powell NB. Maxillofacial surgery and obstructive sleep apnea syndrome. Otolaryngol Clin North Am 1990;23:809–26.

89. Li KK, Powell NB, Riley RW, et al. Long-term results of maxillomandibular advancement surgery. Sleep Breath 2000;4:137–9.

90. Conradt R, Hochban W, Brandenburg U, et al. Long term results after surgical treatment of obstructive sleep apnea by maxillomandibular advancement. Eur Respir J 1997;10:123–8.
91. Riley RW, Powell NB, Guilleminault C. Inferior sagittal osteotomy of the mandible with hyoid myotomy-suspension: a new procedure for obstructive sleep apnea. Otolaryngol Head Neck Surg 1986;94:589–93.
92. Prinsell JR. Maxillo-mandibular advancement surgery for obstructive sleep apnea syndrome. J Am Dent Assoc 2002;133(11):1489–97.
93. Li KK, Riley RW, Powell NB, et al. Obstructive sleep apnea and maxillomandibular advancement: an assessment of airway changes using radiographic and nasopharyngoscopic examination. J Oral Maxillofac Surg 2002;60:526–30.
94. Neruntarat C. Genioglossus advancement and hyoid myotomy under local anesthesia. Otolaryngol Head Neck Surg 2003;129:85–91.
95. Lee RN. Genioglossus muscle advancement techniques for obstructive sleep apnea. Oral Maxillofac Surg Clin North Am 2002;14:337–84.
96. Riley RW, Powell NB, Guilleminault C. Obstructive sleep apnea syndrome: a review of 306 consecutively treated surgical patients. Otolaryngol Head Neck Surg 1993;108:117–25.
97. Li KK, Riley RW, Powell NB, et al. Obstructive sleep apnea surgery: genioglossus advancement revisited. J Oral Maxillofac Surg 2001;59:1181–4.
98. Lee NR, Givens CD Jr, Wilson J, et al. Staged surgical treatment of obstructive sleep apnea syndrome: a review of 35 patients. J Oral Maxillofac Surg 1999;57:382–5.
99. Bettega G, Pepin J, Veale D, et al. Obstructive sleep apnea syndrome: fifty-one consecutive patients treated by maxillofacial surgery. Am J Respir Crit Care Med 2000;162:641–9.
100. Hsu PP, Brett RH. Multiple level pharyngeal surgery for obstructive sleep apnoea. Singapore Med J 2001;42:160–4.
101. Riley RW, Powell NB, Guilleminault C. Obstructive sleep apnea and the hyoid: a revised surgical procedure. Otolaryngol Head Neck Surg 1994;111:717–21.
102. Cistulli PA, Richards GN, Palmisano RG, et al. Influence of maxillary constriction on nasal resistance and sleep apnea severity in patients with Marfan's syndrome. Chest 1996;110:1184–8.
103. Timms DJ. Rapid maxillary expansion in the treatment of nocturnal enuresis. Angle Orthod 1990;60:229–33.
104. Kurol J, Modin H, Bjerkhoel A. Orthodontic maxillary expansion and its effect on nocturnal enuresis. Angle Orthod 1998;68:225–32.
105. Seto BH, Gotsopoulos H, Sims MR, et al. Maxillary morphology in obstructive sleep apnea syndrome. Eur J Orthod 2001;23:703–14.
106. Cistulli PA, Palmisano RG, Poole MD. Treatment of obstructive sleep apnea syndrome by rapid maxillary expansion. Sleep 1998;21:831–5.
107. Pirelli P, Saponara M, Guilleminault C. Rapid maxillary expansion in children with obstructive sleep apnea syndrome. Sleep 2004;27:761–6.
108. Guilleminault C, Li KK. Maxillomandibular expansion by distraction osteogenesis for the treatment of sleep-disordered breathing: preliminary results. Laryngoscope 2004;114:893–6.

Index

Note: Page numbers of article titles are in **boldface** type.

Oral Maxillofacial Surg Clin N Am 23 (2011) 189–192
doi:10.1016/S1042-3699(11)00009-4

oralmaxsurgery.theclinics.com

Moving?

Make sure your subscription moves with you!

To notify us of your new address, find your **Clinics Account Number** (located on your mailing label above your name), and contact customer service at:

Email: journalscustomerservice-usa@elsevier.com

800-654-2452 (subscribers in the U.S. & Canada)
314-447-8871 (subscribers outside of the U.S. & Canada)

Fax number: 314-447-8029

Elsevier Health Sciences Division
Subscription Customer Service
3251 Riverport Lane
Maryland Heights, MO 63043

*To ensure uninterrupted delivery of your subscription, please notify us at least 4 weeks in advance of move.

ELSEVIER

Printed and bound by CPI Group (UK) Ltd, Croydon, CR0 4YY
03/10/2024
01040358-0016